CHILDHOOD LEUKEMIA

A Guide for Families, Friends & Caregivers

Second Edition

Nancy Keene

O'REILLY®

Beijing • Cambridge • Farnham • Köln • Paris • Sebastopol • Taipei • Tokyo

Childhood Leukemia: A Guide for Families, Friends & Caregivers, Second Edition
by Nancy Keene

Copyright © 1999, 1997 O'Reilly & Associates, Inc. All rights reserved.
Printed in the United States of America.

Published by O'Reilly & Associates, Inc., 101 Morris Street, Sebastopol, CA 95472.

Editor: Linda Lamb

Production Editor: Claire Cloutier LeBlanc

Printing History:

> June 1997:   First Edition
>
> October 1999:   Second Edition

This book is meant to educate and should not be used as an alternative for professional medical care. Although we have exerted every effort to ensure that the information presented is accurate at the time of publication, there is no guarantee that this information will remain current over time. Appropriate medical professionals should be consulted before adopting any procedures or treatments discussed in this book.

Library of Congress Cataloging-in-Publication Data:

Keene, Nancy, 1954– .
    Childhood leukemia: a guide for families, friends, & caregivers / Nancy Keene. —
2nd ed.
        p. cm. — (Patient-centered guides)
    Includes bibliographical references and index.
    ISBN 1-56592-632-3 (pbk.)
    1. Leukemia in children. I. Title. II. Series.
    RJ416.L4K44 1999
    618.92'99419—dc21
                                                    99-39059
                                                    CIP

[6/00]

[M]

To my daughters
Katy and Alison

Table of Contents

Foreword

EVERY YEAR IN THE UNITED STATES approximately 11,000 children and adolescents under the age of twenty years are diagnosed with cancer. Of these children, approximately 2,500 will be afflicted with acute lymphoblastic leukemia and 500 with other types of childhood leukemia. Significant progress has been made in the treatment of childhood cancer over the past four decades, best illustrated by the dramatically improved cure rate for children diagnosed with acute lymphoblastic leukemia. A leading textbook on childhood cancer published in 1960[1] described leukemia in childhood as being "incurable." Today, the cure rate for children diagnosed with acute lymphoblastic leukemia is 70 percent overall, and over 85 percent in certain groups of children with particular types of leukemia.

Not every child with acute lymphoblastic leukemia, however, is guaranteed a cure, and progress in the treatment of other types of leukemia, such as the myeloid leukemias and other types of cancer, has been definite but slow. Long-term effects following childhood cancer and its treatment are now common as more children are cured of cancer. Thus the diagnosis of any form of cancer in a child remains devastating to a family suddenly thrust into a foreign and threatening world of new and frightening words, medical tests and treatments, uncertainty about the future and, perhaps worst of all for parents, loss of control in guiding their child's life.

The best resource to help survive this new world is knowledge. Nancy Keene has taken her experience following the diagnosis of leukemia in her three-year-old daughter, Katy, melded this with the experiences of more than thirty other families, and produced an invaluable source of knowledge for parents of children diagnosed with cancer. Although the book focuses on leukemia, it contains information that will prove extremely helpful to parents and

---

[1] Ariel, I.M., and A.T. Pack, eds. *Cancer and Allied Diseases of Infancy and Childhood.* Boston: Little, Brown & Company, 1960.

families coping with any type of childhood cancer. Keene writes in her introduction, "I wanted to provide the insight and experiences of veteran parents who have all felt the hope, helplessness, anger, humor, longing, panic, ignorance, warmth, and anguish of their children's treatment for cancer. I wanted parents to know how other children react to treatment, and I wanted to offer tips to make it easier." She has clearly succeeded.

This most complete parent guide available covers not only detailed and precise medical information about leukemia and the various treatment options from chemotherapy to bone marrow and stem cell transplantation, but also day-to-day practical advice including how to handle procedures, hospitalization, family and friends, school, social and financial issues, communication, feelings and, if therapy is not successful, the difficult issues of death and bereavement. The cumulative experiences of so many families who have faced the entire spectrum of what can happen in caring for a child with leukemia, and the comprehensive bibliographies make this such a unique and helpful resource.

This book, however, is not only for parents. It will prove equally instructive for anyone, but particularly for all healthcare professionals involved in the treatment of children with cancer. The honest and candid opinions expressed by children being treated for cancer, their siblings, and parents serve as a reminder of the continual need for the highest standards of competence and compassion in helping families manage the difficult and sometimes overwhelming physical, emotional, social, and financial burdens they face. Chapter 6, *Forming a Partnership with the Medical Team*, is an especially important chapter because it is this partnership and honest sharing of knowledge which returns as much control as possible to parents in making necessary decisions about the care of their child. Every child is different, as is every hospital, and not every physician or medical center will necessarily follow all of the guidelines described in the book. Treatments evolve and change. Nonetheless, the knowledge gained by reading this book will enable parents to ask the right questions and to become an integral part of the partnership in their child's treatment.

We still strive for the universally "truly cured child." As described by Dr. Jan van Eys, a pioneer in childhood cancer treatment: "Truly cured children are not just biologically cured, free of disease, but developmentally on a par with their peers and at ease with their experience of having had cancer."[2] Parents who read this book will have the opportunity to ensure that, as much as possible, they can give their child the very best opportunity to be "truly cured."

—F. Leonard Johnson, MD
The Robert C. Neerhout Professor of Pediatrics,
Chief, Division of Pediatric Hematology/Oncology,
Oregon Health Sciences University
Director, The Kenneth W. Ford Northwest Children's Cancer Center,
Doernbecher Children's Hospital,
Portland, Oregon

---

[2] Van Eys, J., ed. *The Truly Cured Child: The New Challenge in Pediatric Cancer Care.* Baltimore: University Park Press, 1977.

Introduction

We are all in the same boat, in a stormy sea,
and we owe each other a terrible loyalty.

—G. K. Chesterton

MY LIFE ABRUPTLY CHANGED on Valentine's Day, 1992, when my three-year-old daughter was diagnosed with acute lymphoblastic leukemia (high risk). At the time, I was the full-time mother of two small daughters, Katy, three years old, and Alison, eighteen months.

The phone call from my pediatrician informing me of Katy's probable diagnosis began my transformation into a "hospital mom." On the two-hour trip to the nearest children's hospital, I naively thought that my background would equip me to deal with the difficulties ahead. I had a degree in biology, and had worked my way through the university in a series of hospital jobs. I had experience in the blood bank, the emergency room, the coronary care unit, and the IV (intravenous) team. After college, I was a paramedic with a busy rescue squad and for several years taught emergency medical technician courses at the local community college. I understood the science and could speak the jargon; I thought I was prepared.

I was wrong. Nothing prepares a parent for the utter devastation of having a child diagnosed with cancer. My brain went on strike. I couldn't hear what was being said. I felt like I was trapped in a slow-motion horror movie.

I came home from Katy's first hospitalization with two shopping bags full of booklets, pamphlets, and single sheets containing information on a wide variety of topics. I didn't know how to prioritize what I needed to learn, so I started by researching everything that I could about leukemia. With the help of my wonderful family and hardworking friends, I began to rapidly fill several file cabinets with information on the medical aspects of the disease.

Emotionally, however, I felt lost. Since most of Katy's treatment was outpatient, I lived too far away to benefit from the hospital's support group, and I

knew no local parents whose child had leukemia. I felt isolated. Then I discovered Candlelighters (see Appendix C, *Resource Organizations*). This
marked a turning point in my ability to deal effectively with my daughter's
disease. I began networking with the parents and made marvelous friends. I
soon realized that we shared many of the same concerns and were dealing
with similar problems. Advice from "veteran" parents became my lifeline.

Why I wrote this book

As I approached the end of Katy's treatment, I realized that I had amassed
not only a library of medical information, but scores of first-person accounts
of how individual parents coped. It saddened me to think that most parents
of children with leukemia would, like me, have to expend precious time and
energy to collect, assess, and prioritize information vital to their child's well-
being. After all, parents are busy providing much of the treatment that their
child receives. They make all appointments, prepare their child for procedures, buy and dispense most medicines, deal with all of the physical and
emotional side effects, and make daily decisions on when the child needs
medical attention. In a sense, this book grew out of my concern that other
overwhelmed parents should not have to duplicate my efforts to gather and
organize information.

What this book offers

This book is not intended to be autobiographical. Instead, I wanted to blend
basic technical information in easy-to-understand language with stories and
advice from many parents and survivors. I wanted to provide the insight and
experiences of veteran parents, who have all felt the hope, helplessness,
anger, humor, longing, panic, ignorance, warmth, and anguish of their children's treatment for cancer. I wanted parents to know how other children
react to treatment, and I wanted to offer tips to make the experience easier.

Obtaining a basic understanding of topics such as medical terminology, common side effects of chemotherapy, and how to interpret blood counts can
only improve the quality of life for the whole family suffering along with
their leukemic child. Learning how to develop a partnership with your
child's physician can vastly increase your family's comfort and peace of mind.
Hearing parents describe their own emotional ups and downs, how they
coped, and how they molded their family life around hospitalizations is a

tremendous comfort. Just knowing that there are other kids on chemotherapy who refuse to eat anything but tacos or who have frequent rages makes one feel less alone. My hope is that parents who read this book will encounter medical facts simply explained, will find advice that eases their daily life, and will feel empowered to be a strong advocate for their child.

The parent stories and suggestions in this book are absolutely true, although some names have been changed to protect children's privacy. Every word has been spoken by the parent of a child with cancer, a sibling of a child with cancer, or a childhood cancer survivor. There are no composites, no editorializing, and no rewrites—just the actual words of people who wanted to share what they learned with others.

How this book is organized

I have organized the book sequentially in an attempt to parallel most families' journeys through treatment. We all start with diagnosis, learn about leukemia, try to cope with procedures, adjust to medical personnel, and deal with family and friends. We all seek out various methods of support, and struggle with the strong feelings of our child with cancer and our other children. We try to work with our child's school to provide the richest and most appropriate education for our ill child. And, unfortunately, we must grieve, either for our child or for the child of a close friend we have made in our new community of cancer.

Because it is tremendously hard to focus on learning new things when you are emotionally battered and extremely tired, I have tried to keep each chapter short.

The first time I introduce a medical term, I define it in the text. If you do not read the book sequentially and encounter an undefined term, it will be explained in the glossary at the end of the book.

Since half of the children diagnosed with leukemia are boys, and half girls, I did not adopt the common convention of using only masculine personal pronouns. Because I do not like using he/she, I have alternated personal pronouns within chapters. This may seem awkward as you read, but it prevents half of the parents from feeling that the text does not apply to their child.

All of the medical information contained in this book is current for 1999. As treatment is constantly evolving and improving, there will inevitably be changes. However, most of the medicines now in use have been used for many years. Their use in combination and changes in dosages have accounted for the tremendous increase in treatment effectiveness in the last two decades. Scientists are currently studying some biological agents, however, that may dramatically improve treatment for leukemia. You will learn in this book how to discover the newest and most appropriate treatment for your child.

To meet some of the children you will read about in this book, and to give you more places to find help for your cancer journey, I have included four appendixes for reference: a photo gallery of children during and after treatment, blood counts and what they mean, resource organizations, and books and online sites. In addition, bound in the book is an indispensable health record to be filled out at the end of treatment and copied and given to each subsequent caregiver for the rest of your child's life. This personal long-term follow-up guide educates healthcare providers about the types of treatment given and the follow-up schedule necessary to maintain optimum health.

How to use this book

While researching this book, I was repeatedly told by parents to "write the truth." Because the "truth" varies for each person, more than eighty parents, children with leukemia, and siblings share portions of their experiences. This book is full of such snapshots in time, some of which may be hard to read, especially by those families of children newly diagnosed. Here are my suggestions for a positive way to use the information contained in this book:

- Consider reading only sections that apply to the present or immediate future. Even if your child's prognosis indicates a high probability of cure, reading about relapse or death can be emotionally difficult.

- Realize that only a fraction of the problems that parents describe will affect your child. Every child is different; every child sails smoothly through some portions of treatment while encountering difficulties in others. The more you understand about the variability of cancer experiences, the better you will be able to cope with your own situation as well as be a good listener and helpful friend to other families you meet with differing diagnoses and circumstances.

- Take any concerns or questions that arise to your oncologist and/or pediatrician for answers (or more questions). The more you learn, the better you can advocate for your family and others.

- I have struggled to keep each chapter short and the technical information easy to read. If you want to delve into any topic in greater depth, Appendix D, *Books and Online Sites*, is a good place to start. It contains a short list of pamphlets and books for parents as well as children of all ages. Reading tastes are a very individual matter, so if something suggested in the bibliography is not helpful or upsets you, put it down. You will probably find something else on the list that is more appropriate for you. (If you are interested in more technical information, a bibliography of medical journal articles can be found online at *http://www.patient-centers.com/leukemia.*)

- Share the book with family and friends. Usually they desperately want to help and just don't know how. This book not only explains the disease and treatment but also offers dozens of concrete suggestions for family and friends.

Best wishes for a smooth journey through treatment and a bright future for the entire family.

• • • • •

Katy finished her treatment in May 1994, rapidly regained her strength, and started kindergarten that fall. She is now a rosy-cheeked fifth grader, who enjoys artwork, writing, and playing the piano and cello. Each new school year, we watch her stride off with hope in our hearts and tears in our eyes.

Acknowledgments

This book is truly a collaborative effort for, without the help of many, it would simply not exist. My heartfelt thanks to my family and friends who supported and encouraged me while I wrote both editions of this book. I would especially like to thank my children—Kathryn and Alison—for the joy they bring to my life each day and their patience when I work long hours in my home office. Special thanks to my editor, Linda Lamb, whose creative instinct and gentle guidance shaped this book from its inception; to Carol Wenmoth, for her attention to detail and unfailing good cheer; and to Tim O'Reilly for his belief and support of the patient-centered guides. The entire staff at O'Reilly & Associates has been not only knowledgeable and efficient, but dedicated in their effort to make this a comprehensive, up-to-date resource for those affected by childhood leukemia.

Many well known and respected members of the pediatric oncology community, and professionals in related fields, graciously carved time out of busy schedules to make invaluable suggestions and to ensure that the material contained in this book is factually correct. I especially appreciate the patient and thoughtful answers to my many phone calls and emails. Thank you: Peter C. Adamson, MD; Nancy Bunin, MD; William Carroll, MD; Barbara Clark, MD; Lynne Conlon, PhD; Max Coppes, MD, PhD; Debra Ethier, RTT; Debra Friedman, MD; Daniel Fiduccia, BA; Mark Greenberg, MD; Wendy Hobbie, RN, MSN, PNT; JoAnne Holt, MA; F. Leonard Johnson, MD; Anne Kazak, PhD; Susan J. Leclair, MS, CLS (NCA); Grace Ann Monaco, JD; Mark Newman, MD; Ann Newman, RN; Mary Riecke, pharmacist; Sheryl Lozowski Sullivan, MPH; Heidi Suni, MSW; and David Unger, MD.

The text of *Childhood Leukemia: A Guide for Families, Friends & Caregivers* was read by many people of disparate backgrounds, whose comments proved extremely helpful. Thank you, Belinda Buescher, Wendy Corder Dowhower, Mary Ellen Keene, Patricia Keene, Cynthia Krumme, Christina O'Reilly, Hazel Reed, Donna Santora Vovcsko, Ralene Walls, and the many parents of children with cancer who graciously took time from their families to review and improve this book. In addition, my family of cyber-friends on PEDONC and ALL-KIDS supplied innumerable suggestions, great stories, and years of both support and fun. Thank you all.

To all of the parents, children with cancer, and their siblings, whose words form the heart and soul of this book, thank you: Brenda Andrews, Robin B., Jan Barber, Barbara Bradley, Sue Brooks, Michelle Caldwell, Edie Cardwell, Ricky Carroll, Alicia Cauley, Naomi Chesler, Priscilla Cooperman, Allison E. Ellis, Lisa N. Ellis, E.B. Engelmann, Dana Erickson, Mel Erickson, Patty Feist-Mack, Alana Freedman, Jenny Gardner, Shirley Enebrad Geller, Denise M. Glassmeyer, Roxie Glaze, Melanie Goldish, Kris H., Lisa Hall, Erin Hall, Kathryn G. Havemann, Connie Herron, Douglas L. Herstrom, Connie Higbee-Jones, Honna Janes-Hodder, Ruth Hoffman, Margaret Huhner, Chris Hurley, Cheryl Putnam Jagannathan, Theresa T. Jeniene, Karen and Brian Jordan, Fr. Joseph, Susan Kalika, Winnie Kittiko, Cynthia Krumme, Madeline LaBonte, Missy Layfield, Pat Lee, Suzanne Lee, Kathryn C. Lim, Wies and Julie Matejko, Caitlin McCarthy-King, Deirdre McCarthy-King, Sara McDonnall, Wendy Mitchell, Amanda Moodie, Jean Morris, Leslee Morris, Laura Myer, M. Clare Paris, Jeff Pasowicz, Donna Phelps, Bev Phipps, Mary Riecke, Jennifer M. Rohloff, Steve and Shirlene S., Carole Schuette, Donna Schumacher, Judith Mravetz Schumann, Sharon A. Schuster, Susan Sennett,

Lori Shipman, Mark A. Simmons, DDS, Lorrie Simonetti, Cathi Smith, Carl and Diane Snedeker, Anne Spurgeon, Anabel Stehli, Becky Stephan, Kim Stimson, Dawni Summitt, Gigi N. Thorsen, Lisa Tignor, Laura Todd-Pierce, Kathleen Tucker, Brigit Tuxen, Annie Walls, Tami Watchurst, Helen Wilder, Jean Wilkerson, Erika Zignego, Ellen Zimmerman, and those who wish to remain anonymous.

Thank you to Mitzi Waltz. Some of the material in Chapter 15, *School*, was adapted from her book, *Pervasive Developmental Disorders: Finding a Diagnosis and Getting Help* (O'Reilly & Associates, Inc., 1999).

Despite the inspiration and contributions of so many, any errors, omissions, misstatements, or flaws in the book are entirely my own.

CHAPTER 1

Diagnosis

A journey of a thousand leagues begins
with a single step.

—Lao-tzu

"WE HAVE THE RESULTS of the blood work back. I'm afraid it's bad news. Your child has leukemia." For every parent who has heard those words, it is a moment frozen in time. In one shattering instant, life forever changes. Many parents equate cancer with death and are staggered by the thought of losing their beloved child. Strong emotions will batter every member of the family. However, with time and the knowledge that most children survive childhood leukemia, hope will grow.

Signs and symptoms

Leukemia is cancer of the spongy blood-forming tissues that make up the bone marrow inside large bones. The diseased bone marrow floods the body with abnormal white cells. These cells do not perform the infection-fighting functions of healthy, mature white cells. Moreover, production of red cells, which carry oxygen, and platelets, which help prevent bleeding, is decreased. Chapter 2, *Leukemia*, provides an in-depth explanation of the various leukemias, their causes and treatments.

Diagnosis of leukemia is extremely difficult because many symptoms mimic those of normal childhood illnesses. The onset of the disease can be slow and insidious or very rapid. Initially, children begin to tire easily and rest often. Frequently, they have a fever which comes and goes. Interest in eating gradually diminishes, but only some children lose weight. Parents usually notice pale skin and occasional bruising. Some children develop back, leg, and joint pain which makes it difficult for them to walk. Often lymph nodes in the neck or groin become enlarged, and the upper abdomen protrudes due to enlargement of the spleen and liver. Children become cranky and irritable, and occasional nosebleeds develop.

Usually parents have an uneasy feeling that something is wrong, but cannot pinpoint the cause for their concern:

> Preston (ten years old) had an incredible diagnosis. We were very lucky. We were at our beach cabin for Thanksgiving. Preston was tired and listless and had a low-grade fever (99–100°) that had persisted for several days. We were bringing his younger sister into town to attend a birthday party, so we decided to bring Preston in to have him checked by the pediatrician on call. The doctor asked Preston what was wrong, and he said, "I don't know, I just feel awful." The doctor ordered blood work and a chest x-ray, and within thirty minutes I was told that he had a "blood cancer." I wanted to take Preston back to the cabin, but was told we needed to go immediately to the hospital, where Preston was admitted, and treatment began.

Most parents react to their concerns by taking their child to a doctor, as Preston's parents did. Usually, the doctor performs a physical exam and frequently orders blood work, including a complete blood count (CBC). Sometimes the diagnosis is not so easy or fast as Preston's:

> I had been worried about Christine (three years old) for two weeks. She was pale and tired. She ate nothing but toast, and had developed bruises on her shins. At preschool, she was unusually irritable, and would utter a high-pitched scream whenever upset. She told me that she didn't want to go to preschool anymore, and when I asked why, she said, "It's just too much for me, Mommy."
>
> I took her to the doctor on an afternoon when he was very busy. He measured Christine's weight and height, pronounced them normal, and described her lack of appetite as "nothing to worry about." I told him that all she was doing was lying on the couch and asked why she would have bruises on her legs. He said bruises on shins always take a long time to heal. When I pointed out how pale she was, he stated that all children are pale in the winter.
>
> I grew more and more concerned and took her back the next week. The doctor discovered an ear infection and prescribed antibiotics. I asked why her eyelids were puffy and he thought it was from sinuses. When I told him of Christine's withdrawal from preschool, he suggested that I read a book entitled The Difficult Child.

Things continued to deteriorate, and I called three days later to say that she seemed to be sicker. Her prescription for antibiotics was changed without the doctor seeing her. I was starting to feel frantic, and went to talk to my neighbor who had recently retired after forty years of nursing. I told her I was afraid Christine had leukemia, and I cried. She said I should take her back to the doctor and insist on blood work. When I took her in that afternoon, her white count was over 200,000 (normal is 10,000, the rest were cancer cells) and her hematocrit (percentage of oxygen-carrying red cells) was 12, far lower than the normal 36.

Where should your child receive treatment?

After a tentative diagnosis of leukemia, most physicians refer the family for further tests and treatment to the closest major medical center with expertise in treating children with cancer. It is very important that the child with leukemia be treated at a facility that uses a team approach, including pediatric oncologists, oncology nurses, specialized surgeons and pathologists, pediatric nurse practitioners, pediatric radiologists, rehabilitation specialists, education specialists, and social workers. State-of-the-art treatment is provided at these institutions, offering your child the best chance for remission (disappearance of the disease in response to treatment) and ultimately, cure.

When we were told that Katy had leukemia, for some reason I was worried that she would miss supper during the long road trip to Children's Hospital. Why I was worried about this when she wasn't eating anyway is a mystery. The doctor told us not to stop, just to go to a drive-through restaurant. I was so upset that I only packed Katy's clothes; my husband, baby, and I had only the clothes on our backs for that first horrible week.

Usually the child is admitted through the emergency room or the oncology clinic, where a physical exam is performed. An intravenous line (IV) is started, more blood is drawn, and a chest x-ray is obtained. Early in your child's hospitalization, the oncologist will perform a spinal tap to determine if any leukemia cells are present in the cerebrospinal fluid and a bone marrow aspiration to identify the type of leukemia. Details of these procedures are described in Chapter 3, *Coping with Procedures*.

Physical responses

Many parents become physically ill in the weeks following diagnosis. This is not surprising, given that most parents stop eating or grab only fast food, normal sleep patterns are a thing of the past, and staying in the hospital may expose them to illnesses. Every waking moment is filled with excruciating emotional stress, which makes the physical stress so much more potent.

> *The second week in the hospital I developed a ferocious sore throat, runny nose, and bad cough. Her counts were on the way down, and they ordered me out of the hospital until I was well. It was agony.*

· · · · ·

> *That first week, every time my son threw up, so did I. I also had almost uncontrollable diarrhea. Every new stressful event in the hospital just dissolved my gut; I could feel it happening. Thank God this faded away after a few weeks.*

Parental illness is a very common event. To attempt to prevent its occurrence, it is helpful to try to eat nutritious meals, get a break from your child's bedside to take a walk outdoors, and find time to sleep. Care needs to be taken not to overuse drugs, tobacco, or alcohol. Whereas physical illnesses usually end after a period of adjustment, emotional effects continue throughout treatment.

Emotional responses

The shock of diagnosis results in an overwhelming number of intense emotions. The length of time people experience each of these feelings greatly differs, depending on preexisting emotional issues and coping ability. These preexisting states vary from person to person, with some whose worlds are stable and good, better able to move quickly through powerful emotions than those who are also dealing with other crises. Many of these emotions reappear at different times during the child's treatment. Some of the feelings that parents experience are described below.

Confusion and numbness

In their anguish, most parents remember only bits and pieces from the doctor's early explanations about their child's disease. This dreamlike state is an almost universal response to shock. The brain provides protective layers of numbness and confusion to prevent emotional overload. This allows parents to examine information in smaller, less threatening pieces. Oncologists understand this phenomenon and are usually quite willing to repeat information as often as necessary. It is sometimes helpful to write down instructions, record them on a small tape recorder, or ask a friend to help keep track of all the new and complex information.

> The doctor ordered a CBC from the lab. All the while I'm still convinced my son's bleeding gums were caused by his six-year molars. The rest happened so fast it's hard to recount. We ended up at the hospital getting a bone marrow test. My husband and I tried to tell the doctor that we would go home and let Stephen rest and that when we came back in the morning they could do another CBC. We were positive that his cell counts would go up in the morning. He said that we didn't have until morning. He said Stephen was very, very sick. After the bone marrow test, the doctor called us in a room and said that Stephen had leukemia. After that word I couldn't hear a thing. My ears were ringing, and my body was numb. There were tears in my eyes. It was actually a physical reaction. I asked him to stop explaining because I couldn't hear him. I asked for a book and went back to the hospital room to read and to cry.

· · · · ·

> For the longest time (in fact still, three years later) I can hear the doctor's voice on the phone telling me that Brent had leukemia. I remember every tiny detail of that whole day, until we got to the hospital, and then the days blur.

· · · · ·

> I felt like I was standing on a rug that was suddenly yanked out from under me. I found myself sitting there on the floor, and I just didn't know how to get up.

Denial

In the first few days after diagnosis, many parents use denial to shield themselves from the terrifying situation. They simply cannot believe that their child has a life-threatening illness. In order to convince themselves that the diagnosis is not a mistake, some parents find comfort in seeking a second opinion (see Chapter 6, *Forming a Partnership with the Medical Team*). Denial may serve as a useful method to survive the first few days after diagnosis, but a gradual acceptance must occur so that the family can begin to make the necessary adjustments to cancer treatment. Life has dramatically changed. Once parents accept the doctor's encouraging statistics, push their fears into the background, and begin to believe that their child will survive, they will be better able to provide support for their child and family.

> *After our daughter's diagnosis, we had to drive two hours to the hospital. My husband and I talked about leukemia the entire trip, and, I felt, started to come to grips with the illness. However, after the IV, the x-rays, and the blood transfusions, he became extremely upset that they were going to admit her. He thought that we could just go home and it would be finished. I had to say, "This will be our life for years."*

· · · · ·

> *My husband and I sat and waited in silence until the doctor came back with the test results. The next thing I knew we were in his office with a primary nurse, a social worker, and a resident listening to the sickening news that our son had leukemia. I couldn't stop crying, and just wanted to grab my two-year-old son and run far, far away.*

Guilt

Guilt is a common and normal reaction to childhood leukemia. Parents feel that they have failed to protect their child, and blame themselves. It is especially difficult because the cause of their child's cancer cannot be explained. There are questions: How could we have prevented this? What did we do wrong? How did we miss the signs? Why didn't we bring her to the doctor sooner? Why didn't we insist that the doctor do blood work? Did he inherit this from me? Why didn't we live in a safer place? Maybe I shouldn't have let him drink the well water. Was it because of the fumes from painting the house? Why? Why? Why? It may be difficult to accept, but parents need to remember that nothing they did caused their child's illness. One method to reduce the burden of guilt is to seek information about the causes of leukemia from medical staff and books.

Nancy Roach describes some of these feelings in her booklet *The Last Day of April*:

> *Almost as soon as Erin's illness was diagnosed, our self-recrimination began. What had we done to cause this illness? Was I careful enough*

during pregnancy? We knew radiation was a possible contributor; where had we taken Erin that she might have been exposed? I wondered about the toxic glue used in my advertising work or the silk screen ink used in my artwork. Bob questioned the fumes from some wood preservatives used in a project. We analyzed everything—food, fumes, and TV. Fortunately, most of the guilt feelings were relieved by knowledge and by meeting other parents whose leukemic children had been exposed to an entirely different environment.

Some parents want to do everything possible to make sure that the child's environment does not pose additional risk. One mother explained how she checked on the possibility of electromagnetic fields in her home and yard:

We have two transformers on our property. After Preston's diagnosis, I wanted to check for electromagnetic fields (EMFs). I called our power company about the free service they offer to check EMFs in the home and yard of customers. After my call, they came out promptly with testing equipment. Surprisingly, the highest readings that they found were from Preston's alarm clock next to his bed and some baseboard heaters with fans in our kitchen. These emitted far higher EMFs than the transformers did.

And another parent's thought:

A year before my daughter's diagnosis, we moved into a rural area and relied on water from a well. When we moved in, I had the water tested for all known contaminants. However, within a year, both of our dogs became ill, and my daughter was diagnosed with leukemia. I decided that for my peace of mind, we should buy water which had been extensively treated.

Fear and helplessness

A diagnosis of leukemia strips parents of control over their child's daily life. Previously, parents established routines and rules which defined family life. Children woke up, washed and dressed, ate breakfast, perhaps attended day care or school, played with friends, and performed chores. Life was predictable. Suddenly, the family is thrust into a new world populated by an ever-changing cast of characters (interns, residents, fellows, oncologists, IV teams, nurses, social workers) and containing a new language (medical terminology): a new world full of hospitalizations, procedures, and drugs.

Until adjustment begins, parents sometimes feel utterly helpless. Physicians whom they have never met are making life-or-death decisions for their child. Even if parents are comfortable in a hospital environment, feelings of helplessness may develop because there is simply not enough time in the day to care for a very sick child, deal with their own changing emotions, begin to educate themselves about the disease, notify friends and family, make job decisions, and restructure the family to deal with the crisis.

Parents also experience different levels of anxiety, including fear and panic. Many develop problems sleeping and feel overwhelmed by fears of what the future holds. Their world has turned inside out—they have gone from adults in control of their lives to helpless people who cannot protect their child.

Many parents state that helplessness begins to disappear when a sense of reality returns. They begin to make decisions, study their options, learn about the disease, and grow comfortable with the hospital and staff. However, feelings of fear, panic, and anxiety periodically erupt for many parents at varying times throughout their child's treatment.

> A friend who had lost her husband to cancer called soon after my daughter's diagnosis with acute lymphoblastic leukemia (ALL). I told her that I felt helpless, confused, overwhelmed, and teary. I cried, "When will I be my usual competent self again?" She assured me that the beginning was the worst, but to expect to be on an emotional roller coaster for the entire two years of treatment. She was right.

Anger

Anger is a universal response to the diagnosis of cancer.

> We were sent to the emergency room after my son's diagnosis with leukemia. After the inevitable delays, an IV was started and chest x-rays taken. I struggled to remain calm to help my son, but inside I was screaming NO NO NO. A resident patted me on the shoulder and said, "We'll check him out to make sure that everything is okay." I started to sob. She looked surprised and asked what was the matter. I said "He's not okay, and he won't be okay for a long time. He has cancer." I realized later that she was trying to comfort me, but I was very angry. Surprisingly, by the end of my son's hospitalization, we trusted and felt very close to that resident.

It is nobody's fault that children are stricken with cancer. Since parents cannot direct their anger at the cancer, they target doctors, nurses, spouses, sblings, and sometimes even the ill child. Because anger directed at other people can be very destructive, it is necessary to devise ways to express the anger. Some suggestions from parents for managing anger follow.

Anger at healthcare team:

- Talk with one of the nurses
- Discuss feelings with psychologists and/or social workers
- Talk with parents of other ill children

Anger at family:

- Discuss feelings with psychologists and/or social workers
- Run, walk, lift weights, or do other physical exercise
- Do yoga or relaxation exercises
- Keep a journal or tape-record feelings
- Cry in the shower or pound the walls
- Listen to music
- Read other people's stories about cancer
- Talk with friends
- Talk with parents of ill children
- Join or start a support group
- Improve communication within family
- Try individual or family counseling
- Live one day at a time

Anger at God:

- Discuss feelings with clergymen or church members
- Discuss feelings with spouse and/or friends
- Pray

It is important to remember that angry feelings are normal and expected.

Sadness and grief

Parents feel an acute sense of loss when their child is diagnosed with leukemia. They feel unprepared to cope with the possibility of death and fear that they may simply not be able to deal with the enormity of the problems facing the family. Parents describe feeling engulfed by sadness. Grieving for the child is common, even when the prognosis is good. Parents grieve the loss of normalcy, the realization that life will never be the same. They grieve the loss of their dreams and aspirations for their child. Shame and embarrassment are also felt by some parents. Cultural background, individual coping styles, basic temperament, and family dynamics all affect the type of emotions experienced.

> Even though my daughter's prognosis was good, I would find myself daydreaming about her funeral. Certain songs especially triggered this feeling. I invariably burst into tears because I was ashamed to be thinking/planning a funeral when I just could not imagine my life without her. When these feelings washed over me, I could actually feel a physical sensation of my heart ripping.

Cynthia Krumme's book *Having Leukemia Isn't So Bad. Of Course It Wouldn't Be My First Choice* describes a message tacked on the Massachusetts General Clinic bulletin board:

> How do I feel? Don't ask!... aside from nervousness, irritability, exhaustion, faintness, dizziness, tremors, cold sweats, depression, insomnia, muscle pains, mental confusion, internal trembling, numbness, indecisiveness, crying spells, unsocial, asocial, and anti-social behavior...I feel fine....Thank you.

Parents travel a tumultuous emotional path where overwhelming emotions subside only to resurface later. All of these are normal, common responses to a catastrophic event. For many parents, these strong emotions begin to fade as hope grows.

Hope

After being buffeted by illness, anger, fear, sadness, grief, and guilt, most parents welcome the growth of hope. Hope is the belief in a better tomorrow. Hope sustains the will to live and gives the strength to endure each trial. Hope is not a way around, it is a way through. The majority of children conquer childhood leukemia and live long and happy lives. There is reason for hope.

Many families discover a renewed sense of both the fragility and beauty of life after the diagnosis. Outpourings of love and support from family and friends provide comfort and sustenance. Many parents speak of a renewed appreciation for life and consider each day with their child as a precious gift.

A Japanese proverb says: "Daylight will peep through a very small hole."

The immediate future

The next several chapters will provide information to help you deal with immediate decisions that must be made in the first week of treatment: How to get the best doctors and treatment plan, what is leukemia, how (and when) to tell your child, what type of catheter to choose, whether your child should be enrolled in a clinical study, and chemotherapy. Veteran parents will explain what choices they made, how they adjusted, learned, and became active participants in their children's treatment. Sharing experiences with parents and survivors of childhood leukemia may help your family develop its own unique strategy for coping with the challenges ahead.

A Mother's View

Memory is a funny thing. I'd be hard pressed to remember what I had for dinner last night, but like many people, the day of the Challenger explosion and, even further back, the day of John Kennedy's death, are etched in my mind to the smallest detail.

And like a smaller group of people, the day of my child's cancer diagnosis is a strong and vivid memory, even seven years later. Most of the time, I don't dwell on that series of images. It was, after all, a chapter in our lives, and one that is now blessedly behind us. But early each autumn, when I get a whiff of the crisp smell of leaves in the air, it brings back that dark day when our lives changed forever.

Many of the memories are painful and, like my daughter's scars, they fade a little more each year but will never completely disappear. While dealing with the medical and physical aspects of the disease, my husband and I also made many emotional discoveries. We sometimes encountered ignorance and narrow-mindedness, which made me more sad than angry. Mistakes were made, tempers were short, and family relations were strained. But we saw the other side, too. Somehow, our sense of humor held on throughout the ordeal, and when that kicked in, we had some of the best laughs of our lives. There was compassion and understanding when we needed it most. And people were there for us like never before.

I remember two young fathers on our street, torn by the news, who wanted to help but felt helpless. My husband came home from the hospital late one night to find that our lawn had been mowed and our leaves had been raked by them. They had found a way to make a small difference that day.

Another time, a neighbor came to our house bearing a bakery box full of pastries and the message that his family was praying for our daughter nightly around their supper table. The image of this man, his wife, and his eight children joining in prayer for us will never leave me.

A close friend entered the hospital during that first terrible week we were there to give birth to her son. I held her baby, she held me, and we laughed and cried together.

Sometimes, when I look back at that time, I feel as though everything that is wrong with the world and everything that is right is somehow distilled in one small child's battle to live. We learned so very much about people and about life.

Surely people who haven't experienced a crisis of this magnitude would believe that we would want to put that time behind us and forget as much of it as possible. But the fact is, we grew a little through our pain, like it or not. We see through new eyes. Not all of it is good or happy, but it is profound.

I treasure good friends like never before. I view life as much more fragile and precious than I used to. I think of myself as a tougher person than I was, but I cry more easily now. And sure, I still yell at my kids and eagerly await each September when they will be out of my hair for a few hours each day. But I hold them with more tenderness when they hop off *the school bus into my arms. And I like to think that some of the people around us, who saw how suddenly and drastically a family's life can change, hold their children a little dearer as well.*

Do I want to forget those terrible days and nights seven years ago? Not on your life. And I hope the smell of autumn leaves will still bring the memories back when I'm a grandmother, even if I can't remember what I had for dinner last night.

—Kathy Tucker
CURE Childhood Cancer Newsletter
Rochester, NY

CHAPTER 2

Leukemia

The world breaks everyone and afterward
many are strong at the broken places.

—Ernest Hemingway
A Farewell to Arms

THE WORD LEUKEMIA literally means "white blood." Leukemia is the term used to describe cancer of the blood-forming tissues known as bone marrow. This spongy material fills the long bones in the body and produces blood cells. In leukemia, the bone marrow factory creates an overabundance of diseased white cells that cannot perform their normal function of fighting infection. As the bone marrow becomes packed with diseased white cells, production of red cells (which carry oxygen and nutrients to body tissues) and platelets (which help form clots to stop bleeding) slows and stops. This results in a low red blood cell count (anemia) and a low platelet count (thrombocytopenia).

This chapter first looks at the function and composition of blood. Then it examines who gets leukemia, what the signs and symptoms are, how it is diagnosed, and how doctors determine the prognosis. The current treatments for each type of leukemia are outlined. The chapter ends with a discussion of how to talk with your child about his disease.

Leukemia is a disease of the blood

Blood is a vital liquid which supplies oxygen, food, hormones, and other necessary chemicals to all of the body's cells. It also removes toxins and other waste products from the cells. Blood helps the lymph system to fight infection and carries the cells necessary for repairing injuries. Blood also contains important clotting factors.

Whole blood is made up of plasma, which is a clear fluid, and many other components, each with a specific task. The three main elements involved in leukemia are red blood cells, platelets, and white blood cells.

14

Red blood cells (erythrocytes or RBCs) contain hemoglobin, a protein that picks up oxygen in the lungs and transports it throughout the body. RBCs give blood its red color. When leukemia cells in the bone marrow slow down the production of red cells, the child develops anemia. Anemia can cause tiredness, weakness, irritability, pale skin, and headache.

Platelets (thrombocytes) are tiny, disc-shaped cells that help form clots to stop bleeding. Leukemia can dramatically slow down the production of platelets, causing children to bleed excessively from cuts or in some cases from their nose or gums. Children with leukemia can develop large bruises or small red dots (called petechiae) on their skin.

White blood cells (leukocytes or WBCs) destroy foreign substances in the body such as viruses, bacteria, and fungi. WBCs are produced and stored in the bone marrow and are released when needed by the body. If an infection is present, the body produces extra WBCs. There are two main types of WBCs:

- **Lymphocytes**. There are two types that interact to prevent infection, fight viruses and fungi, and provide immunity to disease:
    - T cells attack infected cells, foreign tissue, and cancer cells.
    - B cells produce antibodies which destroy foreign substances.
- **Granulocytes**. There are four types that are the first defense against infection:
    - Monocytes are cells that contain enzymes that kill foreign bacteria.
    - Neutrophils are the most numerous WBCs and are important in responding to foreign bacteria.
    - Eosinophils respond to allergic reactions as well as foreign bacteria and parasites.
    - Basophils are the rarest of the white cells and play a special role in allergic reactions.

The different types of leukemia are cancers of a specific white blood cell type. For instance, acute lymphoblastic leukemia affects only lymphocytes. The specific types of leukemia are explained later in the chapter.

What is a blast?

"Blast" is a short name for an immature white blood cell such as lympho-blast, myeloblast, or monoblast. Normally, less than 5 percent of the cells contained in healthy bone marrow at any one time are blasts. Normal blasts develop into mature, functioning white blood cells, and are not usually found in the bloodstream. Leukemic blasts remain immature, multiply continuously, provide no defense against infection, and may be present in large numbers in the bloodstream.

How does leukemia begin?

When an abnormal population of blasts appear in the bone marrow, they multiply rapidly and lose their ability to grow up into normal white cells. They begin to crowd out the normal cells that usually develop there. After accumulating in the bone marrow, leukemic cells spill over into the blood. Leukemic cells may also cross the blood-brain barrier and invade the central nervous system (brain and spinal cord).

When the leukemic blasts begin to fill the marrow, production of healthy red cells, platelets, and white cells cannot be normally maintained. As the number of normal cells decreases, symptoms appear. Low red cell counts cause fatigue and pale skin. Low platelet counts may result in bruising and bleeding problems. If mature neutrophils and lymphoblasts are crowded out by the blasts, the child will have little or no defense against infections.

Who gets leukemia?

Acute leukemia is the most common childhood cancer. Although generally thought of as strictly a childhood disease, many more adults than children develop leukemia. Each year in the United States, approximately 25,000 adults and 2,500 children are diagnosed with acute leukemia.

Childhood leukemia is most commonly diagnosed at ages two to seven, with the highest incidence at approximately four years of age. In the United States, leukemia is more common in whites than in blacks, and boys have a slightly higher incidence than girls. Children with genetic diseases such as Down syndrome, Bloom's syndrome, or Fanconi's anemia have a higher risk of developing leukemia than the general population. However, most children with these syndromes do not develop leukemia.

Although the exact cause of childhood leukemia is a mystery, certain factors are known to increase the risk of developing the disease.

Genetic factors

It is known that persons with extra chromosomes (genetic material contained in cells) or certain chromosomal abnormalities have a greater chance of developing leukemia. It is uncertain whether this is a cause or merely an association. In cases where one identical twin has leukemia, the other twin has a 25 percent chance of developing the disease within one year, but this risk decreases with an older age at diagnosis and with time. It is not known whether this is caused by an inherited trait or a simultaneous exposure to the same carcinogen. Leukemia is not contagious; it cannot be passed from one person to another.

Environmental factors

Exposure to ionizing radiation and certain toxic chemicals may predispose individuals to leukemia and other problems involving the bone marrow. Many Japanese who were exposed to fallout from the atomic bomb during World War II and some of the people living near the Chernobyl accident in the Ukraine have developed leukemia. Chronic exposure to benzene has been associated with leukemia in adults. However, most children are not exposed to large amounts of radiation or industrial chemicals. The data so far indicates that there is no increased risk of leukemia from exposure to electromagnetic fields. Although scientists are examining associations with many environmental factors, there are no clear environmental causes of childhood leukemia.

Rates of childhood cancer have increased every year for the last three decades. In response to this and other threats to children's health, in 1997 the US formed the Federal Task Force on Protecting Children from Environmental Health Risks and Safety Risks. Information on this task force can be found on the Internet at *http://www.epa.gov/children/six.htm*.

The US Environmental Protection Agency (EPA) has a Children's Health Resources branch that maintains publications on children's health topics, information on hot lines, and links to Internet resources at (888) 372-8255 and on the Internet at *http://www.epa.gov/children/eleven1.htm*.

For information about the US government's electromagnetic field (EMF) research efforts, including public information materials developed by the EMF RAPID program, refer to the EMF RAPID home page on the Internet: *http://www.niehs.nih.gov/emfrapid/home.htm*.

Viral factors

Viruses that cause leukemia in cows, cats, chickens, gibbons, and mice have been found. A T-cell virus has been identified which causes a rare type of leukemia-lymphoma in adults; however, no virus has been found which causes the types of leukemia commonly found in children.

Currently, it is thought that a complex interaction among genetic, environmental, immunologic, and possibly viral factors predispose individuals to leukemia. The most important point for parents to remember is that at present there is no way to predict or prevent leukemia. Nothing that parents did or did not do caused or could have prevented the leukemia.

How is leukemia diagnosed?

A tentative diagnosis is made after a physical examination of the child and microscopic analysis of a blood sample. Physical findings may include pale skin; bruising or unusual bleeding; enlarged liver, spleen, or lymph nodes; ear or other infections (frequently resistant to treatment); weakness; and fever. Parents or children may describe irritability, night sweats, fatigue, bone pain, and loss of appetite. Blood tests may show decreased red cells, decreased platelets, and either abnormally low or high white blood cell counts. There may be blast cells circulating in the blood.

The T-cell type of ALL sometimes involves the thymus gland in the neck. Enlargement of the thymus can pressure the nearby trachea (windpipe), causing coughing or shortness of breath. The superior vena cava (SVC), a large vein that carries blood from the head and arms back to the heart, passes next to the thymus. An enlarged thymus gland may compress the SVC and cause swelling of the head and arms.

Some children with leukemia have the disease in their central nervous system (brain and spinal cord) at diagnosis. Less than 10 percent of children or teens with leukemia have symptoms of CNS disease, including headache, poor work or school performance, weakness, seizures, vomiting, blurred vision, and difficulty in maintaining balance.

Children with AML are sometimes diagnosed after developing a chloroma— a tumor arising from myeloid tissue and containing a pale green pigment. These are most often found under the skin of the skull.

To confirm a diagnosis of leukemia, bone marrow is sampled and tested (see Chapter 3, *Coping with Procedures*). The bone marrow is examined microscopically by a pediatric oncologist and/or a pathologist, a physician who specializes in body tissue analysis. More than 25 percent blasts in the marrow confirms the diagnosis of leukemia. A portion of the bone marrow (and chloroma biopsy if done) is sent to a specialized laboratory that analyzes many other features of the leukemic cells to help determine which type of leukemia is present.

How is leukemia best treated?

At diagnosis, parents are often confused about how to find the best doctors and treatment plan for their child. The best care available in the US and Canada is obtained from institutions who are part of the Children's Cancer Group or the Pediatric Oncology Group (see Chapter 4, *Clinical Trials*). These study groups, composed of pediatric oncologists and surgeons, urologists, radiation oncologists, researchers, and nurses, establish the standard of care for patients in the US and Canada, conduct new studies to discover better therapies or fine tune the old ones, and establish follow-up for survivors. They are in the process of merging into one entity called the Children's Oncology Group (COG). If the treatment center you are referred to is a member of one of these groups, you can rest assured that your child will have access to the best thinking on the treatment of pediatric cancers.

Types of leukemia

The two broad classifications of leukemia are acute (rapid progression) and chronic (slow progression). The acute leukemias are characterized by abnormal numbers of immature white cells (blasts). In chronic leukemia, mature white cells predominate. Chronic leukemia accounts for less than 5 percent of all childhood leukemia.

Acute leukemia is the most common type of cancer found in children. The two most common types of acute leukemia are acute lymphoblastic leukemia (ALL) and acute myeloid leukemia (AML). AML is also known as acute non-lymphoblastic leukemia (ANLL).

Acute lymphoblastic leukemia (ALL)

Seventy-five percent of all children with leukemia have ALL. It is caused by a rapid proliferation of immature lymphocytes, which would normally have developed into mature T cells or B cells. There are several subgroups of ALL based on whether the cancer cells developed from B cells or T cells, or display characteristics of both. The first sample of bone marrow taken from the child is analyzed to identify cellular characteristics to help plan the best therapy as well as predict response to treatment. Each different subgroup has a different response to treatment; some require less chemotherapy, while others require aggressive treatment to achieve a cure.

> I was walking around the hospital looking shellshocked the day after my daughter had been admitted to Children's Hospital with leukemia. One of the other mothers came up, introduced herself, and asked what we were in for. I told her leukemia. She told me that her son had just relapsed again from a brain tumor. She looked wistful and said how much she wished that her son had ALL. She said, "You might think that's strange, but I see those kids come, get better, and go home. We are still here."

Prognosis for the child with ALL

Treatment of childhood ALL is one of the major medical success stories of the last two decades. In the early 1960s, patients with ALL usually lived only for a few months, but by the late 1990s, over 70 percent of children receiving optimal treatment were cured. The appropriate treatment for each child with ALL is determined by analysis of a multitude of clinical and biologic features. Most centers describe the child's risk of relapse as standard or high.

To determine the risk level, the following prognostic factors are considered: initial white blood count; age at diagnosis; CNS leukemia at diagnosis; presence or absence of chromosomal translocations; and how quickly the child enters remission. You can learn about some of these risk factors at the American Cancer Society web site at *http://www.cancer.org*. Once at the site, click on "cancer information," then "leukemia, child," then "detection and symptoms."

Treatment for ALL

ALL is now considered to be one of the most curable forms of childhood cancer. To receive the best available treatment, it is essential that the child with ALL receive treatment at a pediatric medical center from board-certified pediatric oncologists with extensive experience treating acute leukemia. The intense treatment for ALL begins within days of diagnosis and requires aggressive supportive care. The goal of treatment is to achieve a complete remission by obliterating all cancer cells as quickly as possible. Complete remission occurs when all signs and symptoms of leukemia disappear and abnormal cells are no longer found in the blood, bone marrow, and cerebrospinal fluid.

The mainstay of treatment for ALL is chemotherapy—the use of various drugs to treat disease. Radiation of the brain and sometimes spinal cord is administered to some very high-risk patients. Bone marrow or stem cell (e.g., cord blood) transplantation is infrequently used in the treatment of ALL.

For the average-risk patient, treatment is typically divided into phases: induction, central nervous system prophylaxis, consolidation, reinduction, reconsolidation, and maintenance.

Induction

Induction is the most intensive phase of treatment since its purpose is to kill as many abnormal white cells in the shortest amount of time possible. It usually lasts four weeks, and for a portion of that time, children may need to remain hospitalized for monitoring and transfusions. For the remainder of the time, children are treated on an outpatient basis unless a complication arises. Children may need to be readmitted on more than one occasion during induction due to fever and/or infection.

Chemotherapy is most effective if three or four drugs are used simultaneously. In 1999, the majority of standard-risk ALL induction programs include vincristine, prednisone, and asparaginase. Daunomycin is often added to high-risk protocols. Drugs are given intravenously (through a needle or tube in the vein), intramuscularly (injection in muscle), orally (by mouth), or intrathecally (injected into the cerebrospinal fluid). These drugs can cause numerous side effects. See Chapter 10, *Chemotherapy*, for an in-depth discussion of each drug and its side effects.

Ninety-five percent of children with ALL who receive three or more drugs during induction achieve a complete remission.

Children with extremely high white blood cell counts at diagnosis may require leukapheresis (removal of the white blood cells) before treatment with chemotherapy begins.

CNS prophylaxis

The central nervous system (CNS) is composed of the brain and spinal cord, which are bathed in a fluid called cerebrospinal fluid. When cancer invades the brain, cancer cells are found in the cerebrospinal fluid. In most cases of childhood ALL, the leukemia has not penetrated the brain. However, prior to using radiation and injecting chemotherapy drugs directly into the cerebrosinal fluid, the CNS was frequent relapse site. Therefore, CNS prophylaxis (prevention) is an essential component of treatment for ALL. Because a blood-brain barrier exists that prevents chemotherapy drugs from crossing into the CNS to destroy leukemic cells, chemotherapy drugs are injected directly into the cerebrospinal fluid (called intrathecal medication) during spinal taps. Intrathecal medication is given periodically throughout treatment.

Standard-risk patients receive intrathecal methotrexate, or triple intrathecal therapy—methotrexate, hydrocortisone, and cytarabine—for CNS prophylaxis. Whether patients with a high risk of CNS relapse (e.g., high white cell count at diagnosis; T-cell ALL with a high white cell count; older than age ten years; or those with mediastinal mass) require cranial radiation is still controversial. In many protocols, these patients receive 1800 cGy of cranial radiation as well as intrathecal chemotherapy, although those with a rapid early response to therapy may be treated with intrathecal therapy alone.

CNS prophylaxis has been extraordinarily successful in preventing CNS relapse, and is partially responsible for the huge increase in cure rates. Unfortunately, the treatments can sometimes cause long-term disabilities such as decreased attention span, short-term memory problems, and lower ability in spatial and mathematical skills, particularly when radiation is used (see Chapter 15, *School*). Current clinical trials are attempting to determine how much and what type of intrathecal medicine is necessary to prevent relapse while minimizing the chances for long-term side effects and whether intrathecal medication can replace radiation in some high-risk patients.

Consolidation

Consolidation therapy consists of new combinations of drugs to destroy any cancer cells that survived induction. It includes high doses of previously used or new drugs and central nervous system prophylaxis.

In 1999, the most common drugs used in consolidation are: methotrexate, cyclophosphamide (cytoxan or endoxan), cytosine arabinoside (ARA-C),

6-mercaptopurine (6-MP), dexamethasone (decadron), asparaginase, and thioguanine. See Chapter 10 for detailed descriptions of these drugs.

Reinduction and reconsolidation

A second induction (commonly called delayed intensification or reinduction) and a second consolidation are usually administered prior to maintenance.

More intensive regimens

Protocols for high-risk ALL usually contain more drugs at higher doses, and sometimes cranial radiation. This treatment has increased toxicity, but is more effective for the small percentage of children with high-risk features. Infants with ALL are at the highest risk for relapse, and they require individualized protocols and may need a bone marrow transplant.

The researchers studying childhood cancer are increasing their understanding of what types and subtypes of particular cancers require more intensive therapy and for which ones therapy can be less aggressive. If you are at a center associated with the Children's Cancer Group or Pediatric Oncology Group, you can feel comfortable that your pediatric oncologist will not propose an aggressive treatment unless it is your child's best chance for a cure.

Maintenance

Maintenance therapy, the final phase of treatment for ALL, consists of daily lower-dose chemotherapy for two to three years. Its purpose is to kill any remaining cancer cells. This portion of treatment is less toxic and easier to tolerate than induction and consolidation.

In most clinical trials, mercaptopurine (6-MP) administered every evening and methotrexate given weekly are the standard drugs. In addition, other drugs such as vincristine, prednisone, or dexamethasone may be included. Many protocols also give intrathecal methotrexate during maintenance therapy (see Chapter 10, *Chemotherapy*). During maintenance, children must be monitored for drug-related toxicicies as well as compliance.

Bone marrow or stem cell transplantation (BMT)

Bone marrow or stem cell transplants may be recommended after first remission in some children at extremely high risk of relapse. These may include infants less than one year of age with MLL gene rearrangements. Bone marrow or stem cell transplantation may be recommended for children with ALL who have relapsed and have achieved a second remission (see Chapter 20, *Bone Marrow and Stem Cell Transplantation*).

Newest treatment options

To learn of the newest treatments available, call (800) 4-CANCER and ask for the PDQ (Physician Data Query) for ALL. These free statements, also available on the Internet at *http://cancernet.nci.nih.gov*, explain the disease, state-of-the-art treatments, and ongoing clinical trials. There are two versions available: one for patients that uses simple language and contains no statistics, and one for professionals that is technical, thorough, and includes citations to the scientific literature.

Acute myeloid leukemia (AML)

AML (also called acute myelogenous leukemia, acute nonlymphocytic leukemia, or ANLL) is cancer of the bone marrow. The cancer cells are those that would otherwise develop into myeloid cells like granulocytes. Because treatments for AML and ALL are very different, it is crucial that sophisticated laboratory studies are performed on the bone marrow samples to determine whether the child has AML or ALL.

Eight thousand cases of AML are diagnosed in the US each year, most often in adults over forty. It is also seen in infants or older teens, but can strike children at any age. AML accounts for approximately 15 percent of all cases of childhood leukemia. There are eight different classifications or types of AML (M0 to M7) based on appearance of the diseased cells under the microscope.

> *My six-year-old daughter had been getting bad headaches. The school would call me to pick her up, and she would throw up all the way home. She had an appointment with the optometrist who noticed an odd-looking vein in her eye and that she looked pale and had some bruising. He recommended taking her in for blood work. We did, and she was diagnosed with AML type M2.*

Prognosis for the child with AML

Treatment for AML has dramatically improved in the last decade. Today, 75 to 85 percent of children who receive optimal treatment at a major pediatric medical center achieve a complete remission. Of the children who achieve remission, 40 to 50 percent remain in remission for five years, and are considered cured.

Treatment for AML

Treatment for AML lasts about one year and is very intense. Acute complications of treatment are common. Children with this disease need to be treated at a major pediatric hospital with expertise in treating acute leukemias. The goal of treatment is to achieve a complete remission by obliterating all cancer cells as quickly as possible. Complete remission occurs when all signs and symptoms of leukemia disappear, blood counts are rising towards normal, and abnormal cells are no longer found in the blood, bone marrow (less than 5 percent blasts), and cerebrospinal fluid.

Chemotherapy is the primary treatment to induce remission in children with AML. Radiation of the brain and sometimes the spinal cord is also used (rarely) in some protocols. Bone marrow and stem cell transplantation (see Chapter 20) is frequently used to treat childhood AML in first or second remission.

Treatment usually consists of two or three parts: induction (to achieve remission), postremission consolidation, and/or postremission intensification.

Induction

Induction is the most intense part of treatment; its purpose is to quickly kill as many cancer cells as possible. As with ALL, chemotherapy drugs for AML are more successful if three or four are used simultaneously. The most common drugs used to treat AML are: ARA-C (cytarabine), daunomycin (daunorubicin), etoposide, dexamethasone, and thioguanine. Children with acute promyelocytic leukemia (M3) also receive all-trans-retinoic acid (ATRA) to achieve remission followed by chemotherapy. Recently, it has been discovered that arsenic is also a very effective drug in the treatment of this particular type of leukemia.

Chemotherapy can be administered by mouth (orally), intravenously (through the IV), intramuscularly (injection in the muscle), or intrathecally (through a needle in the lower part of the back). Most AML chemotherapy is given IV. See Chapter 10 for an in-depth discussion of each drug, possible side effects, and parent suggestions.

Several weeks of hospitalization are usually required during induction, as the toxic chemotherapy drugs damage normal cells as well as leukemic cells, leaving the child susceptible to infections and excessive bleeding. Bone marrow growth factors such as granulocyte-macrophage colony-stimulating factor or granulocyte colony-stimulating factor are sometimes used to shorten the duration of neutropenia (low white counts). Transfusions (blood and platelets) and intravenous feeding (hyperalimentation) are often necessary.

If the disease has spread to the brain, the child is given intrathecal chemotherapy (cytarabine or methotrexate) and radiation to destroy the cancer cells. Even if leukemia cells have not been found in the brain, most protocols for childhood AML use some form of CNS treatment, usually intrathecal chemotherapy with or without cranial radiation.

During induction, the majority of patients go into remission, and then enter the second phase of treatment.

Postremission therapy

Even when a child is in complete remission, residual cancer cells would multiply rapidly without additional treatment. Consequently, after a short period of recuperation from induction, children with AML receive either a bone marrow or stem cell transplant or more chemotherapy, called postremission therapy.

Postremission therapy consists of two parts: consolidation and intensification. Your child may receive one or both of these phases of treatment. The drugs used during postremission therapy are high-dose cytarabine, etoposide, amsacrine, vincristine, azacytidine, cyclophosphamide, L-asparaginase, and methotrexate.

In the past, another phase of treatment, called maintenance, has been used. This phase consists of low-dose chemotherapy given for a number of years. Studies have shown that additional therapy after intensive induction and consolidation does not lengthen remission for children with childhood AML. At the time of this writing, 1999, there are ongoing clinical trials using immunotherapy (interleukin-2) versus standard follow-up to see if this treatment extends length of remission.

Bone marrow or stem cell transplantation (BMT/SCT)

BMT/SCT is being used increasingly to treat children with AML in first remission. High-dose chemotherapy, with or without total body radiation, is used to destroy the child's bone marrow and any remaining cancer cells. Healthy, matched marrow is taken from another person, usually a family member, and is dripped into the patient's blood intravenously. The new marrow migrates to the bones and replaces the destroyed marrow. This is called an allogeneic transplant. Nearly 60 percent of children with AML with matched donors who undergo a BMT in first remission experience remissions in excess of three years without severe graft-versus-host disease.

Another method sometimes used for children without a matched, or closely matched, donor is called autologous BMT. In this type of transplant, marrow is removed from the child, may be treated chemically to remove all leukemia cells, and frozen. After the child's own diseased marrow has been destroyed, the frozen marrow is thawed and returned to the patient intravenously. The data so far indicates that this is no better than conventional chemotherapy and is inferior to matched allogeneic bone marrow transplantation.

The role of unrelated (from non-family members) BMTs or cord blood BMTs in treating childhood AML in first remission has not yet been established and is currently being studied. These are often used to treat AML in second remission or AML that occurs as a second cancer.

Chapter 20 discusses in detail the types of transplants, procedures, side effects, and coping suggestions from parents and survivors.

Newest treatment options

To learn of the newest treatments available, call (800) 4-CANCER and ask for the PDQ (Physician Data Query) for childhood AML. These free statements, also available on the Internet at *http://cancernet.nci.nih.gov*, explain the disease, state-of-the-art treatments, and ongoing clinical trials. There are two versions available: one for patients that uses simple language and contains no statistics, and one for professionals that is technical, thorough, and includes citations to the scientific literature.

Chronic myelogenous leukemia (CML)

CML is rare in children, accounting for less than 5 percent of all childhood leukemias. This disease is most common in adults, but occasionally is diagnosed in older boys and girls. It is characterized by a very large spleen, high white count of mostly neutrophils and other types of granulocytes, and high platelet count. Other symptoms of CML are fatigue, weakness, headaches, irritability, fevers, night sweats, and weight loss. Some patients have no symptoms and the cancer is diagnosed after a routine blood test done for other reasons. There is no severe anemia or tendency to bleed.

In over 90 percent of patients with CML, analysis of the cells of the bone marrow shows a genetic abnormality called the Philadelphia chromosome. This chromosome contains a "translocation" or swap of genetic material involving chromosomes 9 and 22, abbreviated as t(9;22).

Phases of CML

Despite its name, CML can progress rapidly, but it generally has three phases:

- A chronic phase (less than 5 percent blasts in the peripheral blood or bone marrow), which can last several years.

- An accelerated phase (greater than 5 percent but less than 30 percent blasts in the peripheral blood or bone marrow).

- A blastic phase (greater than 30 percent blasts in the peripheral blood or bone marrow). When more than 30 percent blasts are present and the child or teen has fever, fatigue, and enlarged spleen, it is called blast crisis.

> Leah, eleven years old, enjoyed participating in basketball, soccer, and gymnastics. She developed severe hip joint pain, and we brought her back to the doctor three times in an unsuccessful attempt to find out what was wrong. The last time, my husband had to carry her in because she couldn't walk. They did blood work, and her white count was 176,000 and her platelets were one million. A bone marrow test confirmed that she had CML.

Treatment for children with CML

The goal of initial treatment is to lower the white count and reduce the size of the spleen. This is accomplished by taking oral medications, usually either hydroxyurea or busulphan (also called myleran). Medicines such as hydroxyurea, busulfan, and the biologic agent interferon alfa may be used to delay disease progression. The average length of the chronic phase of CML is three years, although some patients have remained in this phase for up to ten years.

The doctors did not know how long my daughter had had CML prior to diagnosis, so they estimated that she had three days to four years before the blast phase would begin. They told us that if the blast phase started, there was nothing they could do. She needed a bone marrow transplant as soon as possible.

If the spleen does not shrink after treatment with drugs or radiation, surgical removal may be required.

Although chemotherapy and interferon alpha slow the progress of CML, the best hope for cure is bone marrow transplantation. The highest cure rates occur when the patient is transplanted during the chronic phase with marrow from an identical twin, HLA-identical family member, or HLA-identical non-family donor. Refer to Chapter 20 for detailed information.

The second stage or "accelerated phase" is usually brief. The number of both mature white blood cells and blast cells in the bloodstream increases. The number of red blood cells drops and platelets may increase or decrease. In 1999, treatment for this phase includes high-dose cytarabine, hydroxyurea, busulfan, and/or supportive transfusion therapy (see Chapter 10). Occasionally allogeneic transplants are attempted.

During the blastic phase, white blood cells fail to mature and flood the bloodstream. Treatment for this phase can include any of the following:

- Vincristine and prednisone and sometimes daunorubicin
- Allogeneic bone marrow transplantation (successful in less than 20 percent of cases)
- Autologous bone marrow transplantation (may return the child to the chronic phase)
- Clinical trials using combination chemotherapy (such as 5-azacytidine and mitoxantrone)
- High-dose cytarabine
- Hydroxyurea or radiation to bone lesions (sometimes used to make the child more comfortable)

Chronic myelomonocytic leukemia (CMML)

Chronic myelomonocytic leukemia (also called juvenile CML or JCML) usually strikes children under five years of age. The symptoms are similar to those of the acute leukemias: pale skin, bruising, fatigue, headaches, sweating, and recurrent infection. Also usually present are enlarged lymph nodes, enlarged spleen and liver, and low platelet count. Unlike CML, CMML does not have a chronic phase. Once diagnosed, progressive deterioration usually occurs.

Because chemotherapy is not generally a successful treatment for juvenile CML, bone marrow or stem cell transplantation is the best hope for cure. For more information, see Chapter 20. However, chemotherapy is sometimes used to get the disease under control while preparing for transplant.

> My daughter was diagnosed with JCML in 1993 at the age of 27 months. Although it is a chronic leukemia, it is particularly fast moving and there is no treatment besides BMT. It is also vastly different from the adult CML. My daughter had a mismatched (5/6) related (my husband's sister as donor) BMT four months after she was diagnosed. Today, she is six years post-transplant, is in the second grade, and is the absolute joy of my life.

Once parents understand the basics about the type of leukemia their child has, it is time to begin to decide how and when to tell their child the news.

Telling your child

In the first harrowing days after a diagnosis of leukemia, parents must decide when and what to tell their children. Because parents are coping with a bewildering array of emotions themselves, sharing information and providing reassurance and hope may be difficult. In the past, shielding children from the painful reality was the norm. Most experts now agree that children feel less anxiety and cope with treatments better if they have a clear understanding of the disease. It is important to provide age-appropriate information soon after diagnosis and to create a supportive climate so that children feel comfortable asking questions of both parents and the medical team. Sharing strengthens the family, allowing all members to face the crisis together.

When should you tell your child?

As soon as possible. It is impossible to prevent a child from knowing that he is seriously ill. The child has been whisked to an unfamiliar hospital by frightened parents, endured painful tests, received drugs and transfusions. Cards and presents begin to arrive, and friends and siblings are absent or behave in a strange manner.

Delay in providing age-appropriate information escalates the child's fears. Well-meaning parents may cause great anguish by isolating their child in a conspiracy of silence. Parents may delude themselves into thinking that the diagnosis is a secret, but children are extraordinarily perceptive. They frequently keep their thoughts and feelings to themselves in order to protect their parents from more pain. In this case, not only must the child deal with having cancer, but he must do it on his own with no one to console him. Lacking accurate information, children can imagine scenarios far more frightening than the reality.

> We feel that you have to be very honest or the child will not be able to trust you. Meagan (five years old) has always known that she has cancer and thinks of her treatments and medications as the warriors to help the good cells fight the bad cells.

Who should tell your child?

This is purely a personal decision, influenced by ease of communication within the family, age and temperament of the child, religious beliefs, and sometimes physician recommendation. Small children (ages one to three) primarily fear separation from parents. The presence of strangers in an already unfamiliar situation may cause additional fear. Many parents tell their small child in private, while others prefer to have family members, family physician, oncologist, clergyman, or social worker present.

Older children (four to twelve) sometimes benefit from having the treatment team (oncologist, nurse, social worker, or psychologist) present. This may create a feeling that all present will unite to help her get well. Staff members can answer the child's questions and provide comfort for the entire family. Children in this age group frequently feel guilty and responsible for their illness. They may harbor fears that the cancer is a punishment for something that they did wrong. Social workers and nurses can help explore unspoken questions, provide reassurance, and identify the needs of parents, the sick child, and siblings.

My six-year-old son Brent was sitting next to me when the doctor called to tell me that he had leukemia. I whispered into the phone, "What should I tell him?" The doctor said to tell him that he had a disease in his blood and needed to go to a special children's hospital for help. As we were getting ready to go to the hospital, Brent asked if he had AIDS (it was right after Magic Johnson's announcement), if he was going to die, what were they going to do to him. We didn't know how to answer all the questions, but told him that we would find out at the hospital. My husband told him that he was a strong boy and we would all fight this thing together. I was at a loss for words.

At the hospital, they were wonderful. What impressed me the most was that they always talked to Brent first, and answered all his questions before talking to us. When Zac (Brent's eight-year-old brother) came to the hospital two days later, the doctors took him in the hall and talked to him for a long time, explaining and answering his questions.

I was glad that we were all so honest, because Brent later confided to me that he had first thought he got leukemia because he hadn't been drinking enough milk.

Adolescents' need for control and autonomy should be respected. Teenagers sometimes feel more comfortable discussing the diagnosis with their physician in private. At a time when teens' developmental tasks include becoming independent from their families, they are suddenly totally dependent on medical personnel to save their lives and parents to provide emotional support. In some families, a diagnosis of cancer can create an unwelcome dependence on parents and can add new stress to the already turbulent teen years. Other families report that leukemia helped to forge closer bonds between teenagers and their parents.

When my daughter went into the hospital to get the mediastinal mass diagnosis done, I told her doctor if she got a bad report that I wanted him to tell her father and me and not give her any such news. Her doctor, who I really didn't know before this encounter, informed me that she was fifteen years old and would be the one dealing with cancer and it was very necessary that she be told everything and that nothing be kept from her. I thought that was so mean of him, but I liked him and had never shown any disrespect for a doctor before, so I decided since he had dealt with kids with cancer before and I hadn't that he must know something I didn't

*know. He did! There have been so many times I have been so thankful
that he had the wisdom to tell me that right off the bat. My daughter has
continually told me over the years if the doctor had not always talked
with her in our presence, she would have felt like she was dying.*

Children and teens react to the diagnosis of cancer with as wide a range of
emotions as their parents. They may lapse into denial, feel tremendous anger
or rage, or be extremely optimistic. Children, like their parents, will experience a variety of emotions as treatment progresses.

*We've really marveled at watching Joseph go through the stages of
coping with all of this just as an adult might. First of all, when he was
diagnosed in April and May, he was terrified, then in May and June,
alternately angry and depressed (when we talked to him seriously about
the need to work with the doctors and nurses against the cancer, no matter how scary the things they asked him to do were, he looked us right in
the eye and screamed "I'm on the cancer's side!"), then over the course of
a few weeks he seemed to calm down and made the decision to fight it, to
cooperate with all the caregivers as well as he possibly could and to live as
normal a life as he could. It's hard to believe that someone could do that
at four years old, but he did it. By his fifth birthday on July 26th, he'd
made the transition to where he is now: hopeful and committed to "killing
the cancer."*

What to tell your child

Children need to be told that they are seriously ill, that they will be spending some time in the hospital, that the treatment will last for a long time and
is sometimes painful, that the treatments are usually successful, and that the
doctors and nurses are experts and will provide the very best care available.
Depending on the child's age, this could vary from saying, "Part of your
blood is sick and we need to go to the hospital for medicine to make it better" to reading many books together and answering hundreds of questions.

*My daughter Kathleen Rea knew she had cancer when she was three.
She knew that her motor oil wasn't running her engine right—but she
called it cancer.*

Young children need to be reassured that they did nothing to cause the disease. It is important that they understand the disease is not contagious and

they cannot give it to their siblings or friends. They need to have procedures described realistically, so that they can trust their parents and medical team.

> My four-year-old daughter told me very sadly one day, "I wish that I hadn't fallen down and broken inside. That's how the leukemia started." We had explained many times that nothing she did, or we did, caused the leukemia, but she persisted in thinking that falling down did it. She also worried that if she went to her friend Krista's house to play that Krista would catch leukemia.

Children should understand that it is expected they will have many questions throughout their treatment, and they should be assured they will be answered honestly. Parents need to let their children know that being frightened or upset is normal, indeed is felt by parents and children alike. Gentle and honest communication is essential for the child to feel loved, supported, and encouraged.

> When I told Christine (three years old) that she had a disease in her blood, her first concern was that I might leave. Over the years, I have repeated many, many times that I would always be with her and that I would make sure that there were never any surprises (difficult sometimes in the hospital setting, but it can be done). She is very artistic and wanted me to draw a picture of the cells that were a problem. We drew lots of pictures of white cells being carried off by chemo drugs to be "fixed." Although many of the other parents successfully used images of good cells killing off bad cells, I thought that would upset my extremely gentle daughter. So we imagined, drew pictures of, and talked about chemo turning problem cells into helpful cells.

Barbara Sourkes, PhD, explains the importance of first understanding the child's question prior to responding:

> Coping with the trauma of illness can be facilitated by a cognitive understanding of the disease and its treatment. For this reason, the presentation of accurate information in developmentally meaningful terms is crucial. A general guideline is to follow the child's lead: he or she questions facts or implications only when ready, and that readiness must be respected. It is the adult's responsibility to clarify the precise intent of any question and then to proceed with a step-by-step response, thereby granting the child options at each juncture. He or she may choose to continue

listening, to ask for clarification, or to terminate the discussion. Offering
less information with the explicit invitation to ask for more affords a
safety gauge of control for the child. When these guidelines are not fol-
lowed, serious miscommunications may ensue. For example, an adult
who hears "What is going to happen to me?" and does not clarify the
intent of the query may launch into a long statement of plans or elabo-
rate reassurances. The child may respond with irritation, "I only wanted
to know what tests I am going to have tomorrow."

Telling siblings

A diagnosis of cancer is traumatic for siblings. Family life is disrupted, time
with parents decreases, and a large amount of attention is paid to the ill
child. Brothers and sisters need as much knowledge as their sick sibling.
Information provided should be age appropriate, and all questions should be
answered honestly. Siblings can be extremely cooperative if they understand
the changes that will occur in the family and their role in helping the family
cope. However, parents may see behavior changes such as jealousy, regression (bed wetting in potty-trained toddlers), guilt (thinking that they caused
their sibling's illness), school problems, and symptoms of illness to gain
attention. Maintaining open communication about feelings helps siblings
continue to feel loved and secure. Chapter 16, *Siblings*, explores sibling issues
in detail and contains many suggestions from both parents and siblings.

The following passage was written by Jenny Gardner and is reprinted from
Candlelighters Youth Newsletter, Spring 1995, Vol. XVII No. 2. Jenny was
diagnosed with ALL in 1984 and had five years of treatment. A resident of
New Jersey, she is an accomplished horsewoman and also enjoys singing and
acting.

> *When I was diagnosed with leukemia, I felt like I was trapped in a*
> *room with no windows or doors and the walls were closing in on me. I*
> *thought that I would never be able to smell my grandmother's hand*
> *cream, or feel the way my dad's face felt in the morning before he shaves*
> *or the way my mom's silk blouse feels when I hug her. I thought that I*
> *would never have the sensation of turning one year older again. I thought*
> *that I would never again be able to feel how I feel after it rains, when it*

smells so fresh and clean like the whole world just took a bath. I thought that I would never be able to taste my first glass of champagne on New Year's and feel all bubbly and warm like I was flying in a hot-air balloon. And all of a sudden my dream popped, and I realized that this wasn't a dream, it was reality.

Right now there are thousands of kids like me across the country who are feeling the same way I felt eight years ago, and I would just like to wish them good luck. Because it's a long, hard journey full of needles, blood tests, and chemotherapy, but when you finally get to the end, you feel like you've been freed after years and years of darkness, and I'll tell you one thing—that is the greatest feeling you could have!

CHAPTER 3

Coping with Procedures

Mommy, I didn't cry but my eyes got bright.

—Four-year-old with ALL

THE PURPOSE OF THIS CHAPTER IS TO PREPARE both child and parent for several common procedures by providing detailed descriptions of each. Since almost all procedures are repeated frequently during the long treatment for child-hood leukemia, it is important to establish a routine that is comfortable for your child. The procedure itself may hurt, but a well-prepared, calm child fares far better than a frightened one.

Planning for procedures

Procedures are needed to make diagnoses, check for spread of disease, give treatment, and monitor response to treatment. Interventions range from fig-uring out the best way for your child to take numerous pills to having multi-ple spinal taps. Some procedures are pain-free and the family merely needs clear explanations about what to expect. Others can cause both physical and psychological distress. These reactions can be avoided or minimized by learning good coping skills, using medication, or both.

A family-centered approach works best when planning and implementing procedures. The procedures are often as frightening, or more frightening, for parents as for children. Memories of them can be long lasting. For this rea-son, children, parents, and staff should work together to plan for and cope with procedures.

As soon as possible after your child's diagnosis, find out if the hospital has a child life program or other team (nurses, psychologists, social workers) that helps prepare families for procedures. The purpose of these programs is to minimize psychological trauma, promote optimal development, and to main-tain, as much as possible, normal living patterns during hospitalizations.

They attempt to minimize the child's stress by giving him developmentally appropriate explanations of the reasons for procedures and hospital routines.

> Matthew was in sixth grade when he was diagnosed, and he was worried about the surgery for implanting the port. He didn't know what the scar would look like and he was concerned about AIDS, because it had been in the news a lot that year. The child life worker came in and really helped. She showed him what a port looked like; then they explored the pre-op area, the actual surgery room, and post-op. She showed him on a cloth doll exactly where the incision would be and how the scar would look. Then she introduced him to "Fred," the IV pump. She said that Fred would be going places with him, and that Fred would keep him from getting so many pokes. She told Matthew that he could bring something from home to hang on Fred. Of course, he brought in a really ugly stuffed animal. Throughout treatment, she really helped his fears and my feelings about losing control over my child's daily life.

Child life specialists or other team members accompany children to and provide support during procedures. They establish relationships with children based on warmth, respect, empathy, and understanding of developmental stages. They also communicate with the other members of the healthcare team about the psychosocial needs of children and their families.

Your response as well as your child's depends on temperament, age, previous medical or dental experiences, and other factors. Discuss with the child life professional or social worker when and how to prepare for upcoming procedures. Usually, parents need to experiment with how much advance notice to give younger children about procedures. Some children do better with several days to prepare, while others worry themselves sick. Sometimes, needs change over the years of treatment, so good communication and flexibility are essential.

> I started giving my four-year-old daughter two days' notice before procedures. But she began to wake up every day worried that "something bad was going to happen soon." So we talked it over and decided to look at the calendar together every Sunday to review what would happen that week. She was a much happier child after that.

Although it may not always be possible, try to schedule procedures so that the same person does the same procedure each time. Call ahead to check for unexpected changes to prevent any surprises. Repetition can provide comfort and reassurance to children.

Parents can ask for the medical professional with the most experience to perform procedures such as spinal taps. In the hospital hierarchy, attending physicians are above fellows and residents. However, at some large teaching facilities, attending physicians may not do these procedures very often. Many times, the fellow (and in some states where it is allowed, the nurse) is more skilled, because they do the vast majority of these procedures.

> Katy and I wrote down her requests for each procedure that first week in the hospital. For example, during spinal taps she wanted me (not a nurse) to hold her in position, she wanted xylocaine to be given with a needle, not the pneumatic gun, and she had a rigid sequence of songs that I sang.

Parents should have a choice whether to be present or not during a medical procedure. If your child does better if you are not in the room, ask the child life specialist or other member of the healthcare team to be present solely to comfort your child.

> We decided from the very beginning that, even though it's no fun to have a bone marrow or a spinal, we were going to make something positive out of it. So we made it a party. We'd bring pizza, popcorn, or ice cream to the hospital. We helped Kristin think of the nurses as her friends. We'd celebrate after a procedure by going out to eat at one of the neat little restaurants near the hospital.

Oncology clinics usually have a special box full of toys for children who have had a procedure. It sometimes helps for the child to have a treat to look forward to afterward. Some parents occasionally bring a special gift to sneak into the box for their child to find.

If given the chance, children have definite opinions about how they like things to go at the clinic. For instance, *Having Leukemia Isn't So Bad. Of Course It Wouldn't Be My First Choice* describes a list of rules for clinical personnel written by then seven-year-old Catherine Krumme in the car on the way to the hospital:

1. Must have a good sense of humor.

2. Must always do a good lumbar puncture (LP) and bone marrow.

3. Must always remember the toy box.

4. Must tell the truth.

5. Must like people.

6. Must like junk food.

7. Must know a lot about chemotherapy.

8. Must not mind the sight of blood.

9. Must like bald heads.

10. Must never be grumpy.

Pain management

The goal of pediatric pain management should be to minimize discomfort while performing the procedure. The two methods to achieve this goal are psychological (using the mind) and pharmacological (using drugs). These two methods can be used together to provide an integrated mind/body approach.

Psychological method

Preparation for every procedure is essential. Unexpected stress is more difficult to cope with than anticipated stress. If parents and children understand what is going to happen, where it will happen, who will be there, and what it will feel like, they will be less anxious and better able to cope. Methods to prepare children are:

- Verbally explain each step in the procedure.
- If possible, meet the person who will perform the procedure.
- Tour the room where the procedure will take place.
- Small children can "play" the procedure on dolls.
- Older children can observe a demonstration on a doll.
- Adolescents may observe a videotape describing the procedure.
- Encourage discussion and answer all questions.

For my child, playing about procedures helped release many feelings. Parents can buy medical kits at the store or simply stock their own from clinic castoffs and the pharmacy. We had IV bottles made from empty shampoo containers, complete with tubing and plastic needles. Several dolls had accessed ports, and many stuffed animals in our house fell apart after being speared by the pen during countless spinal taps. Katy's younger sister even ran around sometimes with her own pretend port taped onto her chest. Some suggestions for the child's medical kit are: gauze pads, tape, tubing, stethoscope, reflex hammer, pretend needles, syringes, medical chart, and toy box. Of course, lots of dolls or stuffed animal patients are required.

· · · · ·

My daughter (three years old) took an old stuffed animal to the clinic with her. Having the nurse and doctor perform the procedure first on "Bear" helped her immensely.

Hypnosis is a well-documented method for reducing discomfort during painful procedures. If performed by a qualified healthcare professional (psychologist, physician, nurse, social worker, or child life specialist), hypnosis can help your child control painful sensations, release anxiety, and diminish pain. The professional helps guide children or teens into an altered state of consciousness that helps to focus or narrow attention. To locate a qualified practitioner, call the American Society of Clinical Hypnosis at (837) 297-3317.

Imagery is a way to deliberately create a mental image of sights, sounds, tastes, smells, and feelings. It is an active process that helps children or teens feel as if they are actually entering the imagined place. Focusing on pleasant images allows the child to shift attention from the pain. It can also allow the child to actually alter the experience of pain, which simultaneously gives the child control and diminishes pain. Ask if the hospital has someone to teach your child this very effective technique.

The following description of using imagery was written by Jennifer Rohloff when she was seventeen years old, and is reprinted from the *Free to Be Yourself* newsletter of Cancer Services of Allen County, Indiana.

My Special Place

Many people had a special place when they were young—a special place that they still remember. This place could be an area that has a special meaning for them, or a place where they used to go when they wanted to be alone. My special place location is over the rainbow.

I discovered this place when I was twelve years old, during a relaxation session. These sessions were designed to reduce pain and stress brought on by chemotherapy. This was a place that I could visualize in my mind so that I could go there anytime that I wanted to—not only for pain, but when I was happy, mad, or sad.

It is surrounded by sand and tall, fanning palm trees everywhere. The blue sky is always clear, and the bright sun shines every day. It is usually quiet because I am alone, but often I can hear the sounds of birds flying by.

Every time I come to this place I like to lie down in the sand. As I lie there, I can feel the gritty sand beneath me. Once in a while I get up and go looking for seashells. I usually find some different shapes and sizes. The ones I like the best are the ones that you can hear the sound of the ocean in. After a while I get up and start to walk around. As I walk, I can feel the breeze going right through me, and I can smell the salt water. It reminds me of being at a beach in Florida. Whenever I start to feel sad or alone or if I am in pain, I usually go jump in the water because it is a soothing place for me. I like to float around in the water because it gives me a refreshing feeling that nobody can hurt me here. I could stay in this place all day because I do not worry about anything while I am here.

To me this place is like a home away from home. It is like heaven because you can do anything you want to do here. Even though this place may seem imaginary or like a fantasy world to some people, it is not to me. I think it is real because it is a place where I can go and be myself.

Distraction can be used successfully with all age groups, but it should never be used as a substitute for preparation. Babies can be distracted by colorful, moving objects. Parents can help distract preschoolers by showing picture books or videos, telling stories, singing songs, or blowing bubbles. Many youngsters are comforted by hugging a favorite stuffed animal. School-age children can watch videos or TV, or listen to music. Several institutions use interactive videos to help distract older children or teens.

My daughter went through her therapy prior to the days when kids were given any pain medications for procedures. She and I would make up a schedule of songs for me to sing during the spinal tap or bone marrow. I would stroke her skin and sing softly to her. She visibly relaxed, and the staff found it soothing, as well. I'll never forget the time that the oncologist, nurse, and I were all quietly singing "Somewhere Over the Rainbow" during the spinal tap.

Other adjunctive therapies that are used successfully to help deal with medical treatments are relaxation, biofeedback, massage, and acupuncture. Ask the hospital's child life specialist, psychologist, or nurse to discuss and practice different methods of pain management with you and your child.

Pharmacological method

Most pediatric oncology clinics offer the choice of sedation and/or anesthesia for painful procedures; some do not. If you find that your child is distressed by painful procedures (bone marrow aspiration and spinal taps), it is reasonable to explore all available options for pain relief.

One father, a doctor just completing his anesthesia residency, explained:

That first bone marrow was horrible. To have my little three-year-old look up at me with tears in her eyes and ask, "What else are you going to let them do to me, daddy?" was just too much. It was the worst day of my life.

His wife, a nurse, said:

We really made waves by insisting that Meagan be sedated for her spinal taps and bone marrows. It was mostly a logistical problem, but we held firm, and now it has become much more routine for many other kids as well.

The ideal pain relief drug for children should be easy to administer, predictable in effect, provide adequate pain relief, have a short duration, and have minimal side effects. There are two topical anesthetics in wide use for pediatric procedures. EMLA cream (see Chapter 10, *Chemotherapy*) is a cream put on the skin one to two hours prior to the painful procedure. Ethyl chloride spray is used immediately before the procedure to anesthetize the surface skin.

Other drugs for sedation and/or general anesthesia are given intravenously. Some facilities take the child into the operating room (OR) for the procedure, while others use a preoperating area or clinic sedation room and allow the parent to be present the entire time.

Drugs used for pediatric anesthesia during procedures include:

- **Valium or versed plus morphine or fentanyl**. Valium and versed are sedatives which are used with pain relievers such as morphine or fentanyl. These drugs can be given in the clinic, but due to the possibility of slowed breathing, expert monitoring is required and emergency equipment should be present. The combination of a sedative and a pain reliever will result in your child's being awake but sedated. The child may move or cry, but will not remember the procedure. Often, EMLA (an anesthetic in a cream base; see Chapter 10) or lidocaine are also used to ensure that the procedure is pain free.

- **Propofol**. A milky liquid given by IV, propofol has rapid onset with a rapid recovery. Administration and monitoring by an anesthesiologist (doctor who specializes in giving anesthetics) are required. Propofol, a general anesthetic, will cause your child to lose consciousness. At low doses, propofol prevents memory of the procedure, but may not relieve all pain, so it is often used with EMLA or lidocaine.

- **Ketamine**. Ketamine needs expert monitoring. It has a much longer recovery time than the drugs listed above, and upon awakening, up to 30 percent of children may become confused and/or hallucinate. For these reasons, ketamine is no longer in wide use for pediatric sedation for procedures.

Joel was treated from ages fourteen to seventeen. During his LPs he would get versed once he was positioned on the table. I would always sit at his head and keep his shoulders forward while his head rested on my arm. (Kind of a hug.) As the versed took effect, he would look up at me with huge eyes and give me a grin a mile wide, then would say something off the wall. He had to spend an hour flat after the LP. He'd be groggy the whole time, constantly asking me what time it was and how soon we could leave. He'd forget he asked and ask me again five minutes later. This continued for the whole hour. Later, we'd laugh about it. He never remembered anything from the LPs.

· · · · ·

Patrick (twelve years old) hates the lack of control involved when having a procedure and getting propofol. He attempts to regain some control by verbally explaining to the doctors just exactly how he wants it done each time. He has his own little routine—tells them jokes, sings "I Want to Be Sedated" (you know, the Ramones song), etc. Patrick's biggest problem is the taste from the propofol. We have tried so many different things when he wakes up to mask the taste—Skittles, gum, Gatorade. We now have a supply of atomic fireballs. I give him one as soon as they bring him out and he says that really helps cover the taste.

Be aware that there are many types of drugs and several methods used in administering them, from very temporary (ten minutes) mild sedation to full general anesthesia in the operating room. Discuss with your oncologist and anesthesiologist which method will work best for your child.

Let's face it, kids don't care about blasts, lab work, or protocols, they just want to know if they are going to be hurt again. I think that one of our most important jobs is to advocate, strongly if necessary, for adequate pain control. If the dose doesn't work and the doctor just shrugs her shoulders, say you want a different dosage or drug used. If you encounter resistance, ask that an anesthesiologist be consulted. Remember that good pain control and/or amnesia will make a big difference in your child's state of mind during treatment.

Since children with leukemia are treated for years, many children build up a tolerance for sedatives and pain relievers. Often, over time, doses may need to be increased or drugs changed. If your child remembers the procedure, advocate for a change in drug and/or dosage. It is reasonable to request that an anesthesiologist be present to ensure adequate pain relief.

My job as an oral surgery assistant required me to be very familiar with different types of sedation. From the first day of Stephan's diagnosis, I quietly insisted on versed for bone marrows and spinal taps. We have been in treatment for two years, and they still fight me every time, saying that it's just not necessary. When I make the appointment I tell them we want Stephan sedated, and then I call and remind them so that all will go smoothly.

All sedation can result in complications, primarily to the airway. It is imperative that sedation occur under the care of trained, experienced personnel and that the child is monitored until fully recovered from the medications.

Procedures

Understanding what will occur during a procedure and what other parents do to prepare their children will arm you with essential information. Knowing what to expect will lower the anxiety level of both you and your child and lay the foundation for years of tolerable tests. The descriptions of procedures in the rest of the chapter may not exactly mirror your experience. Practices vary by hospital and practitioner and this variability should be expected. What should be the same, however, is your comfort in asking questions and getting the support and help you need to prepare for and cope with your child's procedures.

Questions to ask before procedures

You need information prior to procedures in order to prepare yourself and your child. Some suggested questions to ask the physician are:

- Why is this procedure necessary and how will it affect my child's treatment?

- What information will it provide?

- Who will perform the procedure?

- Will it be an inpatient or outpatient procedure?

- Please explain the procedure in detail.

- Is there any literature available that describes it?

- Is there a child life specialist on staff who will help prepare my child for the procedure?

- Is the procedure painful?

- What type of anesthetic or sedation is used?

- What are the risks, if any?

- What are the common and rare side effects?

- When will we get the results?

Bone marrow aspiration

Protocols for children with leukemia require bone marrow aspirations, a process by which bone marrow is sucked out with a needle. The purpose of the first, or diagnostic, bone marrow aspiration is to see what percentage of the cells in the marrow are abnormal blasts. Then these cells are analyzed microscopically to determine which type of leukemia is present. The next bone marrow aspiration occurs on day seven or fourteen of treatment. At this time it is important to determine how many blasts are still present. This information helps the oncologists decide how intensive treatment should be. For instance, if the marrow shows less than 25 percent blasts, the child might continue on the intermediate-risk protocol. But if the marrow is still crowded with blasts, the child might be described as a "slow responder," who would require a more intensive course of treatment.

> Since the doctors knew that my daughter had leukemia from the blood work, they did her first bone marrow while she was under anesthesia to implant her Port-a-cath. This was a blessing as her marrow was packed tight with blasts.

Most centers require additional bone marrow aspirations at the end of each phase of treatment and at the end of maintenance (or postremission treatment, if your child does not require the maintenance phase).

To obtain a sample of the bone marrow, doctors usually use the iliac crest of the hip (the top of the hip bone in back or front). This bone is right under the skin and contains a large amount of marrow.

The child is placed face down on a table, sometimes on a pillow to elevate the hip. The doctor will feel the site, then wipe it several times with an antiseptic to eliminate any germs. Sterile paper may be placed around the site, and the doctor will wear sterile gloves. Then an anesthetic (usually xylocaine) may be injected into the skin and a small area of bone. This causes a burning and stinging sensation that passes quickly. The physician usually rubs the area to allow the drug to fully anesthetize the area. The physician then pushes a hollow needle (with a plug inside) through the skin into the bone, withdraws the plug, and attaches a syringe. The liquid marrow is then aspirated (sucked out) through the syringe. After a sample is obtained, the needle is removed and a bandage is put on.

If the child or teen is not sedated, removing the marrow can be very painful. Here are some descriptions from children and adult survivors who have experienced it:

> It was the worst thing of all. It felt really, really bad.

• • • • •

> It hurts a lot. It feels like they are pulling something out and then it aches. You know, it hurts so much that now they put the kids to sleep. Boy, am I glad about that.

• • • • •

It feels like they are trying to suck thick Jell-O from inside the bone. Brief but incredible pain.

· · · · ·

I would become very anxious when they were cleaning my skin and laying the towels down. Putting the needle in was a sharp, pressure kind of pain. Drawing the marrow feels tingly, like they hit a nerve. I always asked a nurse to hold my legs because I felt like my legs were going to jump up off the table.

Spinal tap (lumbar puncture or LP)

Due to the blood-brain barrier, systemic chemotherapy usually cannot destroy any blasts in the central nervous system (brain and spinal cord). Chemotherapy drugs must be directly injected into the cerebrospinal fluid in order to kill any blasts present and prevent a possible central nervous system relapse. The drugs most commonly used intrathecally are methotrexate, ARA-C, and hydrocortisone. The number of spinal taps required varies depending on the child's risk level, the clinical study involved, and whether radiation is used.

Some hospitals routinely sedate children for spinal taps, and others do not. If the child is not sedated, EMLA cream is usually prescribed. EMLA is an anesthetic cream put on the spinal tap site one to two hours prior to the procedure. It anesthetizes deep into the tissue, preventing some or all of the pain associated with the procedure.

To perform a spinal tap, the physician or nurse practitioner will ask the child to lie on her side with her head tucked close to the chest and knees drawn up. A nurse or parent usually helps hold the child in this position. The doctor will feel the designated spot in the lower back, and will swab it with antiseptic several times. The antiseptic feels very cold on the skin. A sterile sheet may drape the area, and the doctor will wear sterile gloves. One or two shots of an anesthetic (usually xylocaine) may be injected into the skin and deeper tissues. This causes a painful stinging or burning sensation that lasts about a minute. If EMLA was used, the doctor may still inject anesthetic into the deep tissues. A few minutes' wait is necessary to ensure that the area is fully anesthetized.

My four-year-old daughter had finished eighteen months of her treatment for ALL when EMLA was first prescribed. She had been terrified of going to the clinic. After using EMLA for her next LP, a dramatic change occurred. She was no longer frightened to go for treatment, and her behavior at home improved unbelievably. We use it for everything now: finger pokes, accessing port, bone marrows, even flu shots.

It is essential that the child hold very still for the rest of the procedure. The doctor will push a needle between two vertebrae into the space where cerebrospinal fluid (CSF) is found. The CSF will begin to drip out of the hollow needle into a container. After a small amount is collected, a syringe is attached to the needle in the back and the medicine is slowly injected, causing a sensation of coldness or pressure down the leg. The needle is then removed and the spot bandaged. The CSF is sent to the laboratory to see if any cancer cells are present and to measure glucose and protein. Occasionally, older children and teenagers get severe headaches from spinal taps. These can sometimes be prevented by lying still for up to an hour after the procedure.

During spinals, Brent listens to rock and roll on his Walkman, but he keeps the volume low enough so that he can still hear what is going on. He likes me to lift up the earpiece and tell him when each part of the procedure is finished and what's coming next.

Starting an IV

Most children with leukemia have a permanent right atrial catheter implanted in their chest within a week after diagnosis (see Chapter 8, *Catheters*) to avoid the pain of years of IV sticks. However, some physicians do not recommend catheters, and there are many medical reasons why surgery for a catheter may be postponed. Even if your child has a catheter, there may be times when your child will need an intravenous line started, as well.

Most pediatric hospitals have teams of technicians who specialize in starting IVs and drawing blood. The IV technician will generally use a vein in the lower arm or hand. First, a constricting band is put above the site to make the veins larger and easier to see and feel. The vein is felt by the technician, the area is cleaned, and the needle is inserted. Sometimes a needle is left in place and sometimes it is withdrawn, leaving only a thin plastic tube in the vein. The technician will make sure that the needle (or tube) is in the proper place, then cover the site with a clear dressing and secure it with tape.

Some methods that help when having an IV started are:

- Stay calm. The body reacts to fear by constricting the blood vessels near the skin surface. Small children are usually more calm with a parent present; teenagers may or may not desire privacy. Listening to music, visualizing a tranquil scene (mountains covered with snow, floating in a pool), or using the same technician each time can help.

- Use EMLA cream. EMLA—a cream anesthetic—is applied to the skin one hour prior to the procedure to prevent pain. In some cases, it can constrict the veins, so experiment to see if it works for your child.

- Keep warm. Cold temperatures also cause the surface blood vessels to constrict. Wrapping the child in a blanket and putting a hot water bottle on the arm can enlarge the veins.

- Drink lots of fluids. Dehydration decreases the fluid in the veins, so encourage lots of drinking.

- Let gravity help. If the child is lying in bed, have her hang her arm down over the side to increase the size of the vessels in the arm and hand.

- Let the child be in control. If the child has a preference, let him pick the arm to be stuck. If the child is a veteran of many IVs, let him point out the best vein.

- Stop if problems develop. The art of treating children is lots of time on preparation and not much time on procedures. If a conflict arises, take a time-out and regroup. Children can be remarkably cooperative if their needs are respected and they are given some control over the situation.

> You'll think I'm crazy, but I'll tell you this story anyway. After getting stuck constantly for a year, my daughter (five years old) just lost it one day when she needed an IV. She started screaming and crying, just flew into a rage. I told the tech, "Let's just let her calm down. Why don't you stick me for a change?" She was a sport and started a line in my arm. I told my daughter that I had forgotten how much it hurt and I could understand why she was upset. I told her to let us know when she was ready. She just walked over and held out her arm.

Subcutaneous injections

Some children require medications given by subcutaneous injection during their treatment. For example, Neupogen (G-CSF), a colony-stimulating factor that is often used to boost the white blood cell count, and methotrexate are usually given by injection.

To minimize pain caused by subcutaneous injections, apply EMLA cream one to two hours before administration. Parents can also reduce pain by rubbing ice over the site to numb the area prior to injection.

> We always used EMLA cream before our son needed a subcutaneous injection. I think part of the benefit to him was pharmacological, and part of it was psychological. He just seemed to be more at ease with the injections when he knew the EMLA was applied a few hours before the needle was given.

· · · · ·

> My two boys have ALL. Brian and Kevin both receive[d] IM methotrexate as part of their protocols. Brian, because of his age (twelve), was very macho about it, used "freezy" spray to numb the thigh, then giggled or made funny faces while the methotrexate was pushed. He had no aftereffects. Kevin, only four when they began, still doesn't like them. There were three or four months of overlap, when both boys got shots at the same time every week. This made it easier for Kevin, but he still insisted on an ice pack and freezy spray. Now, he's graduated to doing it alone and uses the spray only.

Blood draws

Frequent blood samples are a part of life during leukemia treatment. A complete blood count (CBC) tells the physician how effective the drugs are and helps determine the child's susceptibility to infection. It is important to measure blood chemistries to make sure that the liver and kidneys are not being damaged by treatment (for a list of normal blood counts, see Appendix B, *Blood Counts and What They Mean*). During induction and consolidation, transfusions are necessary when the red cell count or platelet count gets too low.

Blood specimens are primarily used for three purposes: to obtain a CBC, evaluate blood chemistries, or culture the blood to check for infection. A CBC measures the types and numbers of cells in the blood. Blood chemistries measure substances contained in the blood plasma to determine if the liver and kidneys are functioning properly. Blood cultures help evaluate whether the child is developing a bacterial or fungal infection. If only a CBC is needed, a finger poke will provide enough blood. Blood chemistries or cultures require one or more vials of blood obtained from a vein in the arm or the right atrial catheter.

Blood is usually drawn from the large vein on the inside of the elbow using a procedure similar to starting an IV, except that the needle is removed rather than left in the arm. The advice for starting an IV also applies to drawing blood from the arm.

Catheters

Children with catheters usually have blood drawn from the catheter rather than the arm or finger. These procedures are described in Chapter 8.

Finger pokes

Finger pokes are different from blood draws in several ways. First, EMLA can be used successfully. Put a blob of EMLA on the tip of the middle finger. Cover the fingertip with plastic wrap, and tape it on the finger. Another method is to buy long, thin balloons with a diameter a bit wider than the child's finger. Cut off the open end, leaving only enough balloon to cover the finger up to the first knuckle. Fill the tip of the balloon with EMLA and slide it on the fingertip. EMLA needs to be applied an hour before a finger poke to be effective. At the laboratory, remove the plastic wrap or balloon, wipe off the EMLA, and ask for a warm pack. Wrapping this heated pack around the finger for a few minutes opens the capillaries to allow the blood to flow out more readily. Now the child is ready for a pain-free finger poke.

The technician will hold the finger and quickly stick it with a small sharp instrument. Blood will be collected in narrow tubes or a small container. It is usually necessary for the technician to squeeze the fingertip to get enough blood. If EMLA is not used, the squeezing part is uncomfortable and the finger can ache for quite a while.

> Even though we use EMLA, Katy (five years old) still becomes angry when she has to have a finger poke. I asked her why it was upsetting if there was no pain, and she replied, "It doesn't hurt my body anymore, but it still hurts my feelings."

Blood transfusions

Treatment for leukemia can cause severe anemia (a low number of oxygen-carrying red cells). The normal life of a red cell is three to four months and, as old cells die, the diseased (or suppressed by treatment) marrow cannot replace them. Many children require transfusions of red cells when first admitted, and periodically throughout treatment.

> Whenever my son needed a transfusion, I brought along bags of coloring books, food, and toys. The number of VCRs at the clinic was limited, so I tried to make arrangements for one ahead of time. When anemic (hematocrit below 20 percent), he didn't have much energy, but by the end of the transfusion, his cheeks were rosy and he had tremendous vitality. It was hard to keep him still. After one unit (bag) of red cells, his hematocrit usually jumped up to around 30.

One bag (called a "unit") of red cells takes approximately two to four hours to administer and is given through an IV or catheter. If your child develops chills and/or fever during a transfusion, the nurse should be notified so that the transfusion can be stopped immediately.

There are some risks of infection from red cell transfusions. Since new tests have been devised to detect the AIDS virus, the risk of exposure is minuscule, less than 1 in 450,000. Although there are excellent tests for the various types of hepatitis, exposure to this disease is still possible (the risk is less than 1 in 4,000). Exposure to cytomegalovirus is also a concern. These risks are the reason transfusions are given only when absolutely necessary.

> My daughter received several transfusions at the clinic in Children's Hospital with no problems. After we traveled back to our home, she needed her first transfusion at the local hospital. Our pediatrician said to expect to be in the hospital at least eight hours. I asked why it would take so long when it only took four hours at Children's. He said he had worked out a formula and determined that she needed two units of packed cells. I mentioned that she only was given one unit each time at Children's. He called the oncologist, who said it was better to give the smaller amount. We went to the hospital, where a unit of red cells was given. Then a nurse came in with another unit. I questioned why he was doing that and he said, "Doctor's orders." I asked him to verify that order, as we had already discussed it with the doctor. He went into another room to call the doctor, and came back and said the pediatrician thought my daughter needed 30 cc more packed cells. I called Children's and they said she didn't need more, so I refused to let them administer any more blood. It just wasn't worth the risk of hepatitis to get 30 cc of blood. Even though I was pleasant, the nurses were angry at me for questioning the doctor.

Platelet transfusions

Platelets are an important component of the blood. They help form clots and stop bleeding by repairing breaks in the walls of blood vessels. A normal platelet count for a healthy child is 150,000/mm^3 to 420,000/ mm^3. Chemotherapy can severely depress the platelet count for some children. If a transfusion is not given when counts are very low, uncontrollable bleeding can result. Many centers require a transfusion when the child's platelet count goes below 10,000 to 20,000/mm^3, and sometimes repeat transfusions are required every two or three days until the marrow recovers.

> Brent (six years old) had several platelet transfusions during induction and consolidation. He had no problems and his counts would immediately jump up to around 40,000/mm^3.

· · · · ·

> Three-year-old Matthew had countless platelet transfusions, and only once did he have a reaction. It was an awful thing to watch, but the nurse who was monitoring him was very calm and professional, which helped both of us. Matthew was always premedicated for his platelet transfusions with Benadryl, which made him very drowsy. Most often he would sleep through the entire transfusion.

Infections transmitted by platelets are identical to those of other blood products: hepatitis, cytomegalovirus, and HIV (the virus that causes AIDS). The chance of contracting these infections, although small, is the reason that platelet transfusions are also given only when absolutely necessary. Because uncontrollable bleeding can be life threatening, prevention is paramount.

Taking pills

When giving oral medications, it is essential to get off to a good start and establish cooperation early. In the following suggestions from veteran parents, you may find a technique that works well for your child.

> To teach Brent (six years old) to swallow pills, when we were eating corn for dinner I encouraged him to swallow one kernel whole. Luckily, it went right down and he got over his fear of pills.

· · · · ·

> I wanted Katy (three years old) to feel like we were a team right from the first night. So I made a big deal out of tasting each of her medications

and pronouncing it good. Thank goodness I tasted the prednisone first. It was nauseating—bitter, metallic, with a lingering aftertaste. I asked the nurse for some small gel caps, and packed them with the pills which I had broken in half. I gave Katy her choice of drinks to take her pills with and taught her to swallow gel caps with a large sip of liquid. Since I gave her over 3,000 pills and 1,100 teaspoons of liquid medication during treatment, I'm very glad we got off to such a good start.

Gel caps come in many sizes. Number 4s are small enough for a three- or four-year-old to swallow, but big enough to hold half a 10 mg. prednisone tablet. Dexamethasone also tastes awful to many kids. Most of the other pills can be chewed or swallowed whole without taste problems. Just remember that children develop different taste preferences and aversions to medications, and gel caps are useful for any medication that bothers them.

After much trial and error with medications, Meagan's method became chewing up pills with chocolate chips. She's kept this up for the long haul.

• • • • •

I always give choices such as, "Do you want the white pill or the six yellow pills first?" It gives them a little control in their chaotic world.

For younger children, many parents crush the pills in a small amount of pudding, applesauce, jam, frozen juice concentrate, or other favorite food.

Jeremy was four when he was diagnosed, and we used to crush up the pills and mix them with ice cream. This worked well for us.

• • • • •

We used the liquid form of prednisone for my son, mixed it with a chocolate drink, and followed this with M&Ms. The chocolate seemed to mask the taste.

Most children on maintenance take SMZ-TMP (sulfamethoxazole and trimethoprim) three times a week to prevent pneumonia. The brand names are Bactrim or Septra. They come in liquid or pill form, and are produced by several different manufacturers. Ask your pharmacist (you'll know her quite well after a few years) for a kid taste test. Letting your child choose a medicine that appeals to him encourages compliance.

Whenever my son had to take a liquid medicine, such as antibiotics, he enjoyed taking it from a syringe. I would draw up the proper amount, then he would put it in his mouth and push the plunger.

Since children associate taking medicine with being sick, it is helpful to explain why they must continue taking pills for years after they feel well. Some parents use the Pac-man analogy, "The pills are needed to gobble up the last few bad cells." Others explain that the leukemia can return, so medicine is needed to prevent it from growing again. It is important that parents give children all the required medications; there are many studies showing low compliance results in lower survival rates.

Issues for teenagers about taking pills are completely different from those for young children. The problems with teens revolve around autonomy, control, and feelings of invulnerability. It is normal for teenagers to be noncompliant, and they cannot be forced to take pills if they choose not to cooperate. Trying to coerce teens fuels conflict and tends to frustrate everyone. If you need help, ask for an assessment by the psychosocial team at the hospital to work out a plan for adherence to treatment. Everyone will need to be flexible to reach a favorable outcome.

I think the main problem with teens is making sure that they take the meds. Joel (fifteen years old) has been very responsible about taking his nightly pills. I've tried to make it easy for him by having an index card for the week and he marks off the med as he takes it. I also put the meds on a dry erase board on the fridge as a reminder. As he takes the med, he erases it. That way it's easy for him (and me) to see at a glance if he's taken his stuff. The index card alone wasn't working because he couldn't find a pen or forgot to mark it off.

One of the biggest concerns with teens and maintenance is noncompliance. I think it's a delicate balancing act to allow the teen to be responsible for taking his own meds and yet have some supervision of the process. Our meds are kept in a small plastic basket on the kitchen counter. All meds are taken there. I'd never want him to keep his meds in his room where I would have no idea if he had taken them or not.

On Friday nights when he is to take his weekly methotrexate—a sixteen-pill dose—I will count it out and put it in a medicine cup on the counter. I am not always an awake and alert person when he comes home at midnight on Friday night. When I get up Saturday morning, I know immediately if he's taken his meds.

If he had shown any resistance to taking the meds, or any sign of tell-
ing me that he had taken them when he had not, I'd be doing this differ-
ently. But he's aware of the importance of each dose and the importance of
his participation in the team beating the leukemia.

My only other advice is to be sure and ask the doctors what to do
about a missed dose for each med. In three-plus years of treatment, you
are going to have a missed dose and it helps to know how to handle it.

Taking a temperature

In the years a child is treated for childhood leukemia, fever becomes an
enemy because it may signal the start of an infection. Parents take hundreds
of temperatures, often when their child is not feeling well. Temperatures can
be taken under the tongue, under the arm, or in the ear using a special type
of thermometer. Rectal temperatures are not recommended due to the risk of
tears and infection, especially when the blood counts are depressed. Here are
a few suggestions that might help:

• Use a glass thermometer under the tongue.

• Digital thermometers can be purchased at any drug store. Some have an
alarm that beeps when it is time to remove the thermometer.

> *We bought a digital thermometer that we only use under his arm. It*
> *has worked well for us.*

• Tympanic thermometers measure infrared waves and are very easy to use.

> *When my in-laws asked at diagnosis if there was anything that we*
> *needed, I asked them to try to buy a tympanic (ear) thermometer. The*
> *device cost over a hundred dollars then, but it worked beautifully. It takes*
> *only one second to obtain a temperature. You can even use it when she is*
> *asleep without waking her. They are now sold at pharmacies and drug*
> *stores, and cost much less.*

Before you leave the hospital, you should know when to call the clinic
because of fever. Usually, parents are told not to give any medication for
fever and to call if the fever goes above 101°F (38.5°C). It is especially
important for parents of children with implanted catheters to know when to
call the clinic, as an untreated infection can be life-threatening.

Providing a urine specimen

Chemotherapy requires frequent urine specimens. One way to help obtain a sample is to encourage lots of drinking the hour before or ask the nurse to increase the drip rate on the IV. Explain to the child why the test is necessary. Ask the nurse to show how the dip sticks work (they change color, so they are quite popular with the preschoolers). Use a "hat" under the toilet seat. This is a shallow plastic bucket that fits under the seat and catches the urine.

> Turn on the water while the child sits on the toilet. I don't know why it works, but it does.

As all parents learn, eating and elimination are areas that the child controls. If she just can't or won't urinate in the hat, go out, buy her the largest drink you can find, and wait.

Echocardiogram

Several drugs used to fight leukemia can damage the muscle of the heart, decreasing its ability to contract effectively. Many protocols require a baseline echocardiogram to measure the heart's ability to pump before any chemotherapy drugs are given. Echocardiograms are then given periodically during treatment and after treatment ends to see if any heart muscle damage has occurred.

An echocardiogram uses ultrasound waves to measure the amount of blood that leaves the heart each time it contracts. This percentage (blood ejected during a contraction compared to blood in the heart when it is relaxed) is called the ejection fraction.

The echocardiogram is performed by a technician, nurse, or doctor. The child or teen lies on a table and has conductive jelly applied to the chest. Then the technician puts a transducer (which emits the ultrasound waves) on the jelly and moves the device around on the chest to obtain different views of the heart. Pressure is applied on the transducer, and can sometimes cause mild discomfort. The test results are displayed on a videotape and photographed for later interpretation.

> Meagan used to watch a video during the echocardiogram. Sometimes she would eat a sucker or a popsicle. She found it to be boring, not painful.

MUGA scan

MUGA stands for multiple-gated acquisition scan; a MUGA scan is another way to test cardiac function. Prior to having a MUGA scan, children are sometimes given a sedative to relax and help them stay perfectly still for the fifteen- to twenty-minute test. An injection of red cells or proteins tagged with a mildly radioactive substance (called technetium) is also given. The child lies on a table with a large movable camera above. This special camera records sequential images of the technetium as it moves through the heart. These pictures of the heart's function allow doctors to determine how efficiently the heart muscle is pumping and if any damage to the heart has occurred.

> My three-year-old daughter had a MUGA scan before she received any chemotherapy. They gave her an injection, and she fell asleep. They laid her on her back on a big table and moved a huge contraption around her to take pictures of her heart beating. We watched on a screen, and they printed out a copy on paper for the doctors.

If either the echocardiogram or MUGA scan shows heart damage, the oncologist may reduce the dosage or remove the drug causing the damage from the child's protocol.

> Meagan is scheduled to go off therapy this May. She's doing well and is very happy. A father at our support group was reminding a new set of parents to remember to view life from the child's perspective; he said that, especially with little ones, parents sometimes agonize more than the child. He said that at the end of the first year of treatment he and his wife were reflecting on how much misery their child had endured, and then she piped up and said, "This has been a great year for me!" Meagan is the same. When I have bad days and get preoccupied with the uncertain future, I see Meagan skipping along and saying as she frequently does, "I'm such a happy girl."

CHAPTER 4

Clinical Trials

The challenge in pediatric oncology remains
clear: to strive for the cure and health of all
children through the development of more
effective yet less damaging treatment
for our young patients.

—Daniel M. Green, MD
 and Giulio J. D'Angio, MD
 Late Effects of Treatment
 for Childhood Cancer

WITHIN DAYS OF ARRIVING at a major pediatric medical center with a newly diagnosed leukemic child, parents may be asked to enroll their child in a clinical trial. A clinical trial is a research study that uses human volunteers to answer specific scientific questions. In order to accurately evaluate any new treatment, large numbers of patients are needed in each clinical trial.

Pediatric clinical trials are all directed toward improving upon existing treatments. A trial can involve a totally new approach that is thought to be promising, fine-tune existing treatments, improve the results or reduce the toxicity of known treatments, or develop new ways to discern response to treatments. More than half of all children with cancer in North America are enrolled in clinical trials for part or all of their treatment.

Making an informed judgment on whether to participate is crucial, as it will determine what treatment your child will receive in the years to come. This chapter describes clinical trials and protocols and gives examples of how different parents made decisions on this important issue.

Enrollment in clinical trials

The enormous improvements in treating childhood leukemia have been the direct result of clinical trials. Because clinical trials offer the most up-to-date treatment available, children who participate in a clinical trial may benefit from the newest research. Most parents derive comfort from knowing that the knowledge gained will make an important contribution to medical science and may help other children with cancer.

Standard treatment

Standard treatment is the best treatment known for a specific type of cancer. For instance, in 1999, the standard treatment for intermediate-risk ALL is combination chemotherapy for two to three years. The standard treatment for high-risk ALL includes more drugs and may include cranial radiation and/or bone marrow transplant for very high-risk groups.

As results from ongoing and completed clinical trials are analyzed, more knowledge is accumulated and standard treatments evolve. In the 1980s, most children with ALL received cranial radiation as standard care. Carefully controlled clinical trials established that the majority of children with ALL do not require cranial radiation. The standard care was changed.

Most clinical trials divide patients into two or more groups (arms). One arm of the trial is the standard treatment, and the other arms are the experimental portions, which scientists hope will prove to be more effective or less toxic than the standard treatment. Each arm is based on preliminary, but not conclusive, information that it will be beneficial and is carefully reviewed by experts in the field before implementation.

> My daughter's clinical trial for high-risk ALL had three arms. One arm was the standard treatment of four drug rotations of chemotherapy with a delayed intensification and consolidation, and 1,800 rads of cranial radiation. The second arm was identical except radiation was replaced with more frequent doses of intrathecal methotrexate. The third arm was for children who had CNS disease at diagnosis or who were slow responders to initial therapy. They received a very aggressive chemotherapy regimen plus cranial radiation.

> The purpose of the study was to compare response to treatment, duration of disease control, and side effects. The investigators hoped to be able to eliminate radiation from the standard care for high-risk ALL.

Randomization

Some scientific studies require a process called randomization. This means that after parents agree to enroll their child in a clinical trial, a computer will randomly assign the child to one arm of the study. If there are three arms, the parents will not know which of the three (one standard, two experimental) their child will receive until the computer assigns one. One group of patients (the control group) always receives the standard treatment to provide a basis for comparison to the experimental arms. Because neither the physician nor the parents choose the treatment option, a comparable mix of patients is assured.

At the time the clinical trial is designed, there is no conclusive evidence to indicate which arm will prove to be superior. Most arms incorporate standard therapy and only a small portion of the arm contains the experimental agents. "Experimental" drugs have usually been used previously, but their efficacy in a given circumstance may not be known. It is not possible to predict if your child will benefit from participating in the study.

> We decided not to participate in a study for several reasons. One arm would require extra spinal taps, and our son was just so little that we couldn't bear the thought of any more treatments than what was required in the standard arm. Another arm contained a second induction, and since we were on Medicaid, we just didn't feel it was right for the taxpayers to pay for anything extra. We felt we were only entitled to basic healthcare.

· · · · ·

> We had a hard time deciding whether to go with the standard treatment or to participate in the study. The "B" arm of the study seemed, on intuition, to be too harsh for her because she was so weak at the time. We finally did opt for the study, hoping we wouldn't be randomized to "B." We chose the study basically so that the computer could choose and we wouldn't ever have to think "we should have gone with the study." As it turned out, we were randomized to the standard arm, so we got what we wanted while still participating in the study.

Design of clinical trials

In the United States and Canada, there are two primary pediatric research groups that focus on childhood leukemia: Children's Cancer Group (CCG) and the Pediatric Oncology Group (POG). Most large pediatric medical centers work in close cooperation with one of these groups, although there are some centers which design their own clinical trials. Experts from many institutions usually collaborate in the design of clinical trials.

In July 1998, a Pediatric Intergroup Summit was held by the leaders of the pediatric cancer clinical trials cooperative groups (there are also groups that study Wilms tumor and rhabdomyosarcoma). They decided to form a single pediatric cancer clinical trials organization. Unification of these groups will have advantages for children with cancer as well as pediatric cancer researchers. It will pool the intellectual resources of all four groups, allowing research that had not been previously possible. Large population-based studies and coordinated treatment trials will help researchers gather data that will be generalizable to the entire North American population of children with cancer. It is hoped that integration of these groups into the Children's Oncology Group (COG) will be complete by the year 2002.

Supervision of clinical trials

The ethical and legal codes ruling medical practice also apply to clinical trials. In addition, most research is federally funded or regulated (all CCG and POG trials are), with rules to protect patients. CCG and POG also have review boards that meet at prearranged dates for the duration of a clinical trial to ensure that the risks of all parts of the trial are acceptable relative to the benefits. If one arm of the trial is causing unexpected or unacceptable side effects, that portion will be terminated, and the children enrolled will be given the better treatment. If one of the arms appears to be less effective than the standard, it will be terminated. Conversely, if one arm is better than the standard, the trial will also be terminated. Whenever a treatment is proven to be superior, all children receive it.

> When Brian first entered the CCG-1922 protocol, there were four arms. One was to see which had the best response in treatments between prednisone versus decadron and 6MP versus 6TG. After Brian completed this protocol, in December 1996, we were told that the patients that were

on 6MP and prednisone were to be switched to 6MP and decadron. There seemed to be a better outcome.

The results of the CCG-1922 study are not complete. But we were told in the beginning of the protocol that if one arm was doing better than the other arm, the patients would be switched to the better arm.

All institutions that conduct clinical trials also have an Institutional Review Board (IRB) or an ethics committee which reviews and approves all research taking place there. These boards, whose purpose is to protect patients, are made up of scientists, doctors, sometimes clergy, and often citizens from the community.

Questions to ask about clinical trials

To fully understand the clinical trial that has been proposed, here are some important questions to ask the oncologist:

- What is the purpose of the study?
- Who is sponsoring the study? Who reviews it? How often is it reviewed? Who monitors patient safety?
- What tests and treatments will be done during the study? How do these differ from standard treatment?
- Why is it thought that the treatment being studied may be better than standard treatment?
- What are the possible benefits?
- What are all possible disadvantages?
- What are the possible side effects or risks of the study? What are the side effects of the study compared to those of standard treatment?
- How will the study affect my child's daily life?
- What are the possible long-term impacts of the study compared to the standard treatment?
- How long will the study last? Is this shorter or longer than standard treatment?
- Will the study require more hospitalization than standard treatment?
- Does the study include long-term follow-up care?
- What happens if my child is harmed as a result of the research?

- Compare the study to standard treatment in terms of possible outcomes, side effects, time involved, costs, and quality of life.
- Have insurers been reimbursing for care under this protocol?

When discussing the clinical trial with the oncologist, it is perfectly reasonable to ensure that the information will be available for later review. Many parents bring a tape recorder or a friend to take notes. Some parents write down all of the doctor's answers for later reference.

Informed consent

True informed consent is a process—not merely an explanation and signing of documents. Informed consent requires that:

1. All the treatments available to the child have been laid on the table and discussed—not just the treatment available at your hospital or through your doctor, but all the treatments that could be beneficial, wherever they are given.

2. The parents and, to the extent possible, the child, have discussed these options and decided that they want to consider one of them.

3. The option selected is thoroughly discussed, with all its benefits and risks clearly explained.

4. Those aspects of the study that are considered experimental and those that are standard are clearly described.

A fully informed medical decision weighs the relative merits of a therapy after full disclosure of benefits, risks, and alternatives.

During the discussions between the doctor(s) and family, all questions should be answered in language that is clearly understood by the parents, and there should be no pressure to enroll the child in the study. The objective of the informed consent process is that the participants are comfortable that they have made a good choice, one they can comply with and stand behind.

> We had many discussions with the staff prior to signing the informed consent to participate in the clinical trial. We asked innumerable questions, all of which were answered in a frank and honest manner. We felt that participating gave our child the best chance for a cure, and we felt good about increasing the knowledge that would help other children later.

The form that parents sign will have language similar to the following: "The study described above has been explained to me, and I voluntarily agree to have my child participate in this study. I have had all of my questions answered, and understand that all future questions that I have about this research will be answered by the investigators listed above."

> *The study that our institution was participating in at the time of my daughter's diagnosis was attempting to lessen the treatment to reduce neurotoxicity yet still cure the disease. My family began a massive research effort on the issue, and we had several family friends who were physicians discuss the case with the heads of pediatric oncology at their institutions. The consensus was that since my daughter was at the high end of the high-risk description, it was advisable to choose the standard care, which was more aggressive.*

> *Although we believe strongly in clinical trials, we decided to opt for the standard treatment because she had a poor prognosis, and we felt that she would need the cranial radiation, despite the possibility of late side effects.*

Parents are experts on their children, but no matter how much reading they do, they are not experts on cancer. By the time a study is published in the literature, doctors on the cutting edge of treatment are one to three years into improving that treatment or learning of its shortcomings. For this reason, it is best to make decisions in partnership with knowledgeable medical caregivers, rather than in isolation.

No matter how comfortable you are with your child's treating oncologist, it may be helpful to have another medical caregiver help sort out your options. Often, that person will be the family's pediatrician or family doctor. Second opinions can also be arranged through the Childhood Cancer Ombudsman Program, which uses volunteer specialists to provide free help to families considering the range of treatment options and informed consent process. (See Appendix C, *Resource Organizations*, for contact information.)

The protocol

A protocol is a recipe for treating cancer. Just like a recipe for baking a cake, it has ingredients that go in at certain times and in certain ways in order for the recipe to have the best chance for success. The protocol document lists the drugs, dosages, and tests for each segment of treatment. If your child is enrolled in a clinical trial, the protocol will outline the treatment for each arm. For instance, the first page of the protocol for the child with intermediate-risk ALL might list the following for the induction period: two bone marrow aspirations, four doses of vincristine, nine doses of L-asparaginase, two intrathecal doses of methotrexate, and twenty-seven oral doses of prednisone. It will state the dates and dosages for each chemotherapy drug and procedure.

If your child is enrolled in a clinical trial, the protocol will outline the treatment for each arm.

> The clinical trial that my child was enrolled in had three arms—A, B, and C. He was in the A portion, so we only referred to the A section of the protocol, which clearly outlined each procedure and drug to be given for the duration of the trial. It also listed the follow-up care required by that particular clinical trial.

If the family chooses not to enroll in a clinical trial, they will be given a protocol for standard treatment (often the standard arm of the clinical trial).

The portion of the protocol devoted to the schedule may be five to twenty-five pages long, and the family may also be given an abbreviated version (one to two pages) to provide quick and easy reference on a daily basis. This part of the protocol is frequently called the "roadmap." Parents and teenage patients should review these documents carefully with the oncologist so that all portions are understood. It will be the parent's responsibility to make the appropriate appointments and give oral medications at the correct times.

Many parents express anguish when discussing their child's protocol, primarily because it was not clearly explained (or they misunderstood) that the protocol is a guideline. Therapy frequently needs to be modified depending on each child's response to treatment.

> I didn't know what a protocol was when Preston was diagnosed, and I understood from the doctors that this was the "exact" regime which must be followed to cure Preston. It frightened me whenever changes were made in the protocol. After several years, I came to view the protocol as merely a guideline which is individualized for each patient according to his tolerance and reaction to the drugs. We ended up deleting whole sections of Preston's protocol due to extreme side effects. He has been off therapy for five years now with no relapse.

It took me a long time to get over my hang-up that things needed to go exactly as per protocol. Any deviations on dose or days was a major stress for me. It took talking to many parents, as well as doctors and nurses, to realize and feel comfortable with the fact that no one ever goes along perfectly and that the protocol is meant as the broad guideline. There will always be times when your child will be off drugs or on half dose because of illness or low counts or whatever. It took a long time to realize that this is not going to ruin the effectiveness, that the child gets what she can handle without causing undue harm.

• • • • •

I sobbed every night for an entire week when Katy was first taken off chemotherapy for low counts. I was convinced that the immunosuppression was due to a relapse. That was two years ago, and we have changed her dosages almost every two weeks due to erratic counts. I wish I had known how normal it is to go off protocol.

The entire trial document

The roadmap described above is actually a very small portion of an extensive document describing all aspects of the clinical study. The entire document often exceeds 100 pages and covers the following topics: study hypothesis, experimental design, scientific background and rationale with relevant references from the scientific literature, patient eligibility and randomization, therapy for each arm of the study, required observations, pathology guidelines, radiation therapy guidelines (if applicable), supportive care guidelines, specific information about each drug, relapse therapy guidelines, statistical considerations, study committee, record-keeping, reporting of adverse drug reactions, and consent form.

Parents are sometimes not aware that this lengthy document exists. Admittedly, for some parents the full protocol could be overwhelming or boring. There are many parents, however, who throw themselves into research to better understand their child's illness. These parents may benefit from having a copy of the study document for several reasons. First, it provides a description of some of the clinical trials that preceded the present one and explains the reasons the investigators designed this particular study. Secondly, it provides detailed descriptions of drug reactions, which comforts many parents who worry that their child is the only one exhibiting extreme responses to some drugs. Thirdly, motivated parents who have only one protocol to keep track of occasionally prevent errors in treatment. Physicians treat children on many different protocols and sometimes make mistakes. And finally, for parents who are adrift in the world of cancer treatment, it can return a bit of control over their child's life. It gives the parents a job to do: monitor their child's treatment.

> *Since knowledge is comfort for me, I really wanted to have the entire clinical trial document, despite its technical language. Whereas the brief protocol that I had listed day, drug, dose, the expanded version listed the potential side effects for each drug, and what actions should be taken should any occur. I learned the parameters.*

Parents have a right to review all literature and information related to their child's treatment. There are no moral, ethical, or legal restrictions that come into play. If you wish to read all of the details of the study, simply insist that a copy be provided to you.

The following are excerpts from a letter to a doctor sent by a mother who discovered the study document two years into her son's treatment:

> *Until just recently, I thought that high-dose methotrexate was being tested against intrathecal methotrexate to determine if it was more effective in preventing CNS relapse. I believed that high-dose methotrexate was the untested drug. I didn't realize that data was available from a prior protocol showing good results with high-dose methotrexate. It would have been reassuring to me to have known this information earlier in Preston's treatment...*

> *As a parent, I worry more about things I don't know. I have found that the more information I have, the less I worry. Please consider giving parents more information in future protocols about chemotherapy side effects and about the evolution and intent of the protocol...*

> *Thank you for listening to me and thank you for all your efforts which benefit the health of my child and so many others.*

Saying no to a clinical trial

Parents have the legal right to decide not to have their child participate in a clinical trial. If the parents choose not to participate, their decision will be respected. The child will still be treated at the pediatric medical center and given the standard treatment for his type of leukemia.

> *Our son's doctor gave us the paperwork on the clinical trial to read and told us that it was our decision and that he would not pressure us. We really decided not to join the study for financial reasons. My husband was a student and we had no health insurance. One of the parts of the study required more clinic visits, and we just couldn't afford it.*

Removing a child from a clinical trial

Parents can withdraw their child from a clinical trial at any time. Before doing so, however, they should talk over their questions or concerns with their child's doctor. If the problem is not resolved, parents have the legal right to remove their child at any time from a clinical trial. This decision should not be held against the parent, and the child should still receive the best available care for her type of cancer. On the consent form signed by the parent, there will be language similar to this: "You are free not to have your child participate in this research or to withdraw your child at any time without penalty or jeopardizing future care."

> *Jesse was enrolled in a clinical trial to assess long-term neuropsychological consequences of cranial radiation. The testing was free, and we were glad to participate. Unfortunately, the billing department of the hospital continually billed us in error. We tried to correct the problem, but it became such a hassle that we withdrew from the study.*

Pros and cons of clinical trials

Pros of clinical trials are:

- Patients receive either state-of-the-art investigational therapy or the best standard therapy available.

- Clinical trials can provide an opportunity to benefit from a new therapy before it is generally available.

- Information gained from clinical trials will benefit children with cancer in the future.

- Children enrolled in clinical trials may be monitored more frequently throughout treatment.

- The IRB has reviewed the protocol for protection of patient's rights as well as for scientific soundness.
- Review boards of scientists oversee the operation of clinical trials.
- Participating in a clinical trial often makes parents feel that they did everything medically possible for their child.
- Some clinical trials provide all treatment and follow-up care at no cost to the family.

Cons to consider are:

- The experimental arm may not provide treatment as effective as the standard, or it may generate unexpected side effects or risks.
- Not all patients in a study receive the new treatment.
- Some clinical trials require more hospitalizations, treatments, clinic visits, or tests that may be more costly or painful than the standard treatment.
- Some families feel additional stress over which arm is the best treatment for their individual child.
- Participation may generate parental guilt if the child has unacceptable toxicity from the more aggressive experimental arm.
- Insurance may not cover investigational studies. Parents need to carefully explore this issue prior to signing the consent form.

When we were struggling with the decision of whether to join the study, I asked the oncologist how would we ever know if we made the right decision. He said something very wise: "You will never know and you should never second-guess yourself, no matter how the study turns out. Statistics are about large groups of kids, not your child. Your child might relapse no matter which arm she is on and she might be cured on an arm where most of the other kids relapse. Statistics for you will be either one hundred percent or zero because your child will either live or die. I can't tell you which will be the better treatment, that is why we are conducting the study. But no matter what, we will be doing absolutely the best we can."

CHAPTER 5

Family and Friends

Shared joy is double joy,
shared sorrow is half sorrow.

—Swedish proverb

THE INTERACTIONS BETWEEN the parents of a child with cancer and their extended family and friends are complex. Potential exists for loving support and generous help, as well as for bitter disappointment and disputes. The diagnosis of leukemia creates a ripple effect, first touching the immediate family, then extended family, friends, coworkers, schoolmates, church members, and the entire community.

This chapter discusses some of the experiences the family might encounter, as well as scores of ideas for helpful things that family and friends can do. To prevent possible misunderstandings between family members and friends, veteran parents also share ideas on things that do not help.

The extended family

Extended family—aunts, uncles, cousins, grandparents—can cushion the shock of a leukemia diagnosis by loving words and actions. Extended family members sometimes drop their own lives to rush to the side of the child with leukemia, and often remain steadfast for the years of treatment. Regrettably, family members may not be helpful, either from ignorance of what the family needs or simply because they are overwhelmed by events in their own lives.

Notifying the family

Notifying relatives is one of the first painful jobs for the parent of a child newly diagnosed with cancer. In times of crisis, family is refuge, and the news is usually quickly shared. Here are some ways that parents have told their relatives:

I called my mom and told her to make all the phone calls to family and friends. I couldn't choke out the word leukemia yet. Then I called our pastor.

·　·　·　·　·

I called my sister and asked her to take care of telling everyone. She called my other sister, and together they told my frail mother.

·　·　·　·　·

I waited three days after the diagnosis to call anyone. The doctors had trouble determining whether it was ALL or AML, and I wanted to be able to give the prognosis on the first call. I called my mom and asked her to notify everyone else but to request that they not call me for a week. I felt too fragile, and didn't want to continually cry in front of my daughter.

Paradoxically, the family members who potentially may provide the greatest support may also be sources of added stress. Some extended families and even entire communities rally around the stricken family, while support never materializes for others. Several factors affect the strength of support: well-established community ties, good communication within extended family, physical proximity to extended family, and clear exchange of information on the needs of the affected family. If any of these elements are missing, support may evaporate.

We had just moved three thousand miles away from family and friends for my husband to accept a new job. We had no family, no friends. Each family member and some close friends used their vacation to fly out and take two-week shifts at our new house to help out. Thankfully, they got us through the first months, but the two stressful years of maintenance were lonely.

Other well-established families have support throughout treatment:

Shortly after Jesse relapsed, I was praying with my bible study group. With four children aged one to nine, I just didn't know how we would manage with one parent 100 miles away at the hospital and one parent working. The group decided to collect enough money to allow my sister to quit her job and move in to take care of the other three children while I was at the hospital with Jesse. She stayed for eight months. It was such a wonderful thing. They didn't even ask us; they just said they would support her financially so that she could care for my children and keep the household running.

Staying in touch

The most important first step for families is to set up clear communication over what truly will help. Sometimes, the child is too sick or too fatigued for company, and this needs to be expressed. Establishing a telephone chain is a good way to keep family informed of the child's progress. One family member can be delegated as communicator, and this person will relay the information to another person who will then phone another. Some families leave updates on their telephone answering machines. Some send out form letters or emails. Others ask a friend or family member to be the social director. This person can spread the word about your situation and prevent many phone calls. He or she can also organize the many people who want to help but don't know what to do.

Grandparents

Grandparents grieve deeply when a grandchild is diagnosed with leukemia. They are concerned not only for their grandchild, but for their own child (the parent) as well. Cancer wreaks havoc with grandparents' expectations, reversing the natural order of life and death. Grandparents frequently say, "Why not me? I'm the one who is old." Parents express anguish at having to tell the grandparents the grim news. Cancer in a grandchild is a major shock to bear.

Many parents reported that the grandparents responded to the crisis with tremendous emotional, physical, and financial support.

> My mother was a rock. She lived far away, but she put her busy life
> on hold to come help. She took care of the baby and kept the household
> running through both induction and reinduction when I was living at the
> hospital with my very ill child. She was strong, and it gave me strength.

Some parents express tremendous gratitude for the role played by the grandparents in providing much-needed stability to the family rocked by cancer. When the grandparents care for the siblings and run the household, the parents can care for the sick child and return to work.

> Because Judd had no neutrophils at diagnosis, he was put in isolation
> at Children's for a month. I stayed with him full time, and my husband
> took a month off work to be there. Luckily, my mother had moved to our
> town just the year before and was able to immediately move to our house

to take care of Erin, my ten-year-old daughter. Grandma was great because she cooked special meals for Erin and helped with cleaning and transportation.

Other families are not so fortunate. Many grandparents are too old, too ill, or simply unable to cope with a crisis of this magnitude. Some simply fall apart.

My mother became hysterical when my daughter was diagnosed with leukemia. She called every day, sobbing. Luckily, she lived far away, and this minimized the disruption. We had to ask her not to come because we just couldn't handle the catastrophe at home and her neediness too. It hurt her feelings, but we just couldn't cope with it.

Other grandparents allow preexisting problems with their adult child to color their perceptions of what the family needs. Sometimes cancer allows grandparents to renew criticism of the way grandchildren are being raised.

While we stayed at the hospital the grandparents moved into our house to care for our eight-year-old daughter. They decided that this was their chance to "whip her into shape, teach her some manners, and get her room cleaned up." Our daughter was in tears, and we ended up saying, "We appreciate your help, but we will take over."

Sometimes grandparents try to blame the parents for the cancer or make other hurtful comments:

The first day in the hospital my mother told me I had caused the leukemia by coloring my hair blond during the pregnancy. My mother-in-law wasn't helpful either. Throughout the ordeal of treatment, all she did was to tell us to "put it in God's hand."

Grave problems can also result when grandparents try to take charge. Criticizing parents' choice of doctors, hospitals, or treatment can be very disruptive and further stress the family's resources.

Some grandparents simply cannot cope and withdraw from the situation. One mother was eight months pregnant, and her parents were visiting when her two-year-old son was diagnosed:

I will never, ever be able to forget how my mother let me and my son down. She never came to the hospital, saying, "He's too sick for com-

pany." I told her he would love to see her, that his little face just would light up when he had visitors. But she never came. She never offered to help at home when he was so ill. She just disappeared.

It is hard to predict how anyone will react to the diagnosis of childhood leukemia. Grandparents are no exception. Some respond with the wisdom gleaned from decades of living, others become needy, and some withdraw. It is natural in a time of grave crisis to look to your parents for support and help, but it is important to remember that grandparents' ability to respond also depends on events in their own lives. If problems develop, help can be obtained from hospital social workers or through individual counseling.

Helpful things for family to do

Families differ in what is truly helpful for them. The suggestions in this chapter are snapshots of what some families appreciated. True listening and working on maintaining the relationship is paramount. Connections can be made in many different, unique, and personally meaningful ways. Try to support the family in ways that respect their wishes while honoring their privacy:

- Be sensitive to the emotional state of both child and parent. Sometimes parents want to talk about the leukemia; sometimes they just need a hand to hold.

- Encourage all members of the family to keep in touch through visits, calls, mail, videotapes, audiotapes, or pictures. When visits are welcome, make them brief and cheerful. Not only do long visits sometimes distress sick children, but they can also overtax a tired parent.

    Our relatives who lived close to the hospital had teenagers. One was a candy striper at Children's on Saturdays. Judd's aunts, uncles, and cousins came to visit several times a week any time he was in the hospital during his three years of treatment. They were all very supportive, very positive, and fun to be around.

- Be understanding if the parents do not want phone calls in the hospital. Remember that the child can hear all phone conversations when parents talk on the phone in the room.

    The first three days in the hospital I spent much of my time crying on the phone when talking to friends and relatives. Then I realized how frightening this must be to my two-year-old. So I just took the phone off the hook and left it there. Now, each time Jennifer is hospitalized, I call one friend and have her spread the news, then I take the phone off the hook again and concentrate on my daughter.

- A cheerful hospital room really boosts a child's spirits. Encourage sending balloon bouquets, funny cards, posters, toys, or humorous books. Be aware that some hospitals do not allow rubber balloons, only mylar. Flowers are also not allowed in children's rooms.

  We plastered the walls with pictures of family and friends and so many people sent balloons that the ceiling was covered. It was a lovely sight.

- Laughter helps heal the mind and body, so send funny videotapes or arrive with a good joke if you think it is appropriate.

  My brother Bill and his wonderful girlfriend Cathy created an exciting "trip" for my four-year-old daughter. She was bald, big-bellied from prednisone, and her counts were too low to leave the house, but her interest in fashion was as sharp as ever. Bill and Cathy bought ten outfits, rigged up a dressing room, and with Cathy as saleswoman, turned Katy's bedroom into a fashion salon. She tried on outfits, discussed all of their merits and shortcomings, and had a fabulous time. It was a real high point for her.

- Puzzles, games, picture books, coloring books, age-appropriate computer games, and crafts are welcome. Remember that attention spans may be shortened by treatment, so keep it simple.

  A friend who was a nurse came to my son's room shortly before Christmas and brought an entire gingerbread house kit, including confectioner's sugar for the icing. We had a very good time putting it together.

- Offer to give the parent a break from the hospital room. A walk outside, shopping trip, haircut, dinner with spouse, or just a long shower can be very refreshing.

- Donate frequent flyer miles to distant family members who have the time but not the money to help.

  A close friend (who lived three thousand miles away) had just lost her job and wished she could be there for us. My parents gave her their frequent flyer miles. She flew in for three weeks during a hard part of treatment and helped enormously.

- If you don't hear from a family member, call. Often silence means that he doesn't know what to do or say. Cynthia Krumme writes in her book *Leukemia Isn't So Bad*:

    An irony that we felt and others expressed was that the difficulty of living with cancer is sometimes compounded when much of the reassurance must come from the patient and the family toward the rest of the world.

Friends

Like family, friends can cushion the shock of diagnosis and ease the difficulties of treatment with their words and actions.

Notifying friends

The easiest way to notify friends is to delegate one person to do the job. Calling one neighbor or close friend prevents numerous tearful conversations. Most parents are at their child's bedside and want to avoid more emotional upheaval, especially in front of their child. Parents need to recognize that friends' emotions will mirror their own: shock, fear, worry, helplessness. Since most friends want to help but don't know what to do or say, giving cues of what would be helpful are welcome.

Helpful things for friends to do

Mother Theresa once said, "We can do no great things—only small things with great love." It is a given that the family of a newly diagnosed child is overwhelmed. The list of helpful things to do is endless, but here are some suggestions from veteran parents.

Household

- Provide meals.

    One of the nicest things that friends did was to bring us a huge picnic basket full of food to the hospital. We spread a blanket on the floor, Erica crawled out of bed, and the entire family sat down together and ate. Most people don't realize how expensive it is to have to eat every meal at the hospital cafeteria, so the picnic was not only fun, but helped us to save a few dollars.

- Take care of pets or livestock.

- Mow grass, shovel snow, rake leaves, weed gardens.

    We came home from the hospital one evening right before Christmas, and found a freshly cut, fragrant Christmas tree leaning next to our door. I'll never forget that kindness.

- Clean the house.

    My husband's cousin sent her cleaning lady over to our house. It was so neat and such a luxury to come home to find the stove and windows sparkling clean.

- Grocery shop (especially when the family is due home from the hospital).

- Do laundry. Drop off and pick up dry cleaning.

- Provide a place to stay near the hospital.

    One of the ladies from the school where I worked came up to the ICU waiting room where we were sleeping and pressed her house key into my hand. She lived five minutes from the hospital. She said, "My basement is made up, there's a futon, there's a TV, you are coming and staying at my house." I hardly knew her, but we accepted. Every day when we came in from the hospital there was some cute little treat waiting for us like a bowl of cookies, or two packages of hot chocolate and a thermos of hot milk.

Siblings

- Baby-sit whenever parents go to the clinic, emergency room, or for a prolonged hospital stay.

    The mother of a secretary from my office called me, introduced herself, and offered to care for my newborn daughter while I spent time at the hospital. I had never met this woman, but she turned out to be a real lifesaver and a jewel. She would come every day, bathe, dress, and feed my daughter, clean up the house, and stay from morning until evening. She did this for several months. I will never forget her for being so kind. I would not have been able to get through those first few difficult months

without this type of support—and to find it in a complete stranger cer-
tainly renewed my faith in mankind!

- When parents are home with a sick child, take sibling(s) to the park, sports event, or a movie.

- Invite sibling(s) over for meals.

- If you bring a gift for the sick child, bring something for the sibling(s), too.

Friends from home sent boxes of art supplies to us when the whole family spent those first ten weeks at a Ronald McDonald house far from our home. They sent scissors, paints, paper, colored pens. It was a great help for Carrie Beth and her two sisters. One friend even sent an Easter package with straw hats for each girl, and flowers, ribbons, and glue to decorate them with.

- Offer to help sibling(s) with homework.

- Drive sibling(s) to lessons, games, or school.

- Listen to how they are feeling and coping. Siblings' lives have been disrupted, they have limited time with their parents, and they need support and care.

Psychological support

- Call frequently, and be open to listening if the parents want to talk about their feelings. Also talk about non-cancer-related topics such as sharing the neighborhood and school news.

- Visit the hospital and bring fun stuff like bubbles, silly string, water pistols, joke books, funny videotapes, rub-on tattoos, board games.

- Bring lots of prepaid phone cards to the hospital so the family can call distant friends and relatives.

- If one parent had to leave work to stay in the hospital with the sick child, coworkers can send messages by mail or tape.

One very neat thing that was an emotional boost was that my friends and former coworkers from Kansas faxed us messages and pictures and things to Meagan while we were in the hospital. It was very nice to get such fresh messages—it really shortened the miles.

- If you think the family might be interested, call Candlelighters, the American Cancer Society, or the social worker at the local hospital to find out if there are support groups for parents and/or kids in your area.

- Offer to take the children to the support groups or go with the parents. For most families, the parent support group becomes a second family with ties of shared experience as deep and strong as blood relations.

- Drive parent and child to clinic visits.

- Buy books (uplifting ones) for the family if they are readers.

- Send cards or letters.

> Word got around my parents' hometown, and I received cards from many high school acquaintances, who still cared enough to call or write and say we're praying for you, please let us know how things are going. It was so neat to get so many cards out of the blue that said, "I'm thinking about you."

- Baby-sit the sick child so that the parents can go out to eat, exercise, take a walk, or just get out of the hospital or house.

- Donate blood. Your blood will not be used specifically for the ill child, but will replenish the general supply, which is depleted by children with cancer.

- If the child has a type of leukemia that may require a bone marrow transplant, organize a drive to have lots of people typed and entered into the marrow registry. Contact: National Marrow Donor Program, 3433 Broadway St. NE, Suite 400, Minneapolis, MN 55413, (800) 654-1247.

- Give lots of hugs.

> Grandpa Fred is a seventy-one-year-old retiree who has been visiting pediatric oncology patients at Children's for almost twelve years. He begins his day at 9:30 every morning on the teens ward, then he moves on to visit the younger patients, the playroom, and the clinic. Grandpa Fred always takes pictures of his young friends, very good ones, and has filled twenty-three photo albums with them. Fred has two prints made of each picture he takes and gives one to the families. He also helps Santa on Christmas and visits on Halloween. He has been the camp manager at Camp Good Times every summer for eight years. Fred feels that a hug is more important than anything he can say to someone. "Listening and giving a hug," he says, "That's the best I can do."

Financial support

Helping families avoid financial disaster can be the next greatest gift after the life of the child and the strength of the family. It is estimated that even fully insured families spend 25 percent or more of their income on copayments, travel, motels, meals, and other uncovered items. Uninsured or underinsured families may lose their savings or even their house. Most families need financial help. Here are some suggestions:

- Start a support fund.

  A friend of mine called and asked very tentatively if we would mind if she started a support fund. We felt awkward, but we needed help, so we said okay. She did everything herself, and the money she raised was very, very helpful. We did ask her to stop the fund when people started calling us to ask if they could use giving to the fund as an advertisement for their business.

- Help them apply for financial aid from the Leukemia Society by calling (800) 955-4LSA and asking for the "Guidelines for Patient Aid Program Application and Reimbursement Process."

- Share leave. Governments and some companies have leave banks that permit persons who are ill or taking care of someone who is ill to use other coworkers' leave so they won't have their pay docked.

- Job share. Some families work out job-share arrangements in which a coworker donates time to perform part of one job to enable one parent to spend time at the hospital. Job sharing allows the job to get done, keeps peace at the job site, and prevents financial losses for the family. Another possibility would be for one or more friends with similar skills (e.g., word processing, filing, sales, etc.) to rotate through the job on a volunteer basis to cover for the parent of the ill child.

- Collect money at church or work to give informally.

  The day my daughter was diagnosed, my husband's coworkers passed the hat and gave us over $250. I was embarrassed, but it paid for gas, meals, and the motel until there was an opening in the Ronald McDonald House.

· · · · ·

Finances were a main concern for us because I wanted to cut back on work to be at home with Meagan. Sometimes my coworkers would pool money and present it with a card saying, "Here's a couple of days work that you won't have to worry about."

· · · · ·

My husband's coworkers didn't collect money, they did something even more valuable. They donated sick leave hours, so that he was able to be at the hospital frequently during those first few months without losing a paycheck.

- Collect money by organizing a bake sale, dance, or raffle.

    Coworkers of my husband held a Halloween party and charged admission for us. We were very uncomfortable with the idea at first, but they were looking for an excuse to have a party, and it helped us out.

- Keeping track of medical bills is time-consuming, frustrating, and exhausting. If you are a close relative or friend, you could offer to review, organize, and file (or enter into a computer) the voluminous paperwork. Making the calls and writing the letters over contested claims or errors in billing are very helpful.

Help from schoolmates

- Encourage visits (if appropriate), cards, and phone calls from classmates.
- Ask the teacher to send the school newspaper and other news along with assignments.
- Classmates can sign a brightly colored banner to send to the hospital.

    Brent's kindergarten class sent a packet containing a picture drawn for him by each child in the class. They also made him a book. Another time they sent him a letter written on huge poster board. He couldn't wait to get back to school.

Religious support

- If the family goes to church, contact a member of the clergy.
- Arrange for church members and clergy to visit the hospital, if that is what the family wants.

- Arrange prayer services for the sick child.
- Have the child's Sunday school class (or whatever class is appropriate for the family's denomination) send pictures, posters, letters, balloons, or tapes to the sick child.

> The day our son was diagnosed, we raced next door to ask our wonderful neighbors to take care of our dog. The news of his diagnosis quickly spread, and we found out later that five neighborhood families gathered that very night to pray for Brent.

Accepting help

One of the kindest things you can do for your friends is to let them help you. Let them channel their time and worry into things that make your life easier. Think of the many times you have visited a sick friend, made a meal for a new mom, baby-sat someone else's child in an emergency, or just pitched in to do what needed to be done. These actions probably made you feel great and provided a good example for your children. When your child is diagnosed with cancer, both you and your friends will immensely benefit if you let them help you and give them guidance on what you need.

One father's thoughts on accepting help:

> Fathers have a deep-seated need to protect their family. Yet here I was with a child with leukemia, and there wasn't a single thing that I could do about it. The loss of control really bothered me. The very hardest thing that I had to learn was to let go enough to let people help us.

One mother's thoughts on accepting help:

> The most important advice I received as the parent of a child newly diagnosed with cancer came from a hospital nurse whom I turned to when I was overwhelmed with all the advice being offered by family and friends. This wise nurse said, "Don't discount anything. You're going to need all the help you can get." I think it is very important for families to remain open and accept the help that is offered. It often comes when least expected and from unlikely sources. I was totally unprepared at diagnosis for how much help I would need, and I'm glad that I remained open to offers of kindness. This is not the time to show the world how strong you are.

What to say

The following are some suggestions on what to say and how to offer help. Of course, much depends on the type of relationship that already exists, but a specific offer can always be accepted or graciously declined:

- I am so sorry.

- I didn't call earlier because I didn't know what to say.

- Our family would like do your yardwork. It will make us feel as if we are helping in a small way.

- We want to clean your house for you once a week. What day would be convenient?

- Would it help if we took care of your dog (or cat, or bird)? We would love to do it.

- I walk my dog three times a day. May I walk yours, too?

- The church is setting up a system to deliver meals to your house. When is the best time to drop them off?

- I will take care of Jimmy whenever you need to take John to the hospital. Call us anytime, day or night, and we will come pick him up.

Things that do not help

Out of ignorance, people sometimes say hurtful things to parents of children with cancer. If you are a family member or friend of a parent in this situation, please do not say any of the following:

- "God only gives people what they can handle." (Some people cannot handle the stress of childhood leukemia.)

- "I know just how you feel." (Unless you have a child with cancer, you simply don't know.)

- "You are so brave," or "so strong," etc. (Parents are not heroes; they are normal people struggling with extraordinary stress.)

- "They are doing such wonderful things to save children with leukemia these days." (Yes, the prognosis is good, but what parents and children are going through is not wonderful.)

- "Well, we're all going to die one day." (True, but parents do not need to be reminded of this fact.)

- "It's God's will." (This is just not a helpful thing to hear.)
- "At least you have other kids," or "Thank goodness you are still young enough to have other children." (A child cannot be replaced.)

   A woman whom I worked with, but did not know well, came up to me one day and out of the blue said, "When Erica gets to heaven to be with Jesus, He will love her." All I could think to say was, "Well, I'm sorry, but Jesus can't have her right now."

Parents also make the following suggestions of things to avoid doing:

- Do not say, "Let us know if there is anything we can do." It is far better to make a specific suggestion.

   Many well-wishing friends always said, "Let me know what I can do." I wish they had just "done," instead of asking for direction. It took too much energy to decide, call them, make arrangements, etc. I wish someone would have said, "When is your clinic day? I'll bring dinner," or "I'll baby-sit Sunday afternoon so you two can go out to lunch."

- Do not make personal comments in front of the child: when will his hair grow back in, he's lost so much weight, she's so pale, etc.
- Do not do things that require the parent to support you (for example, repeatedly call up, crying).
- Do not talk continually about the cancer; some normal conversations are welcome.
- Do not ask "what if " questions: What if he can't go to school? What if your insurance won't cover it? What if she dies? The present is really all the parents can deal with.
- Stories of children you know who have survived leukemia and are doing fine are welcome. Stories of those who have died or who have long-term side effects should not be shared.

Losing friends

It is an unfortunate reality that most parents of children with leukemia lose friends. For a variety of reasons, some friends just can't cope and either suddenly disappear or gradually fade away. Many times this can be prevented by calling them to keep them involved, but sometimes, they just can't handle the stress.

Except for one good friend, none of my friends called when I was home. It seemed that after the initial three-month crisis, they removed themselves from the situation, as often happens.

• • • • •

I had a friend who really thought herself to be empathetic, except that she just couldn't "deal with" hospitals. She said that they made her uncomfortable, so she wouldn't visit. I also got tired of her talking about the silver lining of the dark cloud that has been hanging over my head. I have a really hard time dealing with that.

• • • • •

Friends? What friends? They disappeared, family, too. No one knew what to say to us.

Evan Handler, who was diagnosed with leukemia as a young adult, wrote a powerful memoir called *Time on Fire* about his experience. In it he discussed what his parents did to keep their friends informed:

They began to distribute a newsletter describing my progress as well as the stresses they were under...I saw it as a brilliant device. The exhaustion that is unavoidable to the parents of a sick child, even an adult child, is enough to overwhelm the strongest individual. My parents were simply accepting the offers coming forth and sharing their burden in a fashion that didn't increase their already superhuman load. By revealing themselves in the newsletter, both the good news and the bad, they gave their friends the option of tuning in or out, without having to suffer the indignity of those who could not cope with what my parents coped with daily.

Restructuring family life

Childhood cancer does not only strike families of brave children and heroic parents. In the United States, the popular press has responded to people's terror of cancer by churning out story after story of people who faced the diagnosis with almost superhuman hope and strength. Families rally round, the community cheers, and human will triumphs over the evil of cancer. This simply is not always the case. Cancer strikes all types of families: single-parent families, those with two parents in the home; financially secure families; those with no insurance; families with strong community ties; those who have just moved to a new community; families of every size, type, and color. Most parents do find unexpected reserves of strength to deal with the crisis. They survive the years of stress and pain, emerging different and sometimes stronger. Still, expectations of heroism are not appropriate.

Keeping the household functioning

Every family of a child with leukemia needs massive assistance. It is important for families to recognize this early and learn not only to accept aid gracefully but also to ask for help when needed. As discussed earlier in the chapter, most family members, friends, neighbors, and church members want to help, but they need direction from the family on what is helpful but not intrusive.

In families where both parents are employed, decisions must be made about the jobs. It is better, if possible, to use all available sick leave and vacation days prior to deciding whether one parent needs to terminate employment. Parents need to be able to evaluate their financial situation and insurance availability. This requires time and clarity of thought, both in short supply in the weeks following diagnosis.

> *I was eight months pregnant when my two-year-old son was diagnosed. I went on maternity leave, but we needed to make arrangements quickly with my husband's employer to allow him time off to care for Carl in the hospital after I had the baby. Even worse, I knew that I would need to deliver by caesarian section. Carl's protocol required him to be in the hospital for one week then home for one week from September through January. My husband worked out a schedule where he worked seventy hours the week that Carl was home, then was off work the week Carl was hospitalized. He then only needed to use ten hours of leave, and was able to stay at the hospital with Carl.*

Family and Medical Leave Act (US)

In August 1993, the Family and Medical Leave Act (FMLA) became federal law. FMLA protects job security of workers in large companies who must take a leave of absence to care for a seriously ill child, to take medical leave because the employee is unable to work because of his or her own medical condition, or for the birth or placement of a child for adoption or foster care. The Family and Medical Leave Act:

- Applies to employers with 50 or more employees within a seventy-five-mile radius.

- Provides twelve weeks of unpaid leave during any twelve-month period to care for seriously ill self, spouse, child, or parent. In certain instances, the employee may take intermittent leave, such as reducing his or her normal work schedule's hours.

- Requires employer to continue to provide benefits, including health insurance, during the leave period.

- Requires employer to return employee to the same or equivalent position upon return from the leave. Some benefits, such as seniority, need not accrue during periods of unpaid FMLA leave.

- Requires employee to give 30-day notice of the need to take FMLA leave when the need is foreseeable.

- Is enforced by complaints to the Wage and Hour Division, US Department of Labor, or by private lawsuit. The nearest office of the Wage and Hour Division may be located by looking in the US Government pages of your telephone directory.

Marriage

Cancer treatment places enormous pressure on a marriage. Couples may be separated for long periods of time, emotions are high, and coping styles and skills differ. Initially, family life may be shattered. Couples must simply survive the first few overwhelming weeks, then work together to rearrange the pieces in a new pattern. Here are parents' suggestions and stories about how they managed:

- Share medical decisions.

My husband and I shared decision-making by keeping a joint medical journal. The days that my husband stayed at the hospital, he would write down all medicines given, side effects, fever, vital signs, food consumed, sleep patterns, and any questions that needed to be asked at the next rounds. This way, I knew exactly what had been happening. Decisions were made as we traded shifts at our son's bedside.

· · · · ·

I made most of the medical decisions. My husband did not know what a protocol was, nor did he ever learn the names of the medicines.

He came with me to medical conferences, however, and his presence gave me strength.

· · · · ·

Curt and I discuss every detail of the medical issues. It is so helpful to hash things over together to get a clearer idea of what our main concerns are.

- Take turns staying in the hospital with the ill child.

We took turns going in with our son for painful procedures. The doctors loved to see my husband come in because he's a friendly, easygoing person who never asked them any medical questions. We shared hospital duty, also. I would be there during any crisis because I was the person better able to be a strong advocate, but he went when our son was feeling better and needed entertaining company. It worked out well.

· · · · ·

My husband fell apart emotionally when our daughter was diagnosed, and he never really recovered. He stayed with her once in the hospital and cried almost the whole time. She never wanted him to go again, so I did all of the hospital duty.

· · · · ·

Whenever Brent was in the hospital, we both wanted to be there. We were able to be there most of the time because our children have a wonderful aunt and uncle who stayed with them when needed. During Brent's second extended stay in the hospital, we both let go a little, and we each took turns sleeping at the Ronald McDonald House. That way we each got a decent night's sleep (or some sleep) every other night.

· · · · ·

My wife took care of most of the medical information gathering because she had a scientific background. But my work schedule was more flexible, so I took my son for almost all of his treatments and hospitalizations. I cherish my memories of those long hours in the car and waiting room, because we were always so very close.

- Share responsibility for home care.

My husband worked long hours, and therefore I had to do almost all of the home care. It was very hard on me, especially in the beginning

*when my daughter was so ill and needed so many medications. I felt like I
was doing all the horrible things to her; I wish that he could have done
some of it.*

. . . . .

*We had a traditional relationship in which I took care of the kids and
he worked. I didn't expect him to cook or clean when I was staying at the
hospital—it was all he could do to ferry our daughter to her various
activities and go to work.*

. . . . .

*We both worked full time, so we staggered our shifts. He worked 7 to
3 during the day: I worked 3 to 11 at night. He did every single dressing
change for the Hickman catheter—584 changes, we counted them up.
Wherever I left off during the day, he took over. He was great, and it
really worked out well for us. We shared it all.*

. . . . .

*My husband really didn't help at all. I couldn't even go out because
he wouldn't give the pills. He kept saying that he was afraid that he would
make a mistake.*

- Accept differences in coping styles.

*We both coped differently, but we learned to work around it. I didn't
want to deal with "what if" questions, but he was a pessimist and constantly asked the fellow questions about things that might happen. I felt
that it was a waste of energy to worry about things that might never happen. I didn't want to hear it and felt that it just added to my burden. It
was all I could do to survive every day. We worked it out by going to conferences together, but I would ask my questions and then leave. He stayed
behind to ask all of his questions.*

. . . . .

*My husband didn't have the desire to read as much as I did. How-
ever, whenever I read something that I felt he should read, he always took
the time to do so and then we discussed it.*

- Seek counseling.

> *I went for counseling because I couldn't sleep. At night, I got stuck thinking the same things over and over and worrying. I ended up spending two years on antidepressants, which I think really saved my life. They helped me sleep and kept me on an even keel. I'm off them now, my son is off treatment, and everything is looking up.*

· · · · ·

> *My husband and I went to counseling to try to work out a way to split up the child rearing and household duties because I was overwhelmed and resenting it. I guess it helped a little bit, but the best thing that came out of it was that I kept seeing the counselor by myself. My son wanted to go to the "feelings doctor," too. I received a lot of very helpful, practical advice on the many behavior problems my son developed. And my son had an objective, safe person to talk things over with.*

Most marriages survive, but some don't. It is usually marriages with serious preexisting problems that are further strained by cancer treatment.

> *My husband had a lot of problems that really brought my daughter and me down. The cancer really opened my eyes to what was important in life. We stayed together through treatment, but we divorced after the bone marrow transplant. I just realized that life is too short to spend it in a bad relationship.*

· · · · ·

> *My husband went to work rather than go with us to Children's when our son was diagnosed. It went downhill from there. He started using drugs and mistreating us, so we divorced.*

Siblings

It takes an entire chapter to deal with the complex feelings that siblings confront when their brother or sister has leukemia. Chapter 16, *Siblings*, provides an in-depth examination of the issues from the perspective of both siblings and parents.

I called a close friend to ask if she could drive our second car the 100 miles to the hospital so that my husband could return in it to work. She came with her family to the Ronald McDonald House with two big bags containing snack foods, a large box of stationery, envelopes, stamps, books to read, a book handmade by her three-year-old daughter containing dozens of cut-out pictures of children's clothing pasted on construction paper (which my daughter adored looking at), and a beautiful, new, handmade, lace-trimmed dress for my daughter. It was full-length and baggy enough to cover all bandages and tubing. She wore it almost every day for a year. It was a wonderful thing for my friend to do.

CHAPTER 6

Forming a Partnership with the Medical Team

It is our duty as physicians to estimate
probabilities and to discipline expectations;
but leading away from probabilities there
are paths of possibilities, toward which it is
our duty to hold aloft the light, and the
name of that light is hope.

—Karl Menninger
The Vital Balance

IT IS VITALLY IMPORTANT that parents and the healthcare team establish and maintain a relationship based on excellent medical care, good communication, and caring. In this partnership, trust is paramount. Unlike children with some other diseases, children with leukemia spend years being treated primarily on an outpatient basis. Physicians rely on parents to make and keep appointments, give the proper medicines at the appropriate times, prepare the child for procedures, and be vigilant in noticing any illness or drug side effect. Parents rely on physicians for medical knowledge, expertise in performing procedures, good judgment, caring, and clear communication. It is a delicate dance that spans years of trauma and emotional upheaval.

A climate of cooperation and respect between the healthcare team and parents allows children to thrive. This chapter explores ways to create and maintain that environment.

The hospital

After diagnosis, a steady parade of anonymous faces enters the life of a child with leukemia. To understand who is responsible for the child's treatment, an explanation of hospital pecking order is necessary.

The doctors

A medical student is a college graduate who is attending medical school. Medical students often wear white coats, but do not have MD after the name on their name tags. They are not doctors.

An intern (also called a first-year resident) is a graduate of medical school who is in her first year of postgraduate training.

A resident is a graduate of medical school in his second or third year of postgraduate training. Most of the residents at pediatric hospitals will be pediatricians upon completion of their residencies.

After residency, if the pediatric resident wishes to further specialize in oncology (the study of cancer), she applies for a fellowship in pediatric oncology. Fellows work only at academic centers with fellowship programs, not all pediatric oncology centers. A fellow who treats children with cancer is a doctor who has completed four years of medical school, one year of internship, and two to three years of residency in pediatrics, and is taking additional specialty training in pediatric oncology. In the US, pediatric residency is three years. In Canada it is four years; however, there is no internship.

Above fellows in the hospital hierarchy are attending physicians (called simply "attendings"). These well-established doctors are hired by the medical center to provide and oversee medical care and to train interns, residents, and fellows. They are frequently also professors on the staff of the medical school.

> *Our medical team was wonderful. They always answered our questions and spent the time with us that we needed. We had a group of doctors who were all working together for the patients. I always felt that we were known by each doctor, and that they were on top of Paige's treatment.*

When a child arrives at a teaching hospital, he is assigned an attending. These physicians provide continuous care throughout treatment. The physician in charge of your child's care should be "board-certified" or have equivalent medical credentials. This means that he has taken rigorous written and oral tests by a board of examiners in his specialty, and meets a high standard of competence. You can call the American Board of Medical Specialties at (800) 776-2378 to find out if your child's physician is board-certified.

While an inpatient, your child will see a large number of other doctors. Residents usually rotate to different services every four weeks, so they are an ever-changing group. If questions arise about your child's treatment or illness that are unable to be answered by the resident, you should ask the fellow or attending assigned to your child.

If your family is insured by a health maintenance organization (HMO), you probably will be sent to the affiliated hospital, which will have one or more pediatric oncologists on staff.

The nurses

An essential part of the hospital hierarchy is the nursing staff. The following explanations will help you understand which type of nurse is caring for your child.

An LPN is a licensed practical nurse. LPNs complete a vocational training program and have a narrow scope of practice. For example, they usually do not start IVs or give IV medications.

An RN is a registered nurse who obtained an AA degree or a BA degree in nursing, and then passed a licensing examination. These medical professionals give medicines, take vital signs (heart rate, breathing rate, blood pressure), monitor IV machines, change bandages, and care for patients in hospitals, clinics, and doctors' offices.

> At our hospital, each of our nurses is different, but each is wonderful. They simply love the kids. They throw parties, set up dream trips, act as counselor, best friend, stern parent. They hug moms and dads. They cry. I have come to respect them so much because they have such a hard job to do, and they do it so well.

A nurse practitioner or clinical nurse specialist is a registered nurse who has completed an educational program that has taught her advanced skills. For example, in some hospitals and clinics, nurse practitioners perform procedures such as spinal taps.

The head or charge nurse is the supervisor of all the nurses on the floor for one shift. If you have any problems with a nurse, your first step in resolving them would be to talk to the nurse involved. If this does not work, a discussion with the charge nurse is necessary.

The clinical nurse manager is the administrator for an entire unit such as an oncology floor or oncology clinic. She is in charge of all of the nurses on the unit.

Finding an oncologist

Norman Cousins wrote in *Head First: The Biology of Hope,* "Few things are more delicate or important in dealing with serious illness than the psychological environment in which the patient is treated." Yet parents do not have the luxury of time in choosing a pediatric oncologist. At diagnosis, the family is usually referred to the nearest pediatric center of excellence. The young patient may be assigned the fellow or attending who happens to be on call at the time of diagnosis.

During induction and consolidation, your child may see a myriad of doctors. A permanent assignment is usually made for all outpatient treatment. Be sure that you are working with an oncologist who works with the Children's Cancer Group (CCG) or the Pediatric Oncology Group (POG). Your child's chance for a cure may depend on getting the most up-to-date treatments available.

Often the assignment of oncologist is a good match, and the family finds the doctor to be easy to communicate with, competent, and caring. If the medical facility allows you to choose your child's oncologist, here are several traits to look for:

- Board-certified in the field of pediatric oncology
- Establishes good rapport with child
- Communicates clearly and compassionately
- Skillful in performing procedures
- Answers all questions
- Consults with other doctors on complex problems
- Uses language that is easy to understand
- Makes available the results of all tests
- Is willing to let parents participate in the decision-making process
- Respects parent's values
- Able to deliver the truth with hope

If you don't develop a good rapport with the physician assigned to you, ask to be assigned to a different physician whom you have met on rounds or during clinic visits. Most parents are accommodated, for hospitals realize the importance of good communication between family and physician. You will, however, still see different physicians, because many institutions have rotating physicians on call.

Choosing a hospital

At diagnosis, if your family is not initially referred to a specific hospital, or if there are several excellent pediatric hospitals in the area to choose from, it may be necessary to choose where you would like your child to be treated. Parents can obtain a free referral to an accredited center from the National Cancer Institute (800) 4-CANCER), the Children's Cancer Group (800) 458-6223), or the Pediatric Oncology Group (312) 482-9944.

Types of relationships

There are primarily three types of relationships that develop between physicians and parents:

- **Paternal**. In a paternal relationship, the parent is submissive, and the doctor assumes a fatherly role. The problem with this dynamic is that although medical personnel never intend harm, they are human and mistakes occur. If parents are not monitoring drugs and treatments, these mistakes may go unnoticed. In addition, parents are the experts in their own child and his reactions to drugs and treatments.

> *After we left Children's and returned home for outpatient treatment, the local pediatrician's nurse called and said, "Doctor wanted me to tell you that the blood results were normal." I thought that unlikely since she was on high-dose chemotherapy, so I politely asked for the actual numbers for my records. She read them off and my daughter's ANC (absolute neutrophil count—see Appendix B, Blood Counts and What They Mean) had dropped far below 500. I said, "Would you tell the doctor that her counts have dropped dramatically from last week?" She said in a frosty voice, "Doctor said they were fine." So I called Children's, and they told me to keep her at home, take her off all medications for a week, and then have her blood retested. I was glad that I paid attention to the counts.*

A surprising number of parents are intimidated by doctors and express the fear that if they question the doctors their child will suffer. This type of behavior robs the child of an adult advocate who speaks up when something seems wrong.

- **Adversarial**. Some parents adopt an "us against them" attitude that is counterproductive. They seem to feel that the disease and treatment are the fault of medical staff, and they blame staff for any setbacks that occur. This attitude undermines the child's confidence in his doctor, a crucial component for healing.

> I knew one family who just hated the Children's Hospital. They called it the "House of Horrors" or the "torture chamber" in front of their children. Small wonder that their children were terrified.

- **Collegial**. This is a true partnership in which parents and doctors are all on the same footing and they respect each other's domains and expertise. Here the doctor recognizes that the parents are the experts on their own child and are essential in ensuring that the protocol is followed. The parents respect the physician's expertise and feel comfortable discussing various treatment options or concerns that arise. Honest communication is necessary for this partnership to work, but the effort is well worth it. The child has confidence in his doctor, the parents have lessened their stress by creating a supportive relationship with the physician, and the physician feels comfortable that the family will comply with the treatment plan giving the child the best chance for a cure.

> We had a wonderful relationship with the oncologist assigned to us. He blended perfectly the science and the art of medicine. His manner with our daughter was warm, he was extremely well qualified professionally, and he was very easy to talk to. I could bring in articles to discuss with him, and he welcomed the discussion. Although he was busy, he never rushed us. I laughed when I saw that he had written in the chart, "Mother asks innumerable appropriate questions."

· · · · ·

> Justin's oncologist had remarkable interpersonal skills. At our first meeting he said, "Justin has leukemia. There are two kinds of leukemia, and both of them are treatable." So right away he emphasized the positive. He then wrote on his notepad what all of Justin's blood counts were, he told us what normal counts were and explained clearly what we said

that it was safe and he would allow his own daughter to have one. He was very reassuring. It has been years since that day, and he has always been very caring. He still frequently calls us on the phone.

Another mother relates a different experience:

We tried very hard to form a partnership with the medical team but failed. The staff seemed very guarded and distant, almost wary of a parent wanting to participate in the decisions made for the child. I learned to use the medical library and took research reports in to them to get some help for side effects and get some drug dosages reduced. Things improved, but I was never considered a partner in the healthcare team; I was viewed as a problem.

Communication

Clear and frequent communication is the lifeblood of a positive doctor/parent relationship. Doctors need to be able to explain clearly and listen well, and parents need to feel comfortable asking questions and expressing concerns before they grow into grievances. Nurses and doctors cannot read parents' minds, nor can a parent prepare her child for a procedure unless it has been explained well. The following are parent suggestions on how to establish and maintain good communication:

• Tell the staff how much you would like to know.

I told them the first day to treat me like a medical student. I asked them to share all information, current studies, lab results, everything, with me. I told them, in advance, that I hoped they wouldn't be offended by lots of questions, because knowledge was comfort to me.

· · · · ·:

If the doctors at Children's told me to do something, I didn't question it. I did it because I trust them.

• Inform the staff of your child's temperament, likes, and dislikes.

Whenever my daughter was hospitalized, I made a point of kindly reminding doctors and nurses that she was extremely sensitive, and would benefit from quiet voices and soothing explanations of anything that was about to occur, such as taking temperatures, vital signs, or adjustments to her IV.

- Encourage a close relationship between doctor, nurse, and child. Insist that all medical personnel respect the young person's dignity. Do not let anyone talk in front of the child as if she is not there. If a problem persists, you have the right to ask the offending person to leave. Marina Rozen observes in *Advice to Doctors and Other Big People*:

> The best part about the doctor is when he gives me bubble gum. The worst part is when he's in the room with me and my mom and he only talks to my mom. I've told him I don't like that, but he doesn't listen.

- Most children's hospitals assign each patient a "primary" nurse who will oversee all care. Try to form a close relationship with your child's nurse. Nurses usually possess vast knowledge and experience about both medical and practical aspects of cancer treatment. Often, the nurse can rectify misunderstandings between doctor and parents.

> The nurses at Children's were splendid. They were gentle with both kids and parents. Once, when I asked to have Christine's spinal done by the fellow rather than the resident, the fellow said in a nasty voice, "Well, we'll see about that!" and he disappeared. He didn't come in for two hours; my child was crying, we missed an appointment with radiation, and everyone was upset. The nurse ran back and forth between the fellow and us trying to get it resolved. In the end—after the resident had done the spinal—she hugged me, and told me that she was going to talk with the fellow because his actions were unacceptable.

- Older children and teenagers should be included as part of the team. They should be consulted about treatments and procedures and be given age-appropriate choices.

- Cooperate. If your hometown pediatrician will handle all of your child's outpatient treatment, find ways to facilitate communication between oncologist and pediatrician.

> Before we left Children's, I called our pediatrician to ask what paperwork he had received and what he needed. He had received nothing, so he gave me a list of what he needed, which I was able to get from the primary nurse and carry home with me.

> When maintenance started, I asked if there was anything that he thought might help keep his staff aware of the cycles of blood work and chemotherapy orders. He asked me to write a letter at the beginning of

every three-month cycle listing the day of the cycle, the date, and the treatment. They put this in the front of her chart, and it helped keep the orders and communication flowing smoothly.

- Go to all appointments with a written list of questions. This prevents the exhausted parent from forgetting something important and saves the staff from numerous follow-up phone calls.

- Ask for definitions of unfamiliar terms. Repeat back the information to ensure that it was understood correctly. Writing down answers or tape recording conferences are both common practices.

We found that sitting down and talking things over with the nurses helped immensely. They were very familiar with each drug and its side effects. They told us many stories about children who had been through the same thing and were doing well years later. They always seemed to have time to give encouragement, a smile, or a hug.

- Some parents want to read their child's medical chart to obtain more details on their child's condition and to help in formulating questions for the medical team. Often, the doctor or nurse will let the parents read it in the child's hospital room or in the waiting room at the clinic. Most states have laws that allow patient access to all records. You may have to write to the doctor asking to review the chart and pay any photocopy costs.

- If you have questions or concerns, discuss them with the resident. If she is unable to provide a satisfactory answer, ask the child's assigned fellow or attending physician.

- The medical team is comprised of many specialists: doctors, nurses, physical therapists, nutritionists, x-ray technicians, radiation therapists, and more. At training hospitals, many of these persons will be in the early stages of their training. If a procedure is not going well, the parent has the right to tell the person to stop, and to request a more skilled person to do the job.

At our hospital, family practice residents rotate through, and are often assigned to do the spinal taps. My son was on a high-dose metho- trexate protocol, which required a rescue drug to be administered at a cer- tain time. Once, the resident tried for an hour to do the tap, and just couldn't do it. My son was very late getting the rescue drug, and I was

*worried. Later, I requested a conference with the oncologist and asked him
to perform the spinal taps in the future to prevent the residents from practicing on my child. He agreed, but I didn't intervene that first time and I
felt very guilty.*

· · · · ·

*While I truly supported the teaching hospital concept, it was difficult
to deal with a first-year resident who couldn't do a spinal tap or insert an
IV. We had a tendency to lose patience rather quickly when our child was
screaming and the doctor was getting impatient. More than once we
requested a replacement and had someone else do the test.*

• Know your rights. Legally, your child cannot be treated without your
permission. If a procedure is proposed that you do not feel comfortable
with, keep asking questions until you feel fully informed. You have the
legal right to refuse the procedure if you do not think that it is necessary.

*One day in the hospital a group of fellows came in and announced
that they were going to do a lung biopsy on Jesse. I told them that I hadn't
heard anything about it from her attending, and I just didn't think it was
the right thing to do. They said, "We have to do it," and I repeated that I
just didn't think it needed to be done until we talked to the attending.
They seemed angry, but we stood our ground. When the attending came
later, he said that they were not supposed to do a biopsy because the surgeon said it was too risky of an area in the lung to get to.*

However, if the hospital feels that you are wrongfully withholding permission for treatment (i.e., you reject standard treatment in favor of an
unproven remedy, or you are so concerned about side effects that you
are endangering the child's chance for cure) they can take you to court.
The child is the important person in this equation, and both the hospital and the parents have input once you step into the legal arena.

• Don't let problems build up until there is a long laundry list of
grievances.

*We had a problem with the pediatrician's office not calling me with
the results of my daughter's blood work in time for me to call the clinic.
This would result in worry for me and a delay in changes of her chemotherapy doses. I told the pediatrician's nurse that I knew how busy they
were and I hated having to keep calling to get the results. I asked her if it*

was possible for them to give the lab authorization to call me with the results. They thought it was a great idea, and it worked for three years. The lab would fax the doctor the results, but call me. Then I would call the clinic and get the dose changes. The clinic would then fax that information to the pediatrician's office. It was a win/win situation: the doctor's office received no interruptions, they got copies of everything in writing, and I got quick responses from the clinic on how to adjust her meds to her wildly swinging blood counts.

- Use "I" statements. For example, "I feel upset when you won't answer my questions," rather than, "You never listen to me."

- If it helps you feel more comfortable, keep track of your child's treatments to check for mistakes.

   A nurse thought Arielle had a double-lumen catheter and put two incompatible drugs through her single lumen line. It immediately turned to concrete. She had to have the line removed. When they took it out, we saw the drugs had precipitated and formed what looked like little tablets. If this had become dislodged into her bloodstream (a very real possibility) it could have been fatal. Scary!

- Be specific and not confrontational when describing problems. Allow room for the staff to save face. For example, "My daughter has to go to radiation after this spinal tap. I want it to go smoothly, so I would appreciate it if Dr. Smith, the attending, does the procedure instead of the intern," rather than, "I'm not going to let that intern near my daughter again." Another example is, "My son gets very nervous the longer we wait for our appointment. We have waited over two hours for our last two appointments. Could we call ahead next time to see if the doctor is on schedule?" rather than, "Do you think your time is more valuable than mine?"

- If you have something to discuss with the doctor that will take some time, request a conference. These are routinely scheduled between parents and physicians, and should allow enough time for a thorough discussion. Grabbing a busy doctor in the hallway is not fair to her, and may not result in a satisfactory answer for you.

- Do not be afraid to make waves if you are right or to apologize if you are wrong.

When Meagan was in the hospital during induction, the nurse came in with two syringes. I asked what they were, and she said immunizations. I said that it must be a mistake, and the nurse said that the orders were in the chart. So I checked Meagan's chart, and the orders were there, but they had another child's name on them.

- Show appreciation.

I sent thank you notes to three residents after my daughter's first hospitalization. The notes were short but sweet. I wanted them to know how much we appreciated their many kindnesses.

. . . . .

I always try to thank the nurse or doctor when they apologize for being late and give the reason. I don't mind waiting if it is for a good cause, and I feel they show respect when they apologize.

. . . . .

Erica's doctor would sometimes call up just to say, "How's my little chickadee?" He really cared. It touched me that he took the time to call, and I told him that I appreciated it.

. . . . .

Early in my daughter's treatment, we changed pediatricians. The first was aloof and patronizing, and the second was smart, warm, funny, and caring. He was a constant bright spot in our lives through some dark times. So every year during my daughter's treatment, she and her younger sister put on their Santa hats and brought homemade cookies to her pediatrician and nurse. This year was the first time she was able to walk in, and she looked them in the eye and sang, "We Wish You a Merry Christmas." Her nurse went in the back room and cried, and her doctor got misty-eyed. I'll always be thankful for their care.

Norman Cousins in his book *Head First: The Biology of Hope* shares portions of his commencement talks at the medical schools of UCLA, Harvard, George Washington University, and Baylor University:

There are qualities beyond pure medical competence that patients need and look for in doctors. They want reassurance. They want to be looked after and not just looked over. They want to be listened to. They

want to feel that it makes a difference to the physician, a very big differ-
ence, whether they live or die. They want to feel that they are in the doc-
tor's thoughts. The physician holds the lifeline. The physician's words and
not just his prescriptions are attached to that lifeline.

This aspect of medicine has not changed in thousands of years. Not
all the king's horses and all the king's men—not all the tomography and
the thallium scanners and two-D electrocardiograms and medicinal mood
modifiers—can pre-empt the physician's primary role as the keeper of the
keys to the body's own healing system.

I pray that you will never allow your knowledge to get in the way of
your relationship with your patients. I pray that all the technological
marvels at your command will not prevent you from practicing medicine
out of a little black bag. I pray that when you go into a patient's room you
will recognize that the main distance is not from the door to the bed but
from the patient's eyes to your own—and that the shortest distance
between those two points is a horizontal straight line—the kind of straight
line that works best when the physician bends low to the patient's loneli-
ness and fear and pain and the overwhelming sense of mortality that
comes flooding up out of the unknown, and when the physician's hand on
the patient's shoulder or arm is a shelter against the darkness.

I pray that, even as you attach the highest value to your science, you
will never forget that it works best when combined with your art, and,
indeed, that your art is what is most enduring in your profession. For,
ultimately, it is the physician's respect for the human soul that determines
the worth of his science.

Getting a second opinion

Conscientious doctors welcome consultations and encourage second opinions. Because there are many gray areas in medicine where judgment and
experience are as important as knowledge, consultations are frequent. Many
insurance companies require second opinions. If, after discussions with the
doctor, you are still uneasy about any aspect of your child's medical care,
you should not hesitate to seek another opinion.

There are two ways to get a second opinion: see another specialist or ask the
child's physician to arrange a multidisciplinary second opinion. Many par-

ents seek a second opinion at the time of diagnosis. Do not do this in secret. Explain to your child's oncologist that before proceeding you would like a second opinion, and ask for his recommendation. The Childhood Cancer Ombudsman Program (see Appendix C, *Resource Organizations*), with dozens of participating board-certified pediatric oncologists, will review your child's treatment plan and offer second opinions without charge. To allow for a thorough analysis, arrange to have copies of all records sent ahead to the physician(s) who will give the second opinion.

Multidisciplinary second opinions incorporate the views of several different specialists. Parents who would like to get various viewpoints can ask to have their child's case discussed at a tumor board, which usually meets weekly at major medical centers. These boards include medical, surgical, and radiation oncologists, as well as fellows and residents. Your child's oncologist will present the facts of your child's case for discussion. Ask him to tell you what was said at the meeting.

Doctors informally seek second opinions all the time. Residents confer with their fellow for complicated situations; fellows might confer with the attending when unusual drug reactions or responses to treatment occur. Attendings call colleagues at other institutions. Parents should feel free to ask their physician if he has conferred with other staff members to gain additional viewpoints.

> Brent developed a seizure disorder after a rare drug reaction, so he was on anticonvulsants as well as chemotherapy for two years. We worried about the interaction of all the drugs, as well as the advisability of his continuing on the more aggressive arm of the protocol. We asked the fellow to arrange a care conference, and she met with the clinic director as well as Brent's neurologist to discuss how best to manage his case.

Parents often fear seeking a second opinion because they are afraid of offending the doctor or creating antagonism. Conscientious doctors will not resent a parent seeking a second opinion. If she does resist, consider changing doctors. Cancer is life or death, and you won't have a second chance.

Two opinions that agree are all that parents should require before proceeding. Treatment for the leukemia should begin within days of diagnosis. Parents who drag their child from doctor to doctor are denying the gravity of the situation; they hope that someone will give them more favorable news. But the longer they delay treatment, the worse the possible outcome.

Conflict resolution

Conflict is a part of life. In a situation where a child's life is threatened, such as childhood leukemia, the heightened emotions and constant involvement with the medical bureaucracy guarantee conflict. Because clashes are inevitable, resolving them is of paramount importance. A speedy resolution might result if you adopt Henry Ford's motto, "Don't find fault; find a remedy."

Following are some suggestions from parents on how to resolve problems:

• Treat the doctors with respect, and expect respect from them.

> *I always wanted to be treated as an intelligent adult, not someone of lesser status. So I would ask each medical person what they wished to be called. We would either both go by first names or both go by titles. I did not want to be called 'Mom.'*

• Expect a reasonable amount of sensitivity from the staff.

> *Soon after my daughter began treatment, I was walking by the open door of the residents' room which was directly across from the nurses' station. Written in large letters on the blackboard were the words "Have a blast of a day!" with a picture of a smiling leukemia blast drawn below. I felt like I had been punched in the stomach. I was too upset to say anything, but I always regretted not complaining.*

• Treat the staff with sensitivity. Recognize that you are under enormous stress, and so are the doctors and nurses. Do not blame them for the disease or explode in anger. Be an advocate, not an adversary.

• If a problem develops, state the issue clearly, without accusations, and then suggest a solution.

> *I found out late in my daughter's treatment that short-acting, safe sedatives were being used for many children at the clinic to prevent pain and anxiety during treatments. Only parents who knew about it and requested it received this service. I felt that my daughter's life would have been incredibly improved if we had been able to remove the trauma of procedures. I was angry. But I also realized that although I thought that they were wrong not to offer the service, I was partially at fault for not expressing more clearly how much difficulty she had the week before and after a procedure. I called the director of the clinic and carefully*

explained that I thought that poor staff/parent communication was creating hardships for the children. I suggested that the entire staff meet with a panel of parents to try to improve communication and to educate the doctors on the impact of pain on the children's daily life. They were very supportive and scheduled the conference. This is a classic example of how something good can come out of a disagreement, if both parties are receptive to solving the problem.

- Recognize that it is hard to speak up, especially if you have never had to be assertive before. But it is very important to solve the problem before it grows and poisons the relationship.

- Most large medical centers have social workers and psychologists on staff to help families. One of their major duties is to serve as mediators between staff and parents. Ask their advice on problem solving.

- Monitor your own feelings of anger and fear. Be careful not to dump on staff inappropriately. On the other hand, do not let a physician or nurse behave unprofessionally toward you or your child. Parents and staff members all have bad days, but they should not take it out on each other.

- Do not fear reprisal for speaking up. It is possible to be assertive without aggression or argument. In *Having Leukemia Isn't So Bad*, Cynthia Krumme reports that one day her daughter Catherine arrived at the hospital at 11 a.m., but:

  > *It was not until after 9:00 that the much-feared spinal tap was administered. We were totally unprepared for the delays and despite our best efforts to remain calm, we were upset… We expressed our impatience with the delay, but we were hesitant to complain out of concern that if we rocked the boat it would come back to haunt us. This is a common fear among parents.*

- There are times when no resolution is possible, but expressing one's feelings can be a great release.

  > *My son and I waited in an exam room for over an hour for a painful procedure. When I went out to ask the receptionist what had caused the delay, she said that a parent had brought in a child without an appointment. This parent frequently failed to bring in her child for treatment, and consequently, whenever she appeared, the doctors dropped everything*

to take care of the child. When the doctor finally came in, an hour and a half later, my son was in tears. The doctor did not explain the delay or apologize, he just silently started the procedure. After it was finished, I went out of the room, found the doctor, and said, "This makes me so angry. You just left us in here for hours and traumatized my son. Our time is valuable, too." He told me that I should have more compassion for the other mother because her life was very difficult. I replied that he encouraged her to not make appointments by dropping everything whenever she appeared. I added that it wasn't fair to those parents who played by the rules; she was being rewarded for her irresponsibility. After we had each stated our position, we left without resolution.

Changing doctors

Changing doctors is not a step to be taken lightly, but it can be a great relief if the relationship has deteriorated beyond repair. It is a good policy to exhaust all possible remedies prior to separating, or the same problems may arise with the new doctor. Communication, verbally or in writing, and mediation, using social service staff, can sometimes resolve the issues and prevent the disruption of changing doctors.

Although there is a myriad of reasons for changing doctors, some of the most common are:

- Grave medical errors made

- Poor communication skills or refusal to answer questions

- Serious clash of philosophy, for example, a paternalistic doctor and a parent who wishes to be informed and share in the decision-making

It is one of life's great struggles to face cancer. If the family has a physician whom they trust, can rely on for the best medical treatment, feel comfortable with, communicate freely with, and can count on for advice and support, the struggle is greatly eased. If, on the other hand, the doctor adds to your discomfort rather than reducing it, change doctors.

Do not change doctors because you're searching for a better diagnosis. If two reputable physicians, or a tumor board, have agreed on the diagnosis and treatment, it is best for the child to immediately begin treatment.

Many parents choose to continue with a physician in whom they have no confidence due to fear of reprisals. This simply doesn't happen at large centers of excellence. While there may be lingering bitterness or anger between parents and doctors, the child will continue to benefit from the best-known treatment. Children may actually suffer more from the additional family stress caused by a poor doctor/parent relationship than from changing doctors.

> *In a small treatment center like Group Health, there are only two pediatric oncologists. When parents change doctors, the situation becomes very tense because the terminated doctor still cares for their child nights, weekends, and when he is on call. I would not recommend changing doctors if there are only two doctors in the clinic. It's probably better to change treatment centers if possible.*

Once the decision is made, parents must be candid. Either verbally or in writing, an explanation should be given for the change and a formal request made to transfer records to the new physician. Physicians are legally required to transfer all records upon written request.

Minna Nathanson, in a statement presented to the President's Commission for the Study of Ethical Problems in Medicine and Biomedical and Behavioral Research, stated:

> *And, finally, I wish that professional care team members would all accept and allow questioning, so that parents would feel more comfortable being participants in the decisions about their child's treatment and assistants in their child's care, and that there would be an understanding that parents who show symptoms of stress are reacting normally, not pathologically. Every parent I have ever talked to about their child's illness and hospitalization—whether it be for childhood cancer, cystic fibrosis, spinal bifida, or even a one-shot surgery—has confirmed that most parents are experts on their own child, and as extra eyes and ears can help to avoid mistakes in treatment and aid in keeping the child more comfortable and emotionally better prepared for treatment. If there are medical care staff who would say that this is the opposite of what they find, I would ask them to search deeply to see if they are treating parents as intruders in the decision-making and caretaking processes.*

CHAPTER 7

Hospitalization

Every day is a journey,
and the journey itself is home.

—Matsuo Basho

THERE ARE FEW THINGS in life worse than arising from a lumpy, pullout couch to face another day of your child's hospitalization for leukemia. Hospitals are noisy bureaucracies that run on a time schedule all their own. For a child, being hospitalized means being separated from parents, brothers, sisters, friends, pets, and the comfort and familiarity of home. A child's hospitalization can rob both parent and child of a sense of control, leaving them feeling helpless. With a little ingenuity, however, you can make the most of the facilities, liven up the atmosphere, and even have some fun.

The room

Hospital rooms are often painted a nauseating shade of gray or green, and somehow, most windows seem to look out over a power plant. Covering the walls with big, bright posters (Disney characters, sports figures, rock groups) can liven up the room immensely.

> *The first thing we put up in Meagan's room was a huge poster of* The Little Engine That Could *saying, "I think I can, I think I can."*

Display cards on the walls, hanging from strings like a mobile, or taped around the windowsills. Put up pictures of the child engaged in her favorite activity, and add photos of friends, too. Most hospitals don't allow flowers (can cause fungal infections) on oncology floors, but it's fun to have bouquets of balloons bobbing in the corners. Younger children derive great comfort from having a favorite stuffed animal, blanket, or quilt on their bed. If it doesn't bother your child, make the room smell good with potpourri or aromatherapy oils.

To personalize the visit of each member of the medical staff, some parents bring a guestbook to sign. Others put up a visitor sign-in poster, which must be signed before examinations begin or vital signs are taken. Another variation of the sign-in poster is to have each staff member outline her hand and write within the print.

> In my position as a parent consultant, I suggest that a journal (some titles are Book of Hope, Book of Sharing, My Cancer Experience, Friends Indeed) be kept in the child's room for any visitor, family member, or medical caregiver to write in at any time. Leaving a message if the child is sleeping or out of the room for procedures can be a nice surprise. Later, a surviving child and her family, or the family of a child who has died, have a memory book of those who have touched their lives.

Bringing music will help block out some of the hospital noise as well as help everyone relax. A small cassette player, Walkman with earphones, or CD boom box is portable and useful.

> My daughter's preschool teacher sent a care package. She made a felt board with dozens of cutout characters and designs that provided hours of quiet entertainment. She also included games, drawings from each classmate, coloring books, markers, get well cards, and a child's tape player with ear phones. Because we had run out of our house with just the clothes on our backs, all of these toys were very, very welcome.

Although many hospitals provide brightly colored smocks for the patients, most children and teens prefer to wear their own clothing if at all possible. This can pose a laundry problem, so check to see if the floor has washers available for families to use.

As soon as possible after admission, ask for a "floor tour." Find out if a microwave and refrigerator are available, learn what the approved parent sleeping arrangements are, and ask about showers and bathtubs for both patients and parents. Obtain a hospital handbook if one is available. These booklets often include information on billing, parking, discounts, and other helpful items.

Many children's hospitals have VCRs available. Sign up for a convenient time and bring in or rent a favorite or funny video. Humor helps. Bring in age-appropriate games, puzzles, and books.

A friend brought in a bag from the local dime store. He included
a water pistol (good for unwelcome visitors or unfriendly interns), play
dough, slinky, checkers, dominos, bubbles, a book of corny jokes, and
puzzles.

Food

Buying meals day after day in the hospital cafeteria is expensive. In addition, many of the food items available in the cafeteria deserve the notorious reputation of "hospital food." Check to see if the floor has a refrigerator for parents' food and stock it from home. Remember to put your name in a prominent place on your containers.

Many hospitals have cooking facilities for families where they can cook or microwave favorite meals brought from home. Ask family and friends to bring food in when they visit, and consider ordering extra items to come up on your child's tray. Ordering out for dinner can also be a nice change of pace for you and your child. As long as there are no medical restrictions, there's no reason why pizza can't be delivered to the hospital. Ask the nurses if they have menus from local restaurants.

Just the smell of food nauseated my daughter. I'll never forget taking
the tray out in the hall and gobbling the food down myself. I always felt so
guilty, and thought that the staff viewed me as that parent who ate her
kid's food. But it saved money and prevented her meals from going to
waste. I also did not want to leave her side for the few minutes it took to
go to the cafeteria, although in hindsight, the walk would have done me
some good.

Parking

Most parents of children with cancer have unpleasant memories of driving around in endless loops looking for a parking space while their child is throwing up in a bucket in the back seat (or even worse when the bucket was left at home). Learn about both long- and short-term parking arrangements. Ask the nurses and other parents if parking passes are available or where the cheapest parking is located.

I had no idea that the hospital gave out free parking passes to their frequent customers. Now I tell every new parent to check as soon as possible to see if they can get a parking pass. It will save them lots of money that they would have spent on meters and parking tickets, and time they would have spent running out to move the car out of the emergency parking spot.

The endless waiting

Parents need to become experts in learning how to wait without losing their minds. They need to expect long waits for everything from blood draws to procedures. Many parents find themselves getting nervous or angry while waiting for the doctors to appear during "rounds" each morning (when the attendings, residents, and interns move from room to room in a large group), then feel let down when the visit lasts only a few moments. If you have questions to ask the doctors, write them down and tell the doctors when they come in that you would like a few moments to discuss concerns or ask questions.

It helps to come prepared for long waits each time that you go to the hospital. Some progressive (and well-funded) institutions have VCRs and games available, but usually you need to bring your own things. Have your child pick out favorite card games, board games, computer games, drawing materials, and books. Remember to bring food and drinks.

Befriending the staff

Hospitals are staffed by many wonderful and some not-so-wonderful people. Many parents find that their heightened stress makes them less tolerant of inefficiency or confusion. As discussed in Chapter 6, *Forming a Partnership with the Medical Team*, working together, rather than becoming adversaries, will provide your child with a sense of security. Doing things like helping change soiled bedding, taking out food trays, and giving baths frees up overworked nurses to take care of medicines and IVs. Nurses really appreciate the help, and usually reciprocate by answering questions or negotiating with the doctors for you.

As soon as possible, learn about the shift changes on the oncology floor. If you need to leave during the day or night, don't leave a request with one nurse if another will be coming on duty soon. If you have a request or reminder, you can post it on the child's door, on the wall above the bed, or on the chart.

> *I always made a point of introducing myself to my daughter's nurse and resident for each shift. I told them my child's name and which room we were in. I told them that I would be there the whole time and I would help as much as I could. I tried to talk to them about non-hospital matters to give them a break from their routine, as well as get to know them. I thanked them for any kindnesses and told them I appreciated how hard their job was. Although I wasn't angling for favors, I found that they soon came to like me and helped me out whenever any difficulty arose. Although there were a few that I didn't care for, on the whole I found the staff to be warm, caring, dedicated people.*

Being an advocate for your child

Hospitals can be frightening places for children. Parents need to provide comfort, protection, and advocacy for their vulnerable child. To fulfill these roles, parents need to be present.

Most pediatric hospitals are quite aware of how much better children do if a parent is allowed to sleep in the room. Sometimes small couches convert into beds, or parents can use a cot provided by the hospital. If hospital policy requires the parent to leave, insist on staying. Geralyn Gaes tells a story in *You Don't Have to Die* about a confrontation at her local community hospital:

> *One night a nurse came into Jason's room and curtly informed me that I would have to leave, since it was past visiting hours. With my son pale and retching from chemotherapy, I was not about to go anywhere. Looking her in the eye, I said, "You can send security after me if you like, but I'm not leaving here." No one disturbed me again.*

Of course, sometimes it isn't possible to stay with your child if you are a single parent or if both parents work full time. Many families have grandparents or close friends who stay with the hospitalized child when the parents cannot be present. Older children and teenagers may not want a parent in the room at night, but they may need an advocate there during the day just as much as the preschoolers.

Whenever my husband couldn't be at the hospital at bedtime, he would bring in homemade tapes of him reading bedtime stories. Our son would drift off to sleep hearing his daddy's voice.

· · · · ·

We were always there with her in the hospital and one of us was always with her with treatments. However, she did not want us going back with her into the examining room, so we respected those wishes. Her doctor was very kind in always coming out and making comments to us also after he had allowed her to come in privately with him and the chemotherapy nurse. He showed her complete respect as a fifteen-year-old and also took time to meet our needs too. She has always been the one keeping up with her own medical reports, concerns, etc., and although her father and I have always been there with her and for her in the background, she has been much more knowledgeable about the whole cancer experience than we have in her treatments, medications, etc. She loves being in charge of her medical needs.

· · · · ·

Brian was twelve and could have stayed alone, but we never left him more than five minutes to run down the hall for coffee, bathroom, etc. Someone—my husband, me, grandparents, aunts, uncles—was always there. If we had needed them, church members and friends had also volunteered, as Kevin was only two at the time. With my husband rotating days at work and the hospital, and me rotating home and hospital, somehow we managed. The shift usually changed mid-day, so we each got a half day at both. A caring employer is essential.

Also, Brian became very familiar with all his drugs, allergies, reactions, doses. Several times he corrected the staff even before I could. We also had errors and near-errors, as I'm sure everyone does, but many fewer, I'm sure, because of the constant presence and watchful eye. When Kevin was diagnosed, we supervised everything even more. Operating room doctors and nurses accessed his line without first swabbing with alcohol. Someone wanted to give ibuprofen for fever. Non-oncology nurses were working the pediatric oncology floor and knew less than we did. Our hospital is now greatly improved, but things like this happen everywhere.

For some families, it is less stressful for all if they do not hover at the bedside. An oncologist made the following suggestion:

When people are subject to stress, some people cope by focusing on all the details. For these people, being there all the time reduces their stress level. In other words, they would be more stressed if they were at home or work because they would be worrying all the time. Other people cope with stress by blocking out the details and trying to make life normal. I think that you need to think about how your family can best cope with this process and make your decisions based on that. Have a family meeting to sort out these issues, and don't feel bad if you decide what is best for your family is different from what other people say you should do.

Whenever a family member cannot be present, children who are old enough should be taught to use the telephone. Tape a phone number nearby where a parent can be reached and have the child call if anyone tries to do procedures that are unexpected. The hospital staff should be informed that any changes in treatment need to be authorized by a parent.

Having cancer strips children of control over their bodies. To help reverse this process, parents can take over most nursing care. Children may prefer parents to help them to the bathroom or to clean up diarrhea or vomit. Making the bed, keeping the room tidy, changing dressings, and giving back rubs helps your child feel more comfortable and lightens the burden of the overworked nurses. However, some children and teens may feel better if the nurses provide these services. Parents should allow the child to express his needs, even if it feels like rejection.

I was embarrassed to have the nurse change the sheets when I had an accident in the bed. I couldn't help it when I was taking the cytoxan, but I was still embarrassed.

Parents can help their child regain some control by encouraging choices whenever possible. Older children should be actively involved in discussions about their treatment, while younger children can decide when to take a bath, which arm to use for an IV, what to order for meals, what position for procedures, what clothes to wear, and how to decorate the room. Some children request a hug or a handshake after all treatments or procedures.

Playing

Children need to play, especially when hospitalized. Ask whether the hospital has a recreation therapy department. Often, a large room is devoted to toys, books, dolls, and crafts, and is staffed by specialists who really know how to play with children. These rooms provide many therapeutic activities such as medical play with dolls, which help children to express fears or concerns about what is happening to them. By encouraging contact with other children in similar circumstances, recreation therapy helps children feel less alone, less different from other children. The rooms are a cheerful change from lying in a hospital bed and are full of fun-filled activities and smiling staff people. If the child is too ill or her counts are too low to go to the play area, arrangements can be made for a recreational therapist to bring a bundle of toys, games, and books to the room. This can give the parent time to go out to eat or take a walk.

> When I wanted to have a conference with the oncologist about Katy's protocol, I called recreation therapy and they sent two wonderful ladies to the clinic. The doctor and I were able to talk privately for an hour, and Katy had a great time making herself a gold crown and decorating her wheelchair with streamers and jewels.

Exercise is important, too. For kids strong enough to walk, exploring the hospital can be fun. Plan a daily excursion to the gift shop or the cafeteria. Go outside and walk the entire perimeter of the hospital if weather and the neighborhood permit. Don't feel limited by an IV pole; it can be pushed or pulled and will feel normal after a while. Many children have been seen standing on the base of the IV pole with a parent pushing them down the hall at breakneck speed. Check to see if the hospital has a swimming pool (for you to swim in, your child probably can't use it).

> In our hospital photos, I have several of a grinning four-year-old, hooked up to an IV, in a hospital bed, with the head raised waaaaaaayyyy up, as she'd slide down to the bottom. Of course I was doing guard duty at the door, to alert the happy child when a nurse was coming and she needed to "cease this unsafe behavior immediately!" Sometimes you have to make memories while you can, wherever you are.

• • • • •

> At Egleston, there was a large metal tricycle with a huge metal basket on the back. I would heplock Kenny, toss him in the back, then we would pedal all over the hospital. There is one part of the hospital called "the tunnel" which connects the children's hospital with Emory Hospital. It is about a mile-long tunnel—all downhill. Man, we would fly—laughing and screaming. Of course, coming back up was pure hell.

Children or teens with low white counts may feel refreshed by going up on the roof just to feel the wind on their faces and the warm sun on their skin. Some hospitals even grant passes to young patients whose white counts are high enough.

Preston left the hospital several times on passes. His IV was capped off and his arm was taped to a board resembling a cast. He attended a birthday party and went Christmas shopping on a pass.

Any action that parents, family members, and friends take to support and advocate for the youngster with cancer buoys up the spirit. Courage is contagious.

Sometimes you can create your own fun with just a little imagination. On one particular occasion, Matthew was feeling especially bored. With a little ingenuity, we soon discovered that four unused IV poles and as many blankets as we could steal from the linen cart made for one pretty cool tent. We then used the mattress from a roll-away cot, and spent the night "camping" in his hospital room. He had a wonderful time.

CHAPTER 8

Catheters

Do what you can, with what you have,
where you are.

—Theodore Roosevelt

MOST CHILDREN WITH LEUKEMIA require intensive treatment, including chemotherapy, intravenous (IV) fluids, IV antibiotics, blood and platelet transfusions, frequent blood sampling, and sometimes IV nutrition. Indwelling catheters have proved to be a very effective method for allowing entry into the large veins for intensive therapy. They eliminate the difficulty of finding veins for IVs and allow drugs to be put directly into a large vessel of the heart where they are rapidly diluted and spread throughout the body.

Other names for indwelling catheters are: venous access device, right atrial catheter, implanted catheter, central venous catheter, central line, Hickman, Broviac, Port-a-cath, Medi-port, or PICC lines.

The three types of indwelling catheters most commonly used in children are the external catheter, the subcutaneous port, and the peripherally inserted central catheter.

External catheter

The external catheter is a long, flexible tube with one end in the right atrium of the heart and the other end outside the skin of the chest. The tube tunnels under the skin of the chest, enters a large vein (external or internal jugular) near the collarbone, and threads inside the vein leading to the heart (see Figure 8-1). Because chemotherapy drugs, transfusions, and IV fluids are put in the end of the tube hanging outside the body, the child feels no pain. Blood for complete blood counts (CBC) or chemistry tests can also be drawn from the end of the catheter.

The main types of external catheters generally used are the Hickman or Broviac. With meticulous daily care, the external catheter can be left in place for years.

How it's put in

External catheters are usually put in under general anesthesia. Once the child is anesthetized, the surgeon makes two small incisions. One incision is near the collarbone over the spot where the catheter will enter the vein, the other is the area on the chest where the catheter exits the body. To prevent the catheter from slipping out, it is stitched to the skin where it comes out of the chest (see Figure 8-1). There is a Dacron cuff around the catheter right above the exit site (under the skin) into which body tissue grows. This further anchors the catheter and helps prevent infection. After healing is complete, normal activities such as swimming and showers can resume.

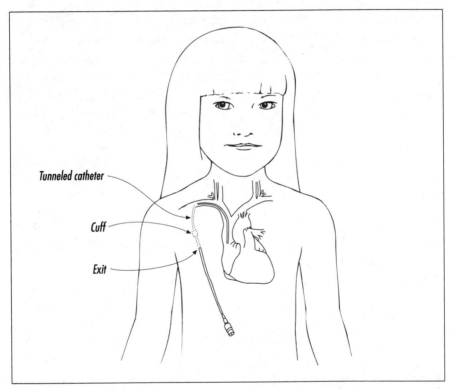

Figure 8-1. External catheter

Daily care

The external catheter requires careful maintenance to prevent infection or the formation of clots. The site where the catheter exits the body must be cleaned frequently and a fresh, sterile dressing needs to be applied and taped in place. The site should be checked for redness, swelling, or drainage. To prevent clots, parents or older patients are taught to flush the line with a heparin solution. Different institutions use different schedules for how often the line should be flushed. Nurses at the hospital instruct parents in catheter care, and plenty of practice should be provided until both parent and child are comfortable with the entire procedure.

> We were very grateful for Matthew's Hickman line. Like a lot of children, he was terribly afraid of needles. The maintenance that was necessary to keep his line working properly became second nature to me. After his diagnosis, and again after his relapse, he had a Hickman implanted. In total, he had his external catheter for more than four years.

Risks

The major complications of using the external catheter are infections—either in the blood or at the insertion site—and the formation of clots in the line or the blood vessel where the catheter is placed. Rare complications are kinking of the catheter or the catheter's becoming dislodged from its proper position.

Infections

Even with the best care, infections are common in children with external lines. Children who are immunosuppressed (have low blood counts) for long periods of time are at risk for developing infections. The need for frequent flushing of the external line also increases the chance for bacteria to enter the catheter. Most infections are caused by a bacterium called staphylococcus epidermidis, although a host of other organisms may also cause infections.

If the child develops a fever over 101°F (38.5°C), redness or swelling at the insertion site, or pain in the catheter area, infection is suspected. To determine if bacteria are present, blood will be drawn from the catheter to culture (grow in a laboratory for 24 to 48 hours). Treatment with antibiotics is usually effective. Treatment will start whenever there is a suspected infection and will end if the culture comes back negative. If the culture is positive, treatment usually continues for ten to fourteen days.

> When my daughter had a line infection, I wanted to use the antibiotic pump at home. It was hard, though. It took two hours per dose, three doses per day, for fourteen days. I would get up at 5 a.m. to hook her up, so that she would sleep through the first dose. The second dose I would

give while she watched a tape in the early afternoon. Then I would hook her up at bedtime so she would sleep through it. I had to wait up to flush and disconnect, so I was very tired by the end of the two weeks.

Some physicians require that the child be hospitalized for antibiotic treatment, while others allow the child to go home. If the infection does not respond to treatment, the catheter may have to be removed.

Clots

Even with excellent daily care, some external lines develop blockages and/or clots. If the catheter becomes blocked, it will be flushed with streptokinase to dissolve the clot. If the line is blocked by a drug precipitate (usually only seen with the drug VM-26), diluted hydrochloric acid may be used to dissolve the blockage.

We had no choice of catheter in 1985, and Judd received the Hickman line from Dr. Hickman himself. We had very little trouble with it until the last six months of the three-year protocol. It was found that Judd had a very large blood clot on the end of the line in his heart, possibly due to being too slow in flushing the line. With only one treatment to go, we had the line removed.

• • • • •

Two months before the end of Kristin's treatment, her line plugged up. We tried several maneuvers at home unsuccessfully. We had to bring her in for the IV team to work on it. I think the bumpy ride to the hospital loosened it because they were able to dislodge the clot just by flushing it with saline.

Kinks and breaks

Rarely, a kink develops in the catheter due to a sharp angle where the catheter enters the neck vein. Some parents and nurses are able to work around this problem by experimenting with different positions for the child when the blood is drawn. Another method is to teach the child a Valsalva maneuver such as bearing down as if to have a bowel movement.

Breaks in the line do happen, but they are very rare. If the break or rupture of the line occurs when it is not in use, only heparin will leak into surrounding tissues. If the break occurs when corrosive chemotherapy drugs are flowing through the catheter, they may leak and cause damage to surrounding tissue. The risk of an internal line leaking is far lower than the chance of leakage from an IV in a vein of the hand or arm.

Other factors to consider

To use an external catheter successfully takes a well-organized and motivated family. The site needs to be cleaned and dressed every other day, and heparin must be injected using sterile technique. Because the dressing must be secured to the skin with a very sticky large tape, if your child is very tape sensitive (cries whenever tape is removed or skin reddens and breaks out), you will need to experiment to find dressings and tape that work for your child.

The external line is a constant reminder of cancer treatment and causes changes in body image. Both parent and child need to be comfortable with the idea of seeing and handling a tube that emerges from the chest. It is noticeable under lightweight clothing and bathing suits. If there is a younger sibling who might pull or yank on the catheter, the Hickman or Broviac might not be the appropriate choice.

On the other hand, the reason external lines are chosen so frequently is that there are no needles and no pain. This is a very important consideration for young children or any person who is frightened of needles, pain, or both. In addition, some protocols require double lumen access and the external catheter is the only appropriate option.

Subcutaneous port

Several different types of subcutaneous (under the skin) ports are used; the Port-a-cath is the most common (see Figure 8-2). The subcutaneous port differs from the external catheter in that it is completely under the skin. A small metal chamber (1" × 1" × 1/2") with a rubber top is implanted under the skin of the chest. A catheter threads from the metal chamber (portal) under the skin to a large vein near the collarbone, then inside the vein to the right atrium of the heart (see Figure 8-3). Whenever the catheter is needed for a blood draw or infusion of drugs or fluid, a needle is inserted by a nurse through the skin and into the rubber top of the portal.

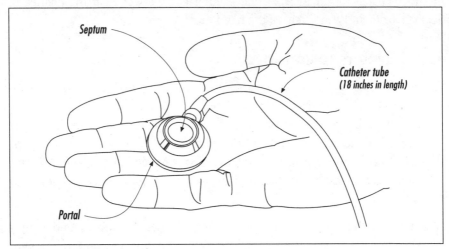

Figure 8-2. Parts of the Port-a-cath

How it's put in

The subcutaneous port is implanted under general anesthesia in the operating room in a procedure that generally takes less than an hour. Sometimes local anesthesia is used for older children or teens. The surgeon makes two small incisions: one in the chest where the portal will be placed, and the other near the collarbone where the catheter will enter a vein (the external or internal jugular) in the lower part of the neck. First, one end of the catheter is placed in the large blood vessel of the neck and threaded into the right atrium of the heart. The other end of the catheter is tunneled under the skin where it is attached to the portal. Fluid is injected into the portal to ensure that the device works properly. The portal is then placed under the skin in the right chest, and stitched to the underlying muscle. Both incisions are then closed. The only evidence that a catheter has been implanted are two small scars and a bump under the skin where the portal rests.

> Before my child's surgery to have a port implanted, I saw other children being wheeled into the operating room screaming and trying to climb off the gurney to return to the parents. It broke my heart. When it was Jennifer's turn, I asked them to give her enough premedication so that she was relaxed and happy to go. I also insisted that I be in the recovery room when she awoke.

· · · · ·

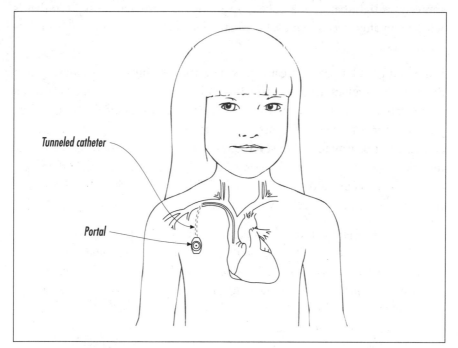

Figure 8-3. Subcutaneous port

Christine had her port surgery late at night. The resident gave her some premedication, then the chief resident ordered him to give her more. She felt so silly that she looked at me, giggled, and said "Mommy has a nose as long as an elephant's." I asked the surgeon if I could be in the recovery room before she awoke, and he said, "Sure." When I told the nurse that I had permission to go in recovery, she refused. When I persisted, she became angry. I told her that my child was expecting to wake up seeing my face, and I intended to be there. I added that she should go in and ask the surgeon to resolve the impasse. When she came out, she let me in the recovery room.

How it works

Because the entire Port-a-cath is under the skin, the device must be accessed in order to use it. To access the catheter, the skin is thoroughly cleansed with antiseptic, then a special needle is inserted through the skin and the rubber top of the portal. The needle is attached to a short length of tubing which hangs down the front of the chest. EMLA cream can be applied one hour prior to the needle poke to anesthetize the skin or ethyl chloride can be sprayed on right before the poke. Subcutaneous ports have a septum that is self-sealing after needle removal, and are designed to withstand years of needle insertions.

If the child is in a part of treatment where the line must be used every day, the nurse will attach the tubing to IV fluids or will close the end off with a sterile cap after flushing with saline solution. A transparent dressing will be put over the site where the needle enters the port. The port can remain accessed in this way for up to seven days. After that time, to avoid the risk of infection, the needle should be removed and the port reaccessed when necessary. If the needle and tubing are to be left in place, it is important to tape them securely to the chest to avoid accidents.

> At the end of delayed intensification while getting cytoxan, Meagan (three years old) got a line infection. Because she hated tape removal, we did not secure the IV tubing to her stomach or chest. On one of her many trips to the potty, we accidentally tugged on the tubing and caused a very small tear in the skin around the needle. It became infected. We did home antibiotics on the pump and felt very fortunate that we were able to clear the line with antibiotics. We were glad our doctor was not too quick to remove the line, but it did require two weeks off chemotherapy.

If the port is only needed infrequently, e.g., during the maintenance phase, this will be the sequence of events: the site will be cleaned, needle put in, line rinsed with saline, drug given or blood drawn, line rinsed with saline, heparin added to line, needle withdrawn, and a Band-Aid placed over the site.Care of the subcutaneous port

The entire port and catheter are under the skin and therefore require no daily care. The skin over the port can be washed just like the rest of the body. Frequent visual inspections are needed to check for swelling, redness, or drainage.

The subcutaneous port must be accessed and flushed with saline and heparin at least once every thirty days, which usually coincides with the monthly clinic visit and blood checks. This procedure is done by a nurse or technician. The port system requires no maintenance by the parent or patient.

Risks

The risks for a subcutaneous port are similar to those for the external catheter: infection, clots, and rarely kinks or rupture. If the needle is not properly inserted through the rubber septum, fluids can leak into the tissue around the portal.

> Brent (eight years old) has had a Port-a-cath for thirty-three months with absolutely no problems. He uses EMLA to anesthetize it prior to accessing. He hates finger pokes so much that he has his port accessed every time he needs blood drawn.

· · · · ·

> We had a few unusual problems in the beginning with the catheter. It was a bit kinked where the catheter went under the clavicle (collarbone) and would not easily draw. This caused more stress than anything in the hospital because their middle-of-the-night blood draws were always an ordeal. They needed to wake her up and try multiple manipulations. Once we were familiar with its idiosyncrasies and were outpatient, we worked it out much better. Then about halfway through maintenance, her catheter broke at the kink and traveled into her heart. To make a long story short, it was retrieved by a cardiologist without major surgery, and she got a new one placed, this time with the catheter going down from her neck. It works like a dream.

Infection

Most studies show that the infection rate of subcutaneous ports is lower than that of external catheters. If the subcutaneous port does become infected, it is treated exactly the same as those in external catheters.

> Katy had two infections in her Port-a-cath during the twenty-seven months of her leukemia treatment. One occurred during reinduction when the tape loosened during a blood transfusion. She developed a fever the next day and required fourteen days of vancomycin. Eighteen months later, we went in for her monthly vincristine, and she became ill in the car on the way home. Her skin became white and clammy, and she felt faint and nauseated. She spiked a 102° temperature which only lasted for two hours. The blood culture both times grew staphylococcus epi.

Kinks, clots, ruptures

These events rarely occur with the subcutaneous port. If they do occur, they are treated as described in the external catheter section.

Peripherally inserted central catheters

A peripherally inserted central catheter is also referred to as a PICC line. This type of catheter is placed in the antecubital vein (a large vein in the inner elbow area) and threaded into a large vein above the right atrium of the heart (see Figure 8-4). Unlike other catheters, a PICC line can be inserted by an IV nurse, rather than a surgeon.

The PICC line can remain in place for many weeks or months, avoiding the need for a new IV every few days. PICC lines can be used to deliver chemotherapy, antibiotics, blood products, other medications, and intravenous nutrition. When the PICC line needs to be accessed, an intravenous (IV) line is connected to the end of the catheter. When it is not in use, the IV is disconnected and the catheter is flushed and capped.

How it's put in

The peripherally inserted central catheter can be inserted in your child's hospital room by a nurse or physician. Your child will be positioned on a flat surface, and she will need to keep her arm straight and motionless during the procedure. An injection to numb the area is given to decrease discomfort during insertion. A special needle is used to place the PICC line into the arm vein. The catheter is then threaded through the needle. Once the line is in place, a chest x-ray is taken to ensure that it is positioned properly.

> Brian had his Hickman pulled when he started maintenance in February 1997, but two weeks later he developed pancreatitis and needed total parenteral nutrition. Since he was still on active treatment, he was given the choice of another Hickman or a PICC, which he decided to try. It was inserted right in our room with no anesthetic other than the morphine pump he was already on for the pancreatitis pain. He pushed his PCA button moments before it was inserted, because he was not sure what to expect. The procedure was uncomfortable, but not terribly painful. They did an x-ray to make sure that it was in the right place. It wasn't, but after some aerobics (moving him into different positions) and lots of flushing, they checked again, and it was.

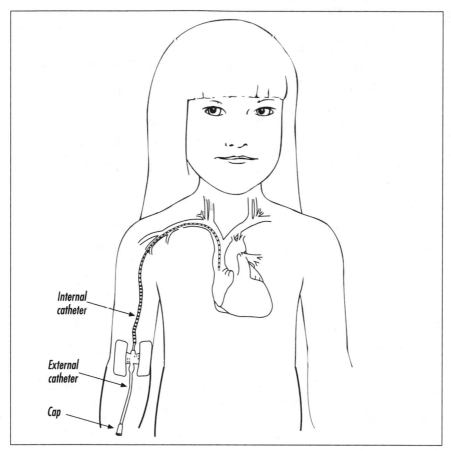

Internal
catheter

External
catheter

Cap

Figure 8-4. PICC line

Care of the peripherally inserted central catheter

The PICC line, like the Hickman catheter, requires meticulous care to prevent problems. You will be taught by the nurses to change the dressing, flush the line, change the injection cap, and inspect the site for possible signs of infection. The dressing covering the exit site is changed on a weekly basis, and changed if it becomes wet or is exposed to the air. The line must be flushed after every use, or every day. You should get plenty of practice under the supervision of a nurse until both you and your child are comfortable with caring for the line. The care required for your child's PICC line may be slightly different from what has been described in this section since institutional preferences vary.

Kelsey had a PICC line in her right arm, and she would not straighten it out, but kept it a little bent. I definitely think she was protecting it, and also I think when she tried to straighten it, it pulled on the suture and on the dressing in an uncomfortable way that could have been painful, so she just wouldn't try. I had to do a heparin flush every day and change the dressing twice a week. She could not tolerate Tegaderm, so we used another kind of porous adhesive bandage, and doused it with Detachol, which dissolved the adhesive within a few minutes, allowing us to get the bandage off quite easily. The Detachol was a godsend for her, as removing the adhesive was like pulling teeth and a source of unnecessary pain.

Risks

The problems associated with a PICC line are similar to those of any external catheter. Veins may become irritated, infection can occur, or the line can be accidentally torn or moved.

Irritated veins

The vein where the catheter is located may become irritated. This is most likely to occur during the first few days after it has been inserted. Signs of irritation include swelling or pain in the area, or the development of small veins near the site. Often, a warm moist cloth placed on the vein will help alleviate discomfort. Raising the arm is also sometimes helpful.

Infection

Meticulous care using sterile techniques is very important to reduce the risk of infection. The dressing exit site should be changed every week, or if it becomes wet or exposed to the air. Injection caps must also be regularly changed using sterile techniques when the line is not in use, and the line must be flushed on a regular basis. Signs of infection include redness, swelling, pain, drainage, or warmth around the exit site. Fever, chills, tiredness, and dizziness may also indicate that the line has become infected. You should notify the doctor if any of these signs are present or if your child has a fever above 101°F (38.5°C).

Torn catheter

Accidents sometimes happen, and it is possible that a hole or tear in the line can occur. The only prevention for this is ensuring that care is taken when handling the catheter. A torn catheter is suspected when fluid leaks out of the line, especially during an injection. If a tear is found, you should find the hole, fold the line above the tear, tape it together and cover it with sterile gauze. You should immediately notify your child's doctor of the problem.

Displacement of the catheter

Like the external catheters discussed earlier in this chapter, it is important that the PICC line is securely taped to the exit site to prevent movement. Signs of a displaced catheter include chest pain, burning or swelling in the arm above the exit site or in the chest, fluid leaking around the catheter, or pain when fluid is injected into the line. If you suspect that the line has moved, you should tape the catheter in place and immediately notify your child's doctor.

Choosing not to use a catheter

Many physicians automatically schedule surgery for catheter implantation as soon as a child is diagnosed with leukemia. Others do not recommend using implanted catheters in their pediatric patients with leukemia, while some physicians only use catheters in high-risk patients. Ask the physician the reason for his recommendation, and request a second opinion if you are uncomfortable with the options presented (see Chapter 6, *Forming a Partnership with the Medical Team*, for methods to obtain second opinions).

> Stephan (six years old) has no catheter. Sometimes I wish he had one. It seems like it would be easier. We were told he didn't need it. He is running out of usable veins and it is getting harder and harder.

Some children and teens prefer IVs to an implanted catheter.

> My son had a port for a very short time, and due to frequent fevers (with no evidence of infection) and because he had a blood clot form in his heart which was probably a result of the port line rubbing against the inferior vena cava, they pulled the port. He had IVs for the remainder of treatment and was much happier with the IVs than with what he called "that foreign object in my chest."

Some physicians recommend trying treatment without a catheter before making a decision.

Our physician gave us the option of using a catheter for our six-year-old daughter with low-risk ALL, but he recommended against it. He said if she could stand the pokes it was better not to use it due to the chance of infections. She had several sessions with the staff psychologist to teach her visualization and imagery which she used successfully to deal with the two years of IVs.

To help you make the best decision for your particular situation, Table 8-1, outlines the pros and cons for each catheter. There is no right or wrong choice; different options are available because each child, each parent, each family, is unique.

Table 8-1. Comparison of Catheters

Things to Consider	External Catheter	Subcutaneous Port	Peripherally Inserted Central Catheter
Infection rate	Higher	Lower	Higher
Maintenance	Daily	Monthly	Daily
Body image	Changes: tube outside body	Minor: lump under skin	Changes: tube outside body
Pain	Dressing changes	Needle poke to access (use EMLA)	Needle poke to insert the line; dressing changes
Anxiety	Low to high	Low to high	Low to high
Cost	More due to daily maintenance	Less; monthly maintenance	More due to daily maintenance
Risk of drugs leaking into tissues	Lowest	Low	Low

The decision: Which catheter for your child?

After reviewing the information presented and the comparison chart, discuss with the doctor his opinion about the merits of each catheter. Talk over the pros and cons with your child if she is old enough. Then make the rounds of the cancer ward, asking both parents and children which type of catheter they chose and why. You will probably hear many strong opinions on the benefits and drawbacks for each catheter.

When we asked one of the young children on the ward which catheter she had, she pulled up her shirt with a big grin to show us her Hickman.

She had a coil of white tubing neatly taped to her chest. My husband's face turned as white as her tubing.

· · · · ·

My four-year-old daughter loved ballet and was extremely interested in her appearance. Her younger sister was very physical, and we were worried that if we chose the Hickman she would grab and pull on the tubing. We chose the Port-a-cath so that she could wear her tutus without reminders of cancer and so that the children could play together without mishap.

· · · · ·

We chose the Hickman for Shawn because we didn't want any needles coming at him. He spent almost the whole first year in the hospital, so it saved him from so many pokes. The line was a blessing. He went three years and three months with no infections. We thought it was just a beautiful thing.

The nurses in the clinic and on the ward are another source of valuable information. They will have seen dozens (or hundreds) of children with catheters, and will be able to give excellent advice, given your family situation. There is no right or wrong choice, just different options for each unique child.

Adhesives

Whether your child has a subcutaneous catheter, external catheter, or PICC line, dressing changes will be necessary. Some children don't mind a bit having the Tegaderm or tape pulled off. For others it is traumatic every time. Parents have many suggestions for ways to make it easier for kids. These suggestions also work for removing tape when using plastic dressings over EMLA:

- Don't use Tegaderm if it bothers your child or reddens the skin. Try plastic wrap cut into a square and use paper tape or tape with perforations in it. Then when it's tape removal time, get some Detachol (an adhesive dissolver) and douse the paper tape with it. The tape will pull off easily with no pain.

- Use Hypafix instead of Tegaderm. It's a dressing retention material that looks like gauze with a sticky side. Usually, several sterile 2 × 2 gauze pads are put over the needle entry site, then Hypafix is applied to hold them in place.

I like Hypafix because when it's time to take it off, you can use the adhesive dissolver where it's stuck to the skin, and even without the dissolver, it comes off easier and gentler than the Tegaderm. The nurses at our oncology clinic use this all the time. Our local clinic and hospital do not use Hypafix, so I bought a roll and take it with me whenever we have to go locally for a port access so we don't have to use the Tegaderm.

• Ask for expert advice.

Apryl has had skin tears and reactions from the adhesives as a result of using Tegaderm. We were using Primapore dressings for a while, but after a year she started with the same reaction. When she had her line replaced, I asked for a consultation with the skincare nurse. She recommended All-Dress. It is a waterproof dressing with non-stick gauze in the center surrounded by Hypafix tape. They are waterproof. Apryl changes hers once every three days, whether it gets wet or not. She also has this pink tape that has zinc oxide in the adhesive to protect the skin. These two have worked out great.

• Negotiate with the nurses to do all tape or Tegaderm removal yourself. Then do it in whatever way is easiest for your child.

Using adhesive dissolver (or peeling off tape or Tegaderm millimeter by millimeter) takes a bit of time—it's not just a swipe and it works. It has to sort of soak in and takes some time to dissolve the sticky stuff. I know the nurses are really busy and under pressure to keep on time lines so it's probably a conflict for them. I deal with this by always being the one to get the Tegaderm off—took some "muscling in" with nurses who were used to doing it, but it works much much better. I try to make a joke of it—"I have a deal with my kid that I'm taking off the Tegaderm. It might take a while and I wouldn't want you to fall asleep waiting on us— how about if I holler out the door when it's off and we're ready?" That way they don't have to stand around and wait, and you don't feel like you need to hurry your child.

Removal of indwelling catheters is explained in Chapter 18, *End of Treatment and Beyond.*

When Scott (age three) was diagnosed, his doctor gave us a choice of which central line we could use. He showed us a mannequin with a Broviac and a Port-a-cath. He also told us the pros and cons of each type, then asked us to decide. We chose the Broviac, and feel it was the best decision for Scott. The day it was installed was the end of a lot of unnecessary pain (from needle sticks) for Scott.

Scott finished all his treatments three months ago, and yesterday he had his Broviac removed. It went extremely smoothly. He had only one cuff and it was halfway out already. And to think, I fretted and worried about the removal all week!

He has lots and lots of energy. His hair is coming back in and he actually has color in his face. He looks so healthy! I love it!

CHAPTER 9

Sources of Support

*The effort to "put up a front" is draining,
isolating, and counterproductive. Support
groups can be a powerful way of letting down
these fronts a bit at a time among people who
understand and feel the same conflicting
pressure—to act as though everything
is all right when it is not.*

—David Spiegel, MD
Living Beyond Limits

THE DIAGNOSIS OF CANCER CAN BE a frightening and isolating experience. Every parent of a child with cancer has a story to tell of lost or strained friendships. Yet we are social creatures, reliant on a web of support from family, friends, neighbors, and church. We need the presence of people who not only care for us, but who try hard to understand what we are feeling. Many parents experience deep loneliness after the first rush of visits, cards, and phone calls end, when the rest of the world goes back to normal life.

Members of families struck by childhood cancer—parents, child with cancer, and siblings—are turning increasingly to support groups and various other forms of psychological help. Families join support groups to dispel isolation, share suggestions for dealing with the illness and its side effects, and talk to others who are living through the same crisis. Individual and family counseling can help address shifting responsibilities within the family, explore methods to improve communication, and help find ways to channel strong feelings constructively.

The various methods of support described in this chapter can help return to families a sense of control over their lives as well as provide a setting for making wonderful new friends.

Hospital social workers

While the need for skilled pediatric social workers is widely recognized, shrinking hospital budgets often prevent adequate staffing. If you bring your child to a children's hospital well-staffed with social workers, child life specialists, and psychologists, consider yourself lucky. Sadly, millions of dollars are spent on technology, while programs that help people cope emotionally are often the first to be discarded. If your pediatric center offers no emotional support, explore the other methods described later in the chapter to get help in dealing with the pain of childhood cancer.

Pediatric social workers usually have a master's degree in social work, with additional training in oncology and pediatrics. They serve as guides through unfamiliar territory by mediating between staff and families, helping with emotional or financial problems, locating resources, and easing the young patient back into school. Many social workers form close, long-lasting bonds with families, and continue to answer questions and provide support long after treatment ends.

> On the day of Carl's diagnosis, we were introduced to a team whom we worked with for the next several years. The team included a primary nurse, a primary oncologist, a first-year resident, second-year resident, third-year resident, and our social worker. I remember that first day her telling us that she was there to help us with anything we needed such as hospital problems, billing, insurance, emotional issues, or behavior issues. She said her job was to be there for us, and she was, whenever we needed her.

· · · · ·

> We went to a children's hospital which was renowned in the pediatric cancer field. The medical treatment was excellent, but psychosocial support was nonexistent. The day after diagnosis, we were interviewed for twenty minutes by a psychiatric resident, and that was it. I never met a social worker, and the physicians were so busy, they never asked anything other than medical questions. If I started crying, they usually left the room. I didn't know Candlelighters existed; I didn't know that there was a local support group; I didn't know that there was a summer camp for the kids. I felt totally isolated.

In addition to social workers, some hospitals have on-staff child life specialists, psychiatric nurses, psychiatrists, psychiatric residents, and psychologists who can help deal with problems while your child is an inpatient.

After Meagan's first bone marrow aspiration, which did not go well and was very painful for her, she stopped talking and she wouldn't even look at us. We couldn't comfort her in any of the normal ways; she didn't want to be held, read to, talked to, sung to. At the time this was more devastating than the leukemia. Anytime somebody would come to the door, she would start shaking. Days into this, we asked, "Isn't there anybody here who helps kids who are feeling his way?" So they sent up a psychiatric nurse, who came once and really worked wonders. However, she never came back, so we made arrangements to see her occasionally on an out-patient basis. When we started getting Meagan anesthesia for her procedures, the withdrawal stopped, and she's a healthy and happy first-grader now.

· · · · ·

After I relapsed, I had a hard time with nausea, so I went to learn self-hypnosis. The doctor who taught the hypnosis also counseled me, and that was very helpful. He was somebody I could relate to and talk to about what was going on. Talking about how I felt about having cancer, and how that affected my life, was very helpful to me.

· · · · ·

We got the most support from our nurse Neva, who accessed Brent's port and gave him his chemotherapy every three weeks. She was always cheerful, concerned, and supportive, not only with Brent, but with the whole family. She listened to us and made valuable suggestions. When she changed job locations, we asked our pediatrician to make arrangements so that we could continue to go to her. He did. Neva was so wonderful that Brent looked forward to his chemotherapy days, just because he would see her. He's been off treatment for over a year, but we still drop by to visit, and he runs up to her, jumps into her arms, and they have a good, long hug.

Support groups for parents

Support groups offer a special perspective for all parents of children with cancer, as well as fill the void left by the withdrawal or misunderstanding of family and friends. Parents in similar circumstances can share practical information learned through personal experience, provide emotional support, give hope for the future, and truly listen. The Seattle Candlelighters sum up their beliefs in the following statement.

> We believe children with cancer are normal children with special needs. We believe a unique bond exists among families who are experiencing childhood cancer that allows for friendship and support through treatment, the uncertainties of daily life, the grief, and the triumphs. We believe in enjoying every day to its fullest and in providing a loving environment to all families facing childhood cancer.

Coping with life-threatening illness requires perspective—the ability to accept the gravity of the situation while not blowing it out of proportion. In support groups, many families find this frame of reference, for there are always those with more severe problems than yours as well as families whose children have completed treatment and are thriving. Just meeting people who have lived through the same situation is profoundly reassuring.

> We hadn't lived here very long when Meagan was diagnosed so we didn't have many friends. So I found that most of my support came from the group. It was really helpful to meet other people who were facing the same problems.

· · · · ·

> The group was a real lifeline for us, especially when Justin was so sick. We looked forward to the meetings and were there for every one. It was a real escape; it was a place to go where people were rooting for us. People from the group would always swing by to see us whenever they were bringing their own kids in for treatment. They always stopped by to visit and chat. We amassed a tremendous library of children's books that the group members would drop off. The support was wonderful.

· · · · ·

> I felt like I was always putting up a front for my family and friends. I acted like I was strong and in control. This act was draining and counterproductive. With the other parents, though, I really felt free to laugh as well as cry. I felt like I could tell them how bad things were without causing them any pain. I just couldn't do that with my family. If I told them what was really going on, they just looked stricken, because they didn't know what to do. But the other parents did.

• • • • •

In the beginning, I was the only father who regularly attended the group. (After three years, I'm happy to report that more fathers now attend.) It made me feel bad that the other fathers didn't come to group. I sometimes wonder how deep their love is for their child if they are not willing to come and learn. I think there are elements of both male pride and fear about sharing feelings that result in their lack of participation. They must think that because they can't protect their child from the cancer, there's nothing they can do. But there is.

• • • • •

Our Tuesday gatherings were an anchor for us. It was a time to meet with parents who truly understood what living with cancer meant. These parents had been in the trenches. They knew the midnight terrors, the frustrations of dealing with the medical establishment; after all, it was an alien world to most of us. They knew about chemo, hair loss, friend loss, and they knew the bittersweet side of cherishing a child more than one thought one could cherish anymore. We gathered to cry, to laugh, to whine, to comfort one another, to share shelter from a frightening world. It was a haven.

Cancer can be a very isolating experience. The issues of all the other moms on the street are light years away from the mother of a kid with cancer. But the moms in the kitchen at a Ronald McDonald house can just look at a child on prednisone wolfing down a complete second dinner, and tell the new mom how fast the appetite goes when the prednisone is tapered. They understand each other's feelings and emotions because they are sharing the same experience. The understanding of a mother or father of a child with leukemia cuts across all social, economic, and racial barriers.

My two-year-old daughter was diagnosed one week after I gave birth to a new baby girl. I remember early in her treatment, I was sitting with Gina on my lap, and my husband sat next to me, holding the new baby. The doctor breezed in and said in a cheerful voice, "How are you feeling?" I burst into sobs and could not stop. He said just a minute and dashed out. A few minutes later a woman came in with her eight-year-old daughter who had finished treatment and looked great. She put her arms around me and talked to me. She told me that everyone feels horrible in the beginning, and it might be hard to believe, but treatment would soon become a way of life for us. She was a great comfort, and of course, she was right.

In addition to Candlelighters—the international support organization—there are dozens of different types of support groups ranging from those with hundreds of members and formal bylaws to three moms who meet for coffee once a week. Some groups deal only with the emotional aspects of the disease, while others may focus on education, advocacy, social opportunities, or crisis intervention. Some groups are facilitated by trained mental health practitioners, while others are self-help groups of parents only. And, naturally, as older members drop out and new families join, the needs and interests of the group may shift.

We have found that it is hard to keep people coming to monthly meetings, even though we have a large membership. We have a fifteen-member board, which meets every month and plans parties and informational meetings with speakers. We have parties for Christmas, Easter, and Halloween, as well as trips to amusement parks and picnics. Our motto is, "If there's food, families will come." We are also lucky to have a full-time staff person who takes care of information, advertising our services, correspondence, and connecting parents with similar needs.

· · · · ·

Our group is very informal. We do have two social workers who are considered the facilitators and are there as resource persons. We just talk about whatever anyone wants to discuss. Occasionally we have invited speakers in. I remember having a psychiatrist discuss stress management, and we also had a talk on therapeutic massage. We have formed close friendships from the group, and we still go twice a month even though our daughter is a year off treatment and doing great. I think our presence comforts the new families.

· · · · ·

I live in a rural area, over 100 miles from the group affiliated with the children's hospital. I started a parents' support group in my area for children with any life-threatening illness, and we had a good response initially, but it gradually fizzled out because our issues were just too varied. But I did meet through that group a mother whose son had leukemia, and we have become fast friends. We have a support group of two. We talk on the phone several times a week, and try to go out to dinner or the movies occasionally, just to get a break. The local hospital gives out my name as the parent contact for newly diagnosed children, and I inform them of the local and national resources, and try to visit and answer questions.

One way to thank all of the people who have supported you during your cancer journey is to have a party to celebrate milestones in treatment.

> We had a great time today celebrating the one-year anniversary of Taylor being in remission. We invited all of our friends and family to the park for "Tay's beating leukemia party." We had red and white balloons that we wrote on that said "Healthy red cells" and "Healthy white cells." We also had a round piñata that said "Leukemia" on it and one of the international symbols for "NO" drawn through it. The kids "beat" leukemia with a stick and candy came pouring. We all had a good time. We also had black balloons that were "bad cells" that the kids sat on and popped. It was a well-attended party. We grilled outside, drank sodas, ate watermelon, played a little volleyball, and just had a great time.

Parents from small, isolated communities may have a difficult time finding a support group in their area that fits their needs. For those families, finding emotional support is possible by computer. Several online discussion groups exist for families dealing with childhood cancer. These groups provide parents with the understanding that only another parent of a child with cancer can give. Topics might include various coping skills that have been effective for other families or concern helpful medical information that you can use in your fight against childhood cancer. Participants in online discussion groups, just like those in face-to-face groups, may provide incorrect or upsetting information. Take any concerns or questions you have to your physician or nurse practitioner.

> The support that I have gained through online discussion groups is priceless. I have received a great deal of comfort from my participation in these groups. They have enabled me to connect with families from all over the world, many of which are fighting the exact same disease. I have often come to my computer in the middle of the night, when everyone else in the house is asleep. I can express my fears at 3:00 a.m., and know that someone will always be there to hold my hand and reassure me with the knowledge that they have felt these things, too. That's one of the most beautiful things about these groups. Someone is always there, even in the middle of the night.

· · · · ·

> Going online enabled me to find answers to many questions. I spent countless hours searching out hopeful stories about other kids who had been through what Leeann was dealing with, and walked away with more

optimism. It didn't take me long to realize that I had to be choosy about what information I took to heart and what I should disregard. I found another mother who had posted to one of the groups with a daughter in the same circumstances as Leeann, and we began to write each other about their treatments, day-to-day lives, etc. We became very good friends and still write on a daily basis four years later. She's always picked me up when I've gone into a panic, and her sense of humor and experience grounds me. We've never met in person even though we only live two states apart, but getting input from her means the world to me.

Appendix D, *Books and Online Sites*, contains further information on Internet support groups.

Support groups for children with cancer

Many pediatric hospitals have ongoing support groups for children with cancer. Often these are run by experienced pediatric social workers, who know how to balance fun with sharing feelings. For many children, these groups are the only place where they feel completely accepted, where most of the other kids are bald and have to take lots of medicine. The group is a place where children or adolescents can say how they really feel, without worrying that they are causing their parents more pain. Many children form wonderful and lasting friendships in peer groups.

> *I went to Junior Candlelighters, which was very helpful. The gal who facilitated the group was a survivor of osteosarcoma and had had her leg amputated. Yet, she skied, she drove, she did everything. I always thought, "If Patty can do it, I can, too. If she can live so well without a leg, I should be able to put up with having a cancer in my blood."*

· · · · ·

> *All four of my kids have been going to the support groups for over seven years now. We have one group for the kids with cancer, which is run by a social worker. The siblings group is run by a woman who specializes in early childhood development. Both groups do a lot of art therapy, relaxation therapy, playing, and talking. They meet twice a month, and I will continue to take them until they ask to stop. I think it has really helped all of them. We also have two teen nights out a year. All of the*

teenagers with cancer get together for an activity such as watching a hockey game or basketball game, or going bowling, to the movies, or out for pizza. They also see each other at our local camp for children surviving cancer (Camp Watcha-Wanna-Do) each year.

· · · · ·

Kristin goes to the kids' support group while my wife and I attend the parents' group downstairs. She doesn't talk much about what goes on, but the facilitator keeps the parents apprised of how things are going. One very vocal nine-year-old boy has recently broken the ice with the kids. He really likes to talk about his feelings about having leukemia, and it has prompted the other children to begin to share their thoughts and reactions about the things that have happened to them. They also have lots of fun.

For children who are too ill or shy to join a group, there are alternatives. There are hundreds of kids who use computers to contact and chat with other kids in similar situations. Use Appendix D, to access some of the available computer groups.

Support groups for siblings

Many hospitals have responded to the growing awareness of siblings' natural concerns and worries by creating hospital visiting days for them. This allows not only one-on-one parent time for the siblings, but gives them the opportunity to explore and become familiar with the hospital environment. Sibling days allow interaction with staff, a time to have questions answered and concerns addressed. Some hospital staffs have expanded these one-day programs into ongoing support groups aimed not just at siblings who are having problems, but also at improving communication, education, and support for all siblings.

Both of Shawn's brothers went to the sibling group for years. It seemed to really help them. I don't really know what they did in that room upstairs, but they always came down happy.

· · · · ·

Annie went to Club Goodtimes long after her brother stopped going and attended camp as many years as they would allow. She intends to be on the staff at camp next summer.

Parent-to-parent programs

Some pediatric hospitals, in conjunction with parent support groups such as Candlelighters, have developed parent-to-parent visitation programs. The purpose of these visits is for veteran parents to provide one-on-one support for newly diagnosed families. The services provided by the veteran parent can be informational, emotional, or logistical. The visiting parent can also:

- Empathize with the newly diagnosed parents
- Help notify family and friends
- Help overcome loneliness
- Ease feelings of isolation
- Provide hospital tours
- Write down parents' questions for the medical team
- Advise on sources of financial aid
- Explain unfamiliar medical terms
- Be available by phone for any problems that arise
- Supply lots of smiles and hugs, but most of all, hope

Newly diagnosed families can ask if the hospital has a parent-to-parent program. If not, ask to speak to the parent leader of the local support group. Often, this person will ask a veteran parent to visit you at the hospital. Many, many veteran parents are more than willing to visit, as they know only too well what those first weeks in the hospital are like. They are often accompanied by their child who has completed therapy, rosy-cheeked and full of energy, a living beacon of hope.

> I am the parent consultant for our region. Among the services I provide are: meet with all newly diagnosed families; give a packet of information to each child or teen with cancer; continue to visit the families whenever they return to the hospital; educate families about the various local resources; provide moral support; stay with children during painful procedures if the parents can't; organize and present all of the school programs; liaison with schools for school reentry; organize and send out monthly reminders for Candlelighters meetings, child support group meetings, and sibling group meetings; send out birthday cards to kids on treatment; serve as activities director at the summer camp; and generally try to help out each family in any way possible. My job is a part-time, paid

position funded through the local independent agency, Cancer Services of Allen County, Inc.

For step-by-step suggestions on how to create, organize, recruit volunteers, and work with the hospital to create a parent-to-parent visitation program, obtain the booklet *Making Contact* from Candlelighters (see Appendix D).

Clergy

Religion is a source of strength for many people. Many parents and children find that their faith is strengthened by the cancer ordeal, while some begin to question their beliefs. Others, who have not relied on religion in the past, turn to it now.

Most hospitals have staff chaplains who are available for counseling, religious services, prayer, and other types of spiritual guidance. Often, the chaplain visits families soon after diagnosis and is available on an on-call basis. As with any mental health encounter, some approaches that work well with one family are not welcome with others.

> *The day after my daughter was diagnosed, a chaplain started coming to the room every day. She was very nice, but I felt like she wanted me to talk about the cancer, and I just couldn't. I clearly remember feeling as if my body parts were being held together by the weakest of threads. I felt if I started talking, or even said the word leukemia, that those threads holding me together would break and I would fly apart into a million pieces. So we chatted about inconsequential things until one day I thanked her for coming, but said I felt strong enough to start talking to my family and friends.*

· · · · ·

> *When Shawn was first diagnosed, Father Ron came in, and we all just really bonded with him. Shawn was in the hospital most of the first year, so we had a chance to become very close. Often Shawn would ask for Father Ron before he had to have a painful procedure. Father Ron would talk to him, give him a little stuffed animal and a big hug, and then Shawn would feel fine.*

> *When Shawn was very ill, I began to worry about the fact that he had never been baptized, and I asked Father Ron to baptize him in the*

chapel. We ended up going to his own little church nearby, and we had a private service with just godparents and family because Shawn's counts were so low. It was a wonderful, special service; I'll never forget it.

Parents who were members of a church, synagogue, or mosque prior to the diagnosis of their child's cancer derive great comfort from the clergy and members of their home church. Members of the congregation usually rally around the family, providing meals, baby-sitting, prayers, and support. Regular visits from clergy provide spiritual sustenance throughout the initial crisis and subsequent years of treatment.

We belong to a bible study group that has met weekly for eight years. In our group during that time there have been three cancer diagnoses and one of multiple sclerosis. We have all become an incredibly supportive family, and we share the burdens. I cannot begin to list the many wonderful things these people have done for us. They consistently put their lives on hold to help. They fill the freezer, clean the house, support us financially, parent our children. They do the laundry covered with vomit. They quietly appear, help, then disappear. I can call any one of them at 3:00 a.m. in the depths of despair and find comfort.

Individual and family counseling

Cancer is a crisis of major proportions for even the strongest of families. Parents do not need to face this crisis alone and unassisted. Many find it helpful to seek out sensitive, objective mental health care professionals to explore the difficult feelings—fear, anger, depression, anxiety, resentment, guilt—that cancer arouses. Family responsibilities and authority undergo profound changes when a child is diagnosed with leukemia. Sometimes members of the family have difficulty adjusting to the changes. While some families discuss the uncomfortable changes and feelings openly and agree on how to proceed, many need help.

Seeking professional counseling is a sign of strength, not failure. In dealing with children with cancer, problems often become too complex for families to deal with on their own. Seeking advice sends children a message that the parents care about what is happening to them and want to help face it together.

One of the first questions that arises is, "Who should we talk to?" There are a number of resource people in the community who can make referrals and valuable recommendations, including:

- Pediatrician
- Oncologist
- Nurse practitioner
- Clinic social worker
- School psychologist or counselor
- Health department social worker
- Other parents who have sought counseling

Ask each of the above for a short list of mental health care professionals who have experience working with your issues, for example, traumatized children, marital problems, stress reduction, or family therapy. Generally, the names of the most well-respected clinicians in the community will appear on several of the lists.

> *Choosing to get therapy isn't easy. And going to a psychologist isn't easy. The only way to really work through the emotional pain is to look closely at it. Sometimes they ask hard questions. But it has been very beneficial for me. The best part about therapy is the person you are talking to is impartial. They aren't related to you, don't go to church with you, don't live with you, and have no connection to you or your situation. A totally unbiased perspective can be helpful when it feels like you are at the bottom of the pit, with no handholds, no ladder, but a shovel right beside you to help you dig deeper.*
>
> *If you decide to go with one, do your research. I called and asked for references from a cancer help line and the social worker at the clinic. Then I talked to a couple before I decided which one to go with. She was also willing to work with me on a payment schedule.*

In making your decision, it helps to understand the different levels of training and education of the various types of mental health care professionals. You will be able to choose from individuals trained in one of these four related fields:

- Psychology (EdD, MA, PhD, PsyD). Marriage and family psychotherapists have a master's degree; clinical and research psychologists have a doctorate (in some states, the use of the title "psychologist" may also be allowed for those with only a master's degree).

- Social work (MSW, DSW, PhD). Clinical social workers have either a master's degree or a doctorate in a clinically emphasized program.

- Pastoral care (MA, MDiv, DMin, PhD, DDiv). Laymen or members of the clergy who receive specialized training in counseling.

- Medicine (MD, RN). Psychiatrists are medical doctors (and only they are able to prescribe medications). In addition, some nurses obtain postgraduate training in psychotherapy.

The designations LCSW (Licensed Clinical Social Worker), LSW (Licensed Social Worker), LMFCC (Licensed Marriage and Family Child Counselor), LPC (Licensed Professional Counselor), LMFT (Licensed Marriage and Family Therapist) refer to licensure by state professional boards, not academic degrees. These initials usually follow others that indicate an academic degree. If they don't, inquire about the therapist's academic training.

You may hear all of the above professionals referred to as "counselors" or "therapists." Most states require licensure or certification in order for professionals to practice independently; unlicensed professionals are allowed to practice only under the supervision of a licensed professional (typically as an "intern" or "assistant" in a clinic or licensed professional's private practice).

When you are seeking a counselor for yourself, ask the professional how long she has been in practice. A licensed marriage and family therapist who has been seeing patients for ten years may be a much finer clinician for your needs than a licensed psychologist or psychiatrist in his first year of practice.

Another method to find a suitable counselor is to call the American Association for Marriage and Family Therapy in Washington, D.C. (202) 452-0109. This is a national professional organization of licensed/certified marriage and family therapists. It has more than 20,000 members in the US and Canada, and its membership also includes licensed clinical social workers, pastoral counselors (who are MFCC/LMFTs), psychologists, and psychiatrists.

To find a therapist, first call two or three therapists who appear on several of your lists of recommendations. During your telephone interview, the following are some suggested questions to ask:

- Are you accepting new clients?

- Do you charge for an initial consultation?

- What training and experience do you have working with ill or traumatized children?

- How many years have you been working with families?

- What is your approach to resolving the problems children develop from trauma? Do you use a brief or long-term approach?

- What evaluation and assessment procedures will be used to define the problem?

- How and when will treatment goals be set?

- How will both parents be involved in treatment?

- What are your fees? Will the insurance company be billed directly?

The next step should be to make an appointment with one or two of the therapists who you think might be able to best address your needs. Be honest about the fact that you are interviewing several therapists prior to making a decision. The purpose of the introductory meeting is to see if you feel comfortable with the therapist. After all, credentials do not guarantee that a given therapist will work for you. Compatibility, trust, and a feeling of genuine caring are essential. It is worth the effort to continue your search until you find a good match.

> I called several therapists out of desperation about my daughter's withdrawal and violent tantrums. I made appointments with two. The first I just didn't feel comfortable with at all, but the second felt like an old friend after one hour. I have been to see her dozens of times over the years, and she has always helped me. I wasn't interested in theory; I wanted practical suggestions of how to deal with the behavior problems. My four-year-old daughter asked why I was going to see the therapist, and I said that Hilda was a doctor, but instead of taking care of my body, she helped care for my feelings. She asked to go to the "feelings" doctor, but was concerned about whether her conversations would be private. I asked the counselor to explain about the limits of confidentiality. So that began a very helpful course of therapy for my daughter. To this day I don't know what was said,

nor would I ever ask my daughter or Hilda. I do know that they did a lot of art therapy, and I know that it helped immensely.

· · · · ·

We went to family counseling because I was concerned that my son seemed to be increasingly withdrawn and depressed. It was a disaster. The kids clammed up, I talked too much, and my husband was offended by some of the remarks that the counselor made. She was not a good choice for our family. It's a hard decision to change counselors when you know you need help, but it's better to make a move than to stay in an uncomfortable situation.

· · · · ·

We went into family therapy because every member of my family experienced misdirected anger. When they were angry they aimed it at me—the nice person who took care of them and loved them no matter what. But I was dissolving. I needed to learn to say "ouch," and they needed to learn other ways to handle their angry feelings.

Children need to be prepared for psychological intervention as for any unknown procedure. The following are several parents' suggestions on how to prepare your child:

- Explain who the therapist is, and what you hope to accomplish. If you are bringing your child in for therapy, explain why you think talking to an objective person might benefit him.

- Older children should be involved in the process of choosing a counselor. Younger children's likes and dislikes should be respected. If your young child does not get along well with one counselor, change.

- Make the experience positive rather than threatening.

- Reassure young children that the visit is for talking, drawing, or playing games, not for anything that is physically painful.

- Ask the therapist to explain the rules of confidentiality to both you and your child. Do not quiz your child after a visit to the therapist.

- Make sure that your child does not think that she is being punished; instead assure her that therapists help both adults and children understand and deal with feelings.

- Go yourself for counseling or to support group meetings to model the fact that all ages and types of people need help from time to time.

In the beginning of treatment, my son had terrible problems with going to sleep and then having nightmares, primarily about snakes. We took him to a counselor, who worked with him for several weeks and completely resolved the problem. The counselor had him befriend the snake, talk to it, and explain that it was keeping him awake. He would tell the snake, "I want you to stop bothering me because I need to go to sleep." The snake never returned.

In *Armfuls of Time*, Barbara Sourkes quotes Jonathan, a boy with cancer, who told her, "Thank you for giving me aliveness." She discusses the importance of psychotherapy for the child with a life-threatening illness:

Even when life itself cannot be guaranteed, psychotherapy can at least "give aliveness" to the child for however long that life may last. Through the extraordinary challenges posed by life-threatening illness, a precocious inner wisdom of life and its fragility emerges. Yet even in the struggle for survival, the spirit of childhood shines through.

Camps

Summer camps for children with cancer, and often their siblings as well, are becoming increasingly popular. These camps provide an opportunity for children with cancer and their siblings to have fun, meet friends, and talk with others in the same situation. Counselors are typically cancer survivors and siblings of cancer victims, or sometimes oncology nurses and residents. Supervised by experts, children can have their concerns addressed without involving their parents. These camps provide a carefree time away from the sadness of the family or the all-too-frequent hospital visits.

Of all the ways to get support, I think the camp really helps the most. You are all there together for enough time to break down the barriers. Although camp does not focus on cancer, many times we really got down to talking about how we really felt. I have been a counselor at the camp for eight summers now. Most of the campers know that I relapsed three times and I'm doing great many years later. They see the many other long-term survivors who are counselors, and it gives them what they need the most—hope. The best support is meeting survivors, because nobody else truly understands.

. . . . .

When we went to pick up seven-and-a-half-year-old Kristin from camp, she told us how wonderful it had been and exclaimed, "I want to come back every year until I am old enough to be a counselor." That said it all to me.

．　．　．　．　．

Caitlin went to camp, and this was a dream come true for her. As we pulled into the parking lot, she exhaled a deep breath and said, "I made it, I am finally normal!"

We are one family
you and I—
Not by birth or legal joining
Not by choice, and definitely not by desire
But by a commonality given to us by the unseen
Seeking peace with uncertainty
Needing the support of another
who has known.

We are one family
you and I—
We fight the beast hungry for our child
and battle for their lives
Striving to plan for tomorrow
explaining, educating, researching
Assertiveness and occasional aggression
To fight with
and for
Our child.

We are one family
you and I—
With the same questions and fears
Why my child? Did I do something to cause this horror?
Am I weak because I still cry?
Will the beast return? When?
Am I missing an early sign?
What late effects of this battle will we see?
How do we deal with them? Where do we get help?

What about my other children?
Will the beast find them too?

We are one family
you and I—
We share a bond that we wish did not exist
and yet since it does exist
we are glad it is there
We gather strength
and rejoice in today
We accept the tears, acknowledge the fears
love and are loved
We walk the road together
not knowing where it leads
on our common journey we are not alone,
Thus we are blessed.

We are one family
you and I—
Not by birth or legal joining
Not by choice, and definitely not by desire
But by a commonality given to us by the unseen
Seeking peace with uncertainty
Needing the support of another
who has known.

—Mary Riecke

CHAPTER 10

Chemotherapy

*In the depths of winter I finally learned
there was in me an invincible summer.*

—Albert Camus

THE WORD CHEMOTHERAPY IS DERIVED from the combination of "chemical" and "treatment." It means using drugs, singly or in combination, to destroy or disrupt the growth of cancer cells without permanently damaging normal cells.

This chapter describes the most common drugs that are used to kill cancer cells as well as drugs that prevent nausea and pain. Numerous stories are included that show the range of responses to different chemotherapy drugs.

Reading about potential side effects of chemotherapy can be disturbing. However, it is important to be aware of the possibilities in order to recognize symptoms early and report them to the doctor so that swift action can be taken to make your child more comfortable. On rare occasions, side effects may be life-threatening and some can persist throughout life. However, most are merely unpleasant and subside soon after treatment ends. Remember that your child may experience several, a few, or none of the side effects discussed here.

How do chemotherapy drugs kill cancer cells?

Normal, healthy cells divide and grow in a well-established pattern. When normal cells divide, an identical copy is produced. The body only makes the number of normal cells that it needs at any given time.

Cancer cells, on the other hand, reproduce uncontrollably and grow in an unpredictable way. They invade surrounding tissue and can travel in blood or lymph to lodge in other parts of the body.

All chemotherapy drugs work in some way to interfere with the ability of the cancer cells to live, divide, and multiply. Some of the types of drugs used to treat leukemia are:

- **Alkylating agents.** All cells use building blocks (DNA and RNA) to make exact copies of themselves. Alkylating agents poison cancer cells by interacting with DNA to prevent cell reproduction.

- **Antimetabolites.** These drugs starve cancer cells by replacing essential cell nutrients.

- **Antibiotics.** This type of drug prevents cell growth by blocking reproduction.

- **Alkaloids.** These drugs, derived from plants, interrupt cell division.

- **Hormones.** These drugs create a hostile environment that slows cell growth.

- **Enzymes.** These interfere with cancer cells' ability to reproduce.

How are chemotherapy drugs given?

The five most common ways that drugs are given during treatment for leukemia are:

- **Intravenous (IV).** Medicine is delivered directly into the bloodstream through a semipermanent IV catheter (Port-a-cath or Hickman) or IV needle in the arm or hand.

- **Oral.** Drugs, taken by mouth in liquid, capsule, or tablet form, are absorbed into the blood through the lining of the stomach and intestines.

- **Intramuscular.** Drugs that need to seep slowly into the bloodstream are injected into a large muscle such as the thigh or buttocks.

- **Intrathecal.** Doctors perform a spinal tap and inject the drug directly into the cerebrospinal fluid, circumventing the barrier between the blood and brain.

- **Subcutaneous.** Drugs are injected under the skin.

Dosages

Dosages vary among protocols, however, most are based on your child's weight or body surface area (BSA). BSA is calculated from your child's weight and height and is measured in m² [meters squared].

> My daughter's m² ranged from .55 to .70 over the course of her treatment. During induction, the protocol required 60 mg/m² of prednisone on days 0 to 27. To determine her dose, the doctor calculated .55 × 60 = 33. He then wrote a prescription that she take 33 mg of prednisone a day in three doses of 11 mg each. So I gave her one 10 mg tablet and one 1 mg tablet three times a day.

You do not need to do the calculations, but you need to understand the dosage and how you should give it for each drug. Most families write the dosages on a calendar and cross them out when given to make sure they don't forget a drug.

Chemotherapy drugs and their possible side effects

The following drug information contains not only common and infrequent side effects, but also parent and survivor experiences and suggestions. You may be overwhelmed by reading all of the potential side effects of each drug. Please remember, each child is unique and will handle most drugs without any problems. Most side effects are unpleasant, not serious, and subside when the medication stops. Parent experiences are included to alert new parents to possibilities and provide comfort and suggestions should a child have an unusual side effect. Consult your child's pediatrician or oncologist should any concerns arise from the following information. Appendix D, *Books and Online Sites*, contains resources for obtaining information on drugs not covered here.

Remember to keep all chemotherapy drugs in a locked cabinet away from children and pets.

Questions to ask the doctor

Prior to giving your child any drug, you should be given basic information including answers to the following:

- What is the dosage? How many times a day should it be given?

- What are the common and rare side effects?

- What should I do if my child experiences any of the side effects?

- Will the drug interact with any over-the-counter drugs (e.g., Tylenol) or vitamins? Will it interact with any natural medicines?

- Will my teen be given detailed counseling on avoiding risks such as drinking alcohol, smoking cigarettes or marijuana, and pregnancy?

- What should I do if I forget to give my child a dose?

- What are both the trade and generic names of the drug?

- Should I buy the generic version?

Guidelines for calling the doctor

Sometimes parents are reluctant to call their child's physician with questions or concerns. Here are general guidelines for when calling is necessary:

- Temperature above 101°F (38.5°C)

- Shaking or chills

- Shortness of breath

- Severe nausea or vomiting

- Unusual bleeding, bruising, or cuts that won't heal

- Pain or swelling at chemotherapy injection site

- Any severe pain that cannot be explained

- Exposure to chicken pox, shingles, or measles

- Severe headache or blurred vision

- Constipation lasting more than two days

- Severe diarrhea

- Painful urination or bowel movements

- Blood in urine

- Whenever child appears sick and you are concerned

- Inability to eat or drink

Chemotherapy drug list

Drugs used for chemotherapy are known by a variety of names. You may hear the same drug referred to by its generic name, abbreviation, or one of several brand names, depending on which doctor, nurse, or pharmacist you are talking to. The list below gives the most common names used for chemotherapy drugs, and tells you what name is used in this chapter so you can easily find it on the following pages of detailed information:

Name	Look Under
Adriamycin	Doxorubicin
ARA-C	Cytarabine
Asp	L-Asparaginase
Cerubidine	Daunorubicin
Cyclophosphamide	Cyclophosphamide
Cytarabine	Cytarabine
Cytoxan	Cyclophosphamide
Cytosar	Cytarabine
Cytosine arabinoside	Cytarabine
Daunomycin	Daunorubicin
Daunorubicin	Daunorubicin
Decadron	Prednisone
Dexamethasone	Prednisone
DMR	Daunorubicin
DNR	Daunorubicin
Doxorubicin	Doxorubicin
Elspar	L-Asparaginase
Etoposide	Etoposide
Hydroxyurea	Hydroxyurea
Hydrea	Hydroxyurea
L-Asp	L-Asparaginase
L-Asparaginase	L-Asparaginase
Mercaptopurine	Mercaptopurine
Methotrexate	Methotrexate
Mexate	Methotrexate
MTX	Methotrexate
Oncovin	Vincristine
Prednisone	Prednisone
Purinethol	Mercaptopurine
Rubidomycin	Daunorubicin
VePesid	Etoposide

Name	Look Under
VCR	Vincristine
Vincristine	Vincristine
VP-16	Etoposide
6-MP	Mercaptopurine
6-TG	6-Thioguanine
6-Thioguanine	6-Thioguanine

L-Asparaginase (L-a-SPARE-a-gin-ase), PEG-Asparaginase

Also called: Asp, L-ASP, Elspar

How given: Intramuscular injection

How it works: These drugs are enzymes that block protein production in cancer cells to prevent them from reproducing.

Types: There are two types of L-asparaginase: *E. coli* asparaginase and *Erwinia* asparaginase.

Precaution: Occasionally a child will have a severe allergic reaction to L-asparaginase. It is important that the drug be given by trained medical personnel who have emergency equipment available. The child should be monitored at the clinic for 20 to 30 minutes after receiving the drug in case a reaction occurs. If a child does have a reaction to *E. coli* asparaginase, *Erwinia* asparaginase may be used for the next dose. If a reaction occurs again, asparaginase therapy is usually discontinued.

Common side effects:
- Loss of appetite and weight
- Fatigue
- Headache
- Abdominal cramps
- Nausea and vomiting

Infrequent side effects:
- Allergic reaction, including swelling, difficulty breathing, rash
- Jaundice (yellow skin and eyes)
- Confusion or hallucinations
- Convulsions

- Swelling of feet or legs
- Unusually frequent urination
- High blood pressure
- Kidney or liver damage
- Stroke
- Pancreatitis
- Excessive bleeding
- Blood clots

> Meagan had no problem with the L-asparaginase other than that the shots in her thigh were painful. This was before EMLA was available. I'd recommend that parents put EMLA on two hours before the shot to reduce the pain.

Most children have no serious side effects from asparaginase. But for those who do, it can be both frightening and life-threatening.

> A couple of hours after Preston's third dose of L-asparaginase his leg began to swell up around the injection site. His leg grew to three times its normal size. The doctors switched him to a different kind of L-asparaginase for all subsequent doses, and he had no further problems.

· · · · ·

> A day after Brent received his last L-asparaginase dose, he began to have intense pain in his kidney area and began to pass blood in his urine. After his arrival at the hospital, his kidneys shut down and he stopped breathing. He was in the ICU on a ventilator and received kidney dialysis for a week. The doctors thought that he had a rare reaction to L-aparaginase which caused tiny blood clots in his kidneys. His kidneys function normally now, but he developed a seizure disorder as a result of the trauma to his brain.

Remember: The vast majority of children have no reaction to L-asparaginase.

Cyclophosphamide (Sye-kloe-FOSS-fa-mide)

Also called: Cytoxan, Endoxan

How given: IV injection

How it works: An alkylating agent that disrupts DNA in cancer cells, preventing reproduction.

Precaution: The child should drink lots of water or be given large amounts of IV fluids while taking Cytoxan to prevent damage to the bladder. Mesna may be given as a precaution to prevent bladder irritation. Antinausea drugs should be given before and for several hours after this drug is administered.

Common side effects:

- Myelosuppression (low blood cell counts)
- Nausea and vomiting (often prevented if effective antinausea drugs are given)
- Loss of appetite
- Hair loss

Infrequent side effects:

- Hemorrhagic cystitis causing blood in the urine
- Abdominal pain and diarrhea
- Mouth sores
- Cough or shortness of breath
- Dizziness and difficulty walking
- Skin rash and itching
- Menstrual periods in teenage girls may temporarily stop
- Sterility (rare at routine ALL doses, more common at BMT doses)

> Erica just could not tolerate the Cytoxan. She had continuous vomiting. At one point she had lost more than one third of her body weight. Our HMO wouldn't authorize using ondansetron (a very effective antinausea drug) because it was so expensive.

• • • • •

Christine breezed through the Cytoxan infusions. She would go to Children's in the afternoon, they would give her lots of IV fluids, and then ondansetron a half hour before the Cytoxan. She would sleep through the night with absolutely no nausea because they were so good about giving her the ondansetron all night and the next morning. It was harder on me because I had to wake up every two hours to change her diaper so that the nurse could weigh it to make sure she was passing enough urine.

Cytarabine (Sye-TARE-a-been)

Also called: ARA-C, Cytosar, cytosine arabinoside

How given: IV, intrathecal, or subcutaneous injection

How it works: Kills cancer cells by disrupting DNA.

Common side effects:
- Myelosuppression (low blood cell counts)
- Immunosuppression (low immune function)
- Nausea and vomiting
- Fever or chills
- Diarrhea
- Mouth sores
- Loss of appetite
- Hair loss

Infrequent side effects:
- Jaundice (yellow skin or eyes)
- Joint and bone pain
- Pneumonia
- Rash
- Numbing or tingling in fingers, toes, or face
- Headache
- Seizures
- Temporary loss of balance
- Difficulty breathing

I told my daughter's oncologist how happy I was that she had not had any severe nausea after her first few doses of ARA-C. His only reply was, "It's cumulative." Within an hour, on the long drive home, she was vomiting constantly. We became ensnared in a two-hour traffic jam. She ran out of clean clothes, so for two hours, I repeatedly carried her to the side of the road, a naked, bald, 25-pound four-year-old with tubing hanging from her chest, and supported her as she dry-heaved. The people in the cars around us were in tears, and kept asking if there was anything they could do to help. I just focused on comforting her, and getting her home to that vial of ondansetron in our fridge.

Daunorubicin (Daw-no-ROO-bi-sin)

Also called: Daunomycin, DMN, DNR, Cerubidine, Rubidomycin

How given: IV injection or infusion over several days

How it works: An antibiotic that prevents DNA from forming, thus preventing cancer cells from multiplying.

Precaution: Daunorubicin is a red color, and may turn urine red for a day or two after each dose. This is normal.

Common side effects:

- Myelosuppression (low blood cell counts)
- Nausea and vomiting
- Hair loss
- Mouth sores
- Diarrhea

Infrequent side effects:

- Burning pain and swelling if any drug leaks into skin
- Heart damage at high doses
- Shortness of breath
- Skin rash

My son didn't have any problems from daunorubicin, but I sure worried about heart damage. I went to a conference and learned that the cut-off dose was below what he had on the protocol. I requested an echocardiogram, and his heart function was normal.

Dexamethasone (Dex-a-METH-a-sone)

See Prednisone.

Doxorubicin (Dox-o-ROO-bi-sin)

Also called: Adriamycin, Doxil, Rubex

How given: IV injection or infusion

How it works: An antibiotic that prevents DNA from forming, thus preventing cancer cells from multiplying.

Precaution: Doxorubicin is a red color, and may turn urine red for a day or two after each dose. This is normal.

Common side effects:

- Myelosuppression (low blood cell counts)
- Nausea and vomiting
- Hair loss
- Mouth sores

Infrequent side effects:

- Loss of appetite
- Diarrhea
- Burning pain and swelling if any drug leaks into skin
- Heart damage at high doses
- Shortness of breath
- Fever and chills
- Abdominal pains
- Dark or bloody stools
- Darkening or ridging of nails

> The Adriamycin just burned right through my son. He never got mouth sores, but he sure had problems at the other end. They had him lie on his stomach with the heat lamp on his bare bottom. His whole bottom was blistered so badly that it looked like he'd been in a fire. They used to mix up what they called "Magic Butt Paste," and I'll never forget the rec-

ipe: one tube Nystatin cream, one tube Desitin, and Nystatin powder. It was like spackle that they would just slather on. He had a lot of gastrointestinal bleeding, too, so he was continuously getting platelets. That's when they decided that he wouldn't have the delayed intensification phase.

. . . . .

Other than red urine and the expected low counts, hair loss, and nausea, Christine had no problems from her many doses of Adriamycin.

Etoposide (E-TOE-poe-side)

Also called: VP-16, VePesid

How given: IV injection

How it works: Prevents DNA from reproducing, and also causes death of dividing cells.

Common side effects:

- Myelosuppression (low blood cell counts)
- Loss of appetite
- Nausea and vomiting
- Hair loss
- Fatigue

Infrequent side effects:

- Decreased blood pressure
- Shortness of breath or wheezing
- Difficulty in walking
- Numbness or tingling in fingers or toes
- Fever or chills
- Rash
- New cancers that occur later in life (secondary cancers)

Hydroxyurea (Hi-DROX-ee-yoo-REE-ah)

Also called: Droxia

How given: Pills by mouth

How it works: Drug is thought to work by stopping DNA production.

Common side effects:
- Myelosuppression (low blood cell counts)

Infrequent side effects:
- Nausea and vomiting
- Loss of appetite
- Mouth sores
- Fever and chills
- Rashes
- Drowsiness
- Diarrhea
- Convulsions
- Headache or dizziness
- Stomach pain
- Confusion or hallucinations

> Drew has been on hydroxyurea for about two years. It is a pill that they can take long term. He is being weaned off it now because of sores (mouth and leg). They are very, very slow to heal.

Mercaptopurine (Mer-kap-toe-PYOOR-een)

Also called: 6-MP, Purinethol

How given: Pills by mouth

How it works: An antimetabolite that replaces part of the backbone of DNA.

Common side effects:
- Myelosuppression (low blood cell counts)
- Loss of appetite

Infrequent side effects:

- Nausea and vomiting
- Skin rashes
- Jaundice (yellow skin or eyes)
- Liver damage

> *Christine had no problems with the 6-MP other than low counts. She needed blood work every two weeks and we were constantly cutting her doses in half or stopping the drugs altogether until her ANC recovered.*

Methotrexate (Meth-o-TREX-ate)

Also called: Mexate, MTX

How given: Pills by mouth, IV, or intrathecal injection

How it works: An antimetabolite which replaces folic acid in cells, preventing them from dividing. Children should not be given extra folic acid in vitamins or the methotrexate will not be effective.

Common side effects:

- Myelosuppression (low blood cell counts)
- Sun sensitivity
- Diarrhea
- Fatigue
- Skin rashes
- Headache, backache, spinal cord irritation (when given intrathecally)

Infrequent side effects:

- Mouth sores
- Hair loss
- Nausea and vomiting
- Loss of appetite
- Dry cough caused by lung damage

- Chills and fever
- Dizziness
- Jaundice (yellow skin and eyes)
- Kidney damage
- Liver damage
- Shortness of breath
- Neurotoxicity which can cause learning disabilities

My daughter had serious problems with rashes during maintenance. The doctors thought that she had developed an allergy to the weekly methotrexate. She often would be covered with rashes which looked like small, red circles with tan, flaky skin inside. They were extremely itchy and unattractive. We spent hundreds of dollars at the dermatologist trying various prescription remedies. None worked. In desperation, I went to our local herbalist and asked if she had anything totally nontoxic, which would help the rash but not affect her chemotherapy. She sold me a small tub of salve made from olive oil, vitamin E oil, and calendula flowers. We checked with her oncologist before using it. It totally cured the rash after two days, and worked each time that the rash reappeared. What a relief!

• • • • •

Two years into maintenance, Shawn started throwing up every Friday night after receiving his methotrexate. We started giving him ondansetron before every dose and continued through the weekend.

• • • • •

Carl was on an experimental IV high-dose methotrexate protocol funded through the National Institutes of Health. Side effects ranged from nausea and vomiting to diarrhea, sore bones, mood swings, and disorientation.

• • • • •

My son developed learning disabilities from his high-dose methotrexate protocol. He received tutoring through high school and is doing extremely well in college.

Prednisone (PRED-ni-sone) and
Dexamethasone (Dex-a-METH-a-sone)

These two steroids are grouped together because they are closely related chemically and have similar action and side effects. Dexamethasone is given in high doses as a chemotherapy drug and in low doses to prevent nausea. To see the side effects of dexamethasone when it is used as an antinausea drug, look under "Drugs Given to Prevent Nausea."

Also called: Decadron, Hexadrol

How given: Pills by mouth, liquid by mouth, IV injection

How they work: Hormones that kill lymphocytes.

Precaution: Every parent interviewed described problems that their children had while on prednisone. The side effects ranged from very mild to severe, but were universal. At high doses, prednisone creates major behavioral problems in children, which gradually subside after the drug is stopped.

Common side effects:

- Mood changes
- Increased appetite
- Food obsessions
- Increased thirst
- Indigestion
- Weight gain
- Fluid retention
- Round face and protruding belly
- Sleeplessness
- Nightmares
- Nervousness, restlessness, hyperactivity
- Loss of potassium
- Hypersensitivy to lights, sound, motion
- Extreme irritability

Infrequent side effects:

- Decreased or blurred vision
- Seeing halos around lights
- Increased sweating
- Weakness with loss of muscle mass
- Muscle cramps or pain
- Swelling of feet or lower legs
- High blood pressure
- High blood sugar
- Hallucinations
- Aseptic necrosis (destruction of blood supply to bones)

Judson was a hyper, high-strung child who became extremely hyperactive when he was on prednisone. My recommendation for other parents dealing with this difficult side effect is to run—don't walk—to your nearest library or bookstore and get some books on hyperactive behavior in children. It is important that parents understand this problem and learn to deal with it in a loving way. Remember, too, that this side effect will go away when the prednisone is out of the child's system. Judd would be hyperactive for the entire two weeks, desiring to eat every fifteen minutes or so, making noises constantly, itching all over, sleeping less, having a terrible temper, and losing his fine motor and concentration skills.

During this time he would develop bad behavior because as parents we could not parent him the way we would normally. A few days after his prednisone ended, we would become very firm and structured in our parenting, and he would return to his normal behavior patterns. My son has been in remission ten years, has never exhibited abnormal hyperactivity since ending chemotherapy, and is a well-adjusted teen and an excellent student.

· · · · ·

Meagan is very emotionally labile after only two doses of prednisone. She is very frustrated, quick to anger, hits, screams. For those five days we try to stay home, and this helps to decrease the stimulation. We plot it out on the calendar in advance so that we can plan accordingly. I think the kids deserve some tender, loving care while taking prednisone.

Of course, I don't allow the hitting, but I do try hard not to aggravate the situation when she is on prednisone. I can see how she is uncomfortable being out of control, but she just can't help it.

· · · · ·

Prednisone sends Stephan into a whirlwind of emotions. Sometimes he seems especially happy, and the rest of the time he is in tears at the drop of a hat. We explained to Stephan that the pill can make him feel this way, and it's okay to tell us, "I'm grumpy and I need to be alone for awhile." He gets physical side effects, too. He takes prednisone five days a month, and, like clockwork, on day six he gets itchy, on day seven he aches all over, on day eight he has severe back, chest, arm, and leg pain, and on day nine he starts to feel better.

· · · · ·

Preston didn't act out while on prednisone; instead he became depressed and too compliant. He spent most of his time moodily cooking himself food and eating. We bought a second wardrobe of sweat pants with elastic waists so that he would be comfortable.

· · · · ·

Rachel had a dual personality on prednisone. She would be fine one minute and then fly into a rage. One time, she literally had an argument with herself. She asked to watch a tape, and then for twenty minutes she argued with herself over whether she should watch the tape. It was painful to watch.

· · · · ·

Prednisone and dexamethasone were the worst drugs for Katy. When she was on for a month straight, she hallucinated horrible things. She'd scream that boys were chasing her or that her heart had stopped beating. She'd sob that I was melting and would disappear. She'd dig her fingers into my arm begging me to help her. She sometimes did this all night, and nothing consoled her. She slept very little while taking prednisone. She would eat an entire loaf of bread, and always asked to have "butter spread on it like icing on a cake." She has never once said that since ending treatment.

· · · · ·

Jeremy never slept well when he was on prednisone. He had night-mares of doctors chasing him through the hospital halls. He had a lot of night sweats, and was hungry all night and day. He slept with a loaf of bread, and when we would go places, he always carried a can of Campbell's chicken soup and a can opener. He desperately needed to make sure that he would never be without food.

· · · · ·

Carrie Beth was both hungry and irritable when taking dexametha-sone. I remember once at the Ronald McDonald house a staff member whom she really liked simply said, "Hello, Carrie Beth," and she started to scream. She ended up on the floor kicking and yelling.

· · · · ·

Jody just seemed a little high when on prednisone. He was crazy for food, but didn't have any behavior problems. He had lots of energy.

· · · · ·

Prednisone caused "moon" face, swollen stomach, dark circles under his eyes, and vomiting. Considering Carl was only two and a half when he was going through this, it was difficult to explain the side effects to him. The best we could do was make him as comfortable as possible, stay with him, and make sure he had the blankets and stuffed animals he really loved.

· · · · ·

John began prednisone when he was fourteen months old, and he began to swell immediately. His moods would swing quickly from happy to sad, but he continued to sleep through the night, and he remained a happy child.

6-Thioguanine (Thigh-oh-GWAN-neen)

Also called: 6-TG

How given: Pills taken by mouth

How it works: Antimetabolite that replaces part of the backbone of DNA.

Precaution: In some cases, 6-TG has caused liver problems with rapidly enlarging abdomens. Call your doctor immediately if this occurs.

Common side effects:

- Myelosuppression (low blood cell counts)
- Nausea and vomiting

Infrequent side effects:

- Enlarged liver (venoocclusive disease)
- Jaundice (yellow skin or eyes)
- Stomach pain
- Loss of appetite
- Mouth sores

> Tay's abdomen slowly began to enlarge and then it suddenly went from a little bloated to huge. He looked pregnant and it was rock hard. He gained ten pounds in one day—from 55 to 65 pounds. It affected his white, red, and platelet counts. Tay was taken off all meds, he was given potassium by mouth, albumen IV, and several blood and platelet transfusions. It was very scary! He also ran fever off and on, and we were in the hospital for days. Once his abdomen shrank and his counts stayed steady we went home.

Vincristine (Vin-CRIS-teen)

Also called: Oncovin, VCR

How given: IV injection

How it works: Vincristine is an alkyloid derived from the periwinkle plant. It causes cells to stop dividing.

Note: The side effects of vincristine are most pronounced during induction and consolidation when it is given weekly. It is generally better tolerated during maintenance when it is given monthly.

Common side effects:

- Constipation
- Pain in jaw, face, back, joints, bones; may be severe
- Foot drop (child has trouble lifting front part of foot)
- Numbness, tingling, or pain in fingers and toes
- Extreme weakness and loss of muscle mass

- Blurred or double vision, drooping eyelids
- Hair loss
- Pain and blisters if drug leaks during administration

Infrequent side effects:
- Loss of appetite, sometimes nausea and vomiting
- Weight loss
- Headaches, dizziness, light-headedness
- Convulsions
- Difficulty urinating
- Rashes
- Difficulty sleeping
- Itchiness

Most parents interviewed stated that their children had no difficulties when given vincristine. But some children did develop severe problems.

> *Erica (diagnosed age one) once had a vincristine burn on her arm at the IV site. It was red when we went home from the clinic, but by the second day it was badly burned. She developed a blister as big as a half dollar, which left a bad scar. It hurt and was sensitive for a long time. She also developed severe foot drop (she could not lift up the front part of her foot) and fell a lot.*

· · · · ·

> *Preston (diagnosed age ten) had an awful time from vincristine. He would develop cramping in his lower legs, and would just curl up in bed, in great pain. It would start a couple of days after he received the vincristine, and would last a week. I would massage his legs, use hot packs, and give him Tylenol. I would have to carry him into the clinic because he couldn't walk. I did some research, and discovered that when the bilirubin is high, the child can't excrete the vincristine and therefore the toxicity is increased. We lowered his vincristine dose and got him into physical therapy.*

· · · · ·

Vincristine incapacitated Katy. She couldn't walk, lift her head, open one eyelid. She had trouble swallowing and stayed in bed for weeks during induction and consolidation. I read the package insert for vincristine and discovered that the manufacturer recommended that vincristine be given at least 12 to 24 hours before asparaginase to minimize toxicity. Katy's protocol required that both drugs be given at the same time. I negotiated with the doctors and had her schedule changed so that these two drugs were given on different days. She was soon back on her feet, but still, after a year off treatment, she has generalized muscle weakness and problems with balance.

· · · · ·

Soon after diagnosis at age five and a half, Robby became so weak in the hospital he stopped walking. He did not walk for at least a week, maybe more. When Robby did walk, he was up on his toes. I kept asking the docs about it and was poohpoohed, saying it is just the vincristine. Finally I took Robby to the pediatrician, who was horrified at how bad his feet had gotten. We immediately started daily physical therapy and major exercises and got traction boots to wear at night.

Prophylactic antibiotics

Children and teens on chemotherapy take antibiotics two to three days each week to prevent pneumocystis pneumonia (PCP). They usually continue to take the antibiotics a few months to a year after treatment ends. The prescription of preventative or prophylactic antibiotics is at the discretion of the oncologist. Some children have reactions to the antibiotics, so this may affect the doctor's decision. Also, PCP is less common in some parts of the country.

The antibiotic of choice for PCP prevention is a combination drug containing sulfamethoxazole and trimethoprim; it is sold under the brand names Bactrim and Septra. This antibiotic can cause gastrointestinal upsets, skin rashes, sun sensitivity, and low blood counts. If a substitute is needed, one of the following is used:

- Pentamidine, administered as an aerosol or nebulized (can be difficult for children because it takes twenty minutes and it smells bad), or IV once a month.

- Dapsone, pills given orally every day.

The oncologist explained it this way. Bactrim is the best prophylactic antibiotic for PCP (pneumocystis) but can affect counts. Pentamidine IV can affect counts, but nebulizer treatments (once a month) usually don't. Dapsone can be used, but it can cause anemia.

We just started the Dapsone because Katie was starting to buck the nebulizer treatment (it smells/tastes horrible). The Bactrim costs about $3/month, the Dapsone about $7/month, and the Pentamidine nebulizer treatment is about $300/month!!

Colony-stimulating factors

Colony-stimulating factors are not usually used for ALL, but are used for children with AML or those who have BMTs. High-dose chemotherapy reduces the number of white blood cells used by the body to fight infections. The administration of colony-stimulating factors, such as granulocyte colony-stimulating factor (G-CSF) and granulocyte-macrophage colony-stimulating factor (GM-CSF), can reduce the severity and duration of low white blood counts, lessening the chance of infection.

Kenny was only two years old when he was receiving G-CSF, so he was too young to understand why he needed the shots. He would cry and beg us not to hurt him—that he was sorry. My heart would break, but I would have to stick him. We finally developed a really good system. Right before being discharged after a round of chemo, we would put EMLA on Kenny's arm and then have the nurse place an insulflon. It was a small catheter that Kenny didn't even notice was in his arm. It was good for seven to ten days, which was the duration of his G-CSF for the entire month. We would draw up the amount needed for injection, then place it in the insulflon and inject very slowly. Kenny never felt it and no longer begged us not to do the G-CSF. Oh, how I wished we had done this from the beginning! Kenny's counts would usually start to decline about four days after his chemo. At about day ten the G-CSF would kick in and his counts would skyrocket.

· · · · ·

Katie had GCSF (brand name is Neupogen) after each high-dose Ara-C. But it is in her protocol to give it to her if her other chemotherapy caused a delay of over seven days—and we were pretty close a few times.

She's had no side effects from Neupogen that I can recall. The worst thing about it for us was giving the shots at home. They're subcutaneous, so the needle is short, but Katie still said they hurt, even with EMLA.

Antinausea drugs used during chemotherapy

Antinausea drugs make chemotherapy treatments more bearable, but can potentially cause side effects. The following sections list both common and infrequent side effects of antinausea drugs. There are many more drugs used to prevent nausea that are not described here. Some of these are Marinol, Reglan, Scopolomine patch, and Atarax. You can find books to look up these and other drugs in Appendix D, *Books and Online Sites*.

Antinausea Drug List

As with chemotherapy drugs, several different names can be used to refer to each of the antinausea drugs. The list below will help you find detailed information about each drug on the following pages:

Name	Look Under
Ativan	Lorazepam
Benadryl	Diphenhydramine
Compazine	Prochlorperazine
Decadron	Dexamethasone
Dexamethasone	Dexamethasone
Hexadrol	Dexamethasone
Lorazepam	Lorazepam
Kytril	Granisetron
Ondansetron	Ondansetron
Phenergan	Promethazine
Prochlorperazine	Prochlorperazine
Zofran	Ondansetron

Dexamethasone (dex-a-METH-a-sown)

Also called: Decadron, Hexadrol

How given: IV injection, usually given in combination with other antinausea drugs, or by mouth

Common side effects:

Side effects are different than those experienced when it is given in high doses for long periods of time. When dexamethasone is used to treat nausea, side effects may be:

- Euphoria
- Restlessness
- Confusion

Diphenhydramine (Die-fen-HIGH-dra-meen)

Also called: Benadryl

How given: Liquid by mouth, IV injection

When given: Usually given every six to eight hours.

Common side effects:

- Drowsiness
- Dizziness
- Impaired coordination

Granisetron

Also called: Kytril

How given: IV injection, pills or liquid by mouth

When given: Kytril is usually given one half hour prior to the start of chemotherapy infusion.

Common side effects:

- Headache

Infrequent side effects:

- Diarrhea
- Constipation

> *Sarah got Zofran at first, then the clinic switched to liquid Kytril. Sarah usually hates liquid meds (she much prefers pills), but she loves Kytril. She thinks it's really yummy. And it works, too!*

Lorazepam (lor-AZ-a-pam)

Also called: Ativan

How given: Pills by mouth, IV injection, intramuscular injection

When given: This is a tranquilizer, which is generally given in combination with other antinausea drugs.

Common side effects:

- Drowsiness or sleepiness
- Forgetfulness
- Unsteadiness
- Low blood pressure

Ondansetron (on-DAN-se-tron)

Also called: Zofran

How given: IV injection, liquid by mouth, pills by mouth

When given: Usually 30 minutes prior to chemotherapy drugs, and every four to eight hours until nausea ends, or in a higher dose once a day.

Note: Zofran comes in flavored oral solutions. 1 teaspoon = 4 mg.

Infrequent side effects:

- Mild headache
- Constipation

> *After Jeremy had his first inpatient treatment, he was allowed to go on an outpatient basis, wearing a cad pump at home. He felt fine, but every couple hours he would vomit for no reason. The next morning, when his oncologist asked him how it had gone, Jeremy was hesitant to tell him about the vomiting. When he did, the doctor asked us if the Zofran hadn't helped. I gave him a confused look and asked him what a Zofran was. I can laugh about it now, but it was an oversight. Everyone thought someone else had taken care of it! We rarely had any problems with nausea after that.*

Prochlorperazine (pro-chlor-PAIR-a-zeen)

Also called: Compazine

How given: Pills or long-acting capsule by mouth, rectal suppository, intramuscular injection, IV injection

When given: Used alone if only mild nausea is expected.

Common side effects:

- Drowsiness
- Low blood pressure
- Nervousness and restlessness
- Neck spasms (should be given with Benadryl to avoid this)

Promethazine (Pro-METH-ah-zeen)

Also called: Phenergan

How given: Pills by mouth, rectal suppository, intramuscular injection, IV injection

When given: Usually given every four to six hours.

Common side effects:

- Drowsiness
- Dizziness and inpaired coordination
- Fatigue
- Blurred vision
- Euphoria
- Insomnia
- Neck spasms (should be given with Benadryl to avoid this)

Drugs used to relieve pain

As with other drugs, drugs used for pain relief can be given by various methods and can cause side effects. The following section lists some drugs commonly used to relieve pain. Many other medications are used to relieve pain in children, including Tylenol, Nalbuphrine, Fentanyl, Hydrocodone, and others. You can find books to look up these and other drugs in Appendix D.

Pain medication list

Several different names can be used to refer to each of the pain medications. You may hear the same drug referred to by its generic name or one of several brand names, depending on which doctor, nurse, or pharmacist you are talking to. The list below gives various names of pain medications, and what name to look under in this chapter.

Name	Look Under
Codeine	Codeine
Demerol	Meperidine
Dilaudid	Hydromorphone
Dolophine	Methadone
Methadone	Methadone
Morphine	Morphine
Percocet	Oxycodone

Codeine

How given: Intramuscular injection, pills by mouth, liquid by mouth

How it works: Codeine is an alkaloid obtained from opium.

Common side effects:

- Light-headedness

- Dizziness

- Sedation

- Euphoria

- Constipation

Infrequent side effects:

- Nausea

- Vomiting

Meperidine

Also called: Demerol

How given: Intravenous injection, liquid by mouth, pill by mouth

How it works: Meperidine is a narcotic similar to morphine.

Common side effects:
- Sedation
- Constipation

Infrequent side effects:
- Dizziness
- Nausea and vomiting
- Sweating
- Rashes
- Respiratory depression
- Decreased blood pressure
- Seizures
- Headaches
- Visual disturbances

Hydromorphone

Also called: Dilaudid

How given: IV injection, pill by mouth, rectal suppository

How it works: Hydromorphone is a narcotic pain reliever.

Precautions: Hydromorphone can cause respiratory depression.

Common side effects:
- Light-headedness and dizziness
- Sedation
- Nausea
- Vomiting

- Sweating
- Euphoria
- Alterations of mood
- Headache
- Respiratory depression

Infrequent side effects:
- Circulatory depression
- Hallucinations and disorientation
- Respiratory arrest
- Shock
- Cardiac arrest

Methadone

Also called: Dolophine

How given: IV injection, pill by mouth, liquid by mouth

How it works: Methadone is a narcotic pain reliever.

Common side effects:
- Light-headedness and dizziness
- Sedation
- Nausea and vomiting
- Sweating
- Euphoria
- Anorexia (loss of appetite)

Infrequent side effects:
- Respiratory depression
- Circulatory depression
- Shock

Morphine

How given: IV injection, pill by mouth, liquid by mouth

How it works: Morphine is a narcotic derived from the opium plant.

Common side effects:

- Euphoria
- Nausea and vomiting
- Drowsiness
- Constipation

Infrequent side effects:

- Reduction in body temperature
- Respiratory depression
- Allergic reactions, including hives
- Seizures

Oxycodone

Also called: Percocet, oxycotin

How it works: Oxycodone is a narcotic derived from opium.

Common side effects:

- Light-headedness
- Dizziness
- Sedation
- Nausea and vomiting

Infrequent side effects:

- Respiratory depression
- Skin rash

Local anesthetics to prevent pain

Two products commonly used to prevent pain are EMLA and Numby Stuff.

EMLA cream

How given: Applied to the skin and covered with an airtight dressing one to two hours before procedures such as spinal tap, bone marrow aspiration, or injection.

How it works: Emulsion which contains two anesthetics, lidocaine and prilocaine.

Note: May take longer than an hour to achieve effective anesthesia in dark-skinned individuals.

> We use EMLA for everything: finger pokes, accessing port, shots, spinal taps, and bone marrows. I even let her sister use it for shots because it lets her get a bit of attention, too. Both of my children have sensitive skin which turns red when they pull off tape, so I cover the EMLA with plastic wrap held in place with paper tape. I also fold back the edge of each piece of tape to make a pull tab so the kids don't have to peel each edge back from their skin.

Numby Stuff

How given: Needle-free method of delivering pain medication through the use of low-level electric currents applied to the skin.

How it works: Emulsion which contains two anesthetics, lidocaine and epinephrine.

Note: Anesthetizes skin and tissue in ten to fifteen minutes. Some children and teens do not like the electrical sensation that goes from the site to the battery pack.

Adjunctive treatments

In recent years there has been increasing research on mind-body medicine and its effect on coping with the side effects of illness. Adjunctive therapies are those that can be expected to add something beneficial to the ongoing treatment program. For example, imagery and hypnosis are widely used in established treatment programs to help children and teens prepare for or cope with medical procedures. Other helpful adjunctive therapies are relaxation, biofeedback, massage, visualization, acupuncture, meditation, aromatherapy, and prayer. Chapter 3, *Coping with Procedures*, discusses adjunctive therapies and how to obtain information about them.

Alternative treatments

Alternative treatments can be defined as those that are used in place of conventional medical treatment or, if used in addition to treatment, may have unknown or adverse effects. Sometimes these therapies are illegal or unavailable in the United States or Canada, and patients travel to other countries to obtain them.

Alternative treatments are usually based on word-of-mouth endorsements called anecdotal evidence. Medical therapy is based on scientific studies using large groups of patients. In treating cancer, these large clinical trials have resulted in increases in survival rates in the past three decades.

Many alternative treatments can help parents and children feel that they are aiding the healing process. Even with a good prognosis for your child, it is difficult to ignore the advice of friends and relatives extolling the virtues of various alternative treatments. Parents just want to help their children in every way possible; they often feel helpless, and they agonize over the pain and misery that their child endures for many months or years while on conventional therapy. Conventional treatment can be brutal, but it is effective in most cases.

It is extremely important that any therapy that involves ingestion or injection into the body (herbs, vitamins, special diets, enemas) only be given with the oncologist's knowledge. The involvement of the physician is necessary to prevent giving something to your child that could lessen the effectiveness of the conventional chemotherapy. For instance, folic acid (a type of B vitamin) replaces methotrexate in cells and reduces or eliminates its effectiveness, allowing cancer cells to flourish. The oncologist will be much more knowledgeable about these potential conflicts than a parent, herbalist, or health food store salesperson.

Despite the effectiveness of childhood cancer treatment, you may wish to research alternatives. Parents of children who have relapsed one or more times often are drawn to exploring these treatments. To help you evaluate claims made about alternative treatments, here are several ways to collect enough information to make an educated judgment:

- Go to or call your local American Cancer Society or Canadian Cancer Society's division office and ask for their information on the therapy you are considering. They have compiled information on many therapies describing the treatment, its known risks, side effects, opinion of the medical establishment, and any lawsuits that have been filed. The American Cancer Society has an online database at *http://www.cancer.org* with information about many alternative treatments.

- Check with the National Institutes of Health's Office of Alternative Medicine to see if any scientific evidence exists on the treatment that interests you (301) 443-3170; *http://altmed.od.nih.gov.*

- Check the Web site of the University of Texas Center for Alternative Medicine Research (UT-CAM) at *http://www.sph.uth.tmc.edu/utcam/.*

- Ask specifically what this treatment is expected to do for your child; ask what is in it; ask what tests will be done to determine whether your child needs it and whether your child is benefiting from it.

- Collect and study all available objective literature on the treatment. Ask the alternative treatment providers if they have treated other children with cancer, what results have been achieved, how these results have been documented, and where they have reported their results. Ask for the reports so that your doctor can review them.

- Talk with other people who have gone through the treatment. Inquire about the training and experience of the person administering the treatment. Be sure to find out how much the therapy costs, as your insurance company may not pay for alternative treatments.

- Beware of any practitioner who will give your child the alternative therapy only if you stop taking the child in for conventional treatments.

- Avoid spending outrageous sums of money, as these treatments are often very costly.

- Never inject any alternative product into a central line. Children have developed life-threatening infections and have died from this.

Take all the information you have gathered to your child's oncologist to discuss any positive or negative impact that it may have on your child's current medical treatment. Do not give any alternative treatment or over-the-counter drugs to your child in secret. Some treatments negate the effectiveness of chemotherapy, while other substances, such as those containing aspirin or related compounds, can cause uncontrollable bleeding in children with low platelet counts.

> At one point, we decided to try some alternative therapies with our son. Our plan was to use it in conjunction with his conventional treatment. I scheduled a meeting with his oncologist and discussed the alternatives with him. I wouldn't dare attempt to start anything, not even vitamin supplements, without first talking it over with the doctor, because I was scared that I would cause him more harm than good. I was grateful that he was willing to listen to what I had to say and offer his opinion.

> We both agreed that the alternative therapy we had in mind wouldn't do any damage or interfere with the chemotherapy he was receiving. Two months later, we decided that it was doing absolutely nothing for him, so we stopped. I figured the money would be better spent at the toy store than on a useless alternative therapy. I learned a valuable lesson from that experience. I'm much more skeptical now than I used to be. My new motto is "show me the proof."

· · · · ·

> I gave my son echinacea when he received chemotherapy. I checked with his doctor first. He didn't think it would hurt, but didn't think it would help, either. Still, all the nurses in emergency swore by the stuff. We got good results, too. We started the echinacea after lots of treatment, and it was the first time that he wasn't had to be readmitted three days after chemo for febrile neutropenia. I'm convinced that it helped him during the recovery period when his counts would bottom out.

If, after thorough investigation, you feel strongly in favor of using an alternative treatment in addition to conventional treatment and your child's oncologist adamantly opposes it, listen to his reasoning. If you disagree, go get a second opinion. Remember, the child is the most important person here. Don't give the treatment in secret or your child may be the loser.

My daughter Meagan was diagnosed with average-risk ALL over seven years ago. She had many chemotherapy-related side effects, including severe high blood pressure and ongoing liver problems. We were constantly adjusting her doses or taking her off chemo altogether. I was so obsessed about it that the doctor took me aside and told me that it's easier to treat leukemia than liver failure and he just had to take her off her medications. He told me I had to stop worrying, but I couldn't.

When her hair fell out again during maintenance, I just worried more. I realized that every child seemed to have something that went wrong, but I was amazed at how many different "somethings" there were.

Now she has a head full of gorgeous hair. She was just chosen for the select soccer team and is quite an accomplished skier. She has no long-term effects, and is healthy and happy.

CHAPTER 11

Common Side Effects of Chemotherapy

The first wealth is health.

—Ralph Waldo Emerson

CHEMOTHERAPY DRUGS INTERFERE with cancer cells' ability to grow or reproduce. Because rapidly dividing cells are more susceptible to chemotherapy drugs, cancer cells are severely affected. Unfortunately, healthy cells that multiply rapidly can be damaged as well. These normal cells include those of the bone marrow, mouth, stomach, intestines, hair follicles, and skin. This chapter explains the most common side effects of chemotherapy drugs, and explores ways to effectively deal with them. Chemotherapy side effects that prevent good nutrition are discussed in Chapter 14, *Nutrition*.

Hair loss

Chemotherapy drugs destroy not only cancer cells, but also normal cells that are produced at a rapid rate. Because hair follicle cells reproduce quickly, chemotherapy causes some or all body hair to fall out. The hair on the scalp, eyebrows, eyelashes, underarms, and pubic area may slowly thin out or may fall out in big clumps.

Hair regrowth usually starts one to three months after maintenance starts or intensive chemotherapy ends. The color and texture may be different from the original hair. Straight hair may regrow curly; blond hair may be brown. Toward the end of maintenance, some children's hair begins to thin out again.

The following suggestions for dealing with hair loss come from parents:

- When hair is thin or breaking, use a brush with very soft bristles.

- Avoid bleaches, permanents, curlers, blow dryers, or hair spray, as these may cause additional damage.

- If hair is thin, use a mild shampoo specifically designed for overtreated or damaged hair.

- A flannel receiving blanket placed on the pillow at night will help collect hair that is falling out.

- Recognize that hair loss is traumatic for all but the youngest children. It is especially hard on teenagers.

- Emphasize to your child that the hair loss is temporary and that it will grow back.

- Try to have your child meet children in maintenance or off therapy, so that they can see for themselves that hair will regrow soon.

- Allow your child or teen to choose a collection of hats, scarves, or cotton turbans to wear. These are tax-deductible medical expenses, and may be covered by insurance.

- To order several styles of reversible all cotton headwear for girls seven to twelve and women, contact Just in Time, in Philadelphia, Pennsylvania, (215) 247-8777, or online at *http://www.softhats.com*.

- If your child expresses an interest in wearing a wig, take pictures of her hairstyle prior to hair loss. Also cut snippets of hair to take in to allow a good match of original color and texture. The cost of the wig may be covered by insurance if the doctor writes a prescription for a "wig prosthesis." This should include the medical reason for the wig such as "Alopecia due to cancer chemotherapy." To find a wig retailer, look in the yellow pages of your phone book under "Hair Replacements, Goods, and Supplies." The American Cancer Society, (800) ACS-2345, and some local cancer service organizations offer free wigs in some areas. Another source for a free wig is Hair Club for Kids sponsored by Hair Club for Men in New York City, (212) 462-1400, ext. 3085.

- Advocate that school-age children be permitted to wear hats or other head coverings to school.

- Separate your feelings about baldness from your child's feelings. Many parents rush out to buy wigs and hats without discussing with their child how he wants to deal with his baldness.

- Allow your child to choose whether to wear head coverings or not. Let it be okay to be bald.

Hair loss is quite variable for children being treated for leukemia. Some only lose part of their hair, some have hair that thins out, and some quickly lose every hair on their head.

Preston never completely lost his hair, but it became extremely thin and wispy. When he was first diagnosed, a friend bought him a fly-fishing tying kit, and he became very good at tying flies. He even began selling them at a local fishing shop. When his hair began to fall out, we would gather it up and put it in a plastic bag. He started tying flies out of his hair, and they were displayed in the shop window as "Preston's Human Hair Flies." He was only eleven, but the shop owner hired him to help around the shop. He became very popular with the clientele, because everyone wanted to meet the boy who tied flies from his own hair. He really turned losing his hair into something positive.

. . . . .

Three-year-old Christine's hair started to fall out within three weeks of starting chemo. She had beautiful curly hair, but she never talked about losing it, and I thought it didn't bother her. Occasionally she would wear a hat or the hood of a sweatshirt, but most of the time she went bald. One day, I learned how she really felt. We were talking about the different colors of hair in our family, and she began shouting, "I don't have brown hair! I'm bald, just like a baby."

. . . . .

The chemo greatly affected Meagan's hair. During maintenance, it came back in lush and curly, then after a few months it began falling out again. This was very upsetting. She hasn't gone completely bald again, but it remains very thin and unhealthy hair, while others in the same stage of treatment have beautiful hair back again.

. . . . .

Jeremy, four years old, was great. Once he was watching his brother in a T-ball game when the members of the other team started to point and laugh. One started shouting, "Look at that kid, he's fat and bald." Jeremy just walked right up to him and said, "Do you know why I look this way? Because I have cancer and the chemo made my hair fall out." We bought him hats, but he never wore them.

Nausea and vomiting

The effects of anticancer drugs vary from person to person and dose to dose. A drug that makes one child violently ill often has no effect on other children. Some drugs produce no nausea until several doses have been given, while others cause nausea after a single dose. Because the effects of chemotherapy are so wildly variable, each child's treatment must be tailored to her individual needs. There is no relationship between the amount of nausea and the effectiveness of the medicine.

The following is a list of suggestions for helping children and teenagers cope with nausea and vomiting:

- Give your child antiemetic (antinausea) medications as prescribed. Do not skip any doses.

- Your child should wear loose clothing because it is both more comfortable and easier to remove if soiled.

- Parents should always have at least one change of clothes for their child in the car.

- Carry a bucket, towels, and baby wipes in the car in case of vomiting.

- Try to keep your child in a quiet, well-ventilated room after chemotherapy.

- Smells can trigger nausea. Try not to cook in the house when your child feels ill. If possible, open windows to provide plenty of fresh air.

- If your child is nauseated by smells, use a covered cup with a straw for liquids.

- Do not serve hot foods, as the odor can aggravate nausea.

- Serve dry foods such as toast, pretzels, or crackers in the morning or whenever the child is feeling nauseated.

- Serve several small meals rather than three large ones.

- Have the child keep his head elevated after eating. Lying flat can induce nausea.

- Provide plenty of clear liquids such as water, juice, Gatorade, or ginger ale.

- Avoid giving sweet, fried, or very spicy food. Instead, serve bland foods such as potatoes, cottage cheese, soup, or toast.

- Watch for any signs of dehydration. These include dry skin and mouth, sunken eyes, dizziness, and decreased urination. Call the physician if your child appears dehydrated.

- Use distractions such as TV, videos, music, games, or reading aloud to divert attention from nausea.

- After your child vomits, have him rinse his mouth with water or a mixture of water and lemon juice to remove the taste.

- If your child develops a metallic taste in her mouth, chewing gum or sucking on popsicles may help.

> *Meagan has always had problems in every phase of treatment with stomachaches, especially in the morning. She will often vomit once and then be over it. She is frequently soothed with just rubbing her tummy or laying a hot towel on it.*

If the various antinausea medications do not work well for your child, investigate the FDA-approved Relief Band. This wrist band gives an electrical stimulation (too faint to feel) to an acupuncture point in the wrist that affects the portion of the brain which controls nausea. Information about the band is available toll-free at (888) 297-9728 and online at *http://www.reliefband.com.*

Low blood counts

Bone marrow, the spongy material which fills the inside of the bones, produces red cells, white cells, and platelets. Chemotherapy drugs destroy the cells inside the bone marrow and dramatically lower the number of cells circulating in the blood. Frequent blood tests are crucial in determining whether the child needs transfusions. Most children treated for leukemia require many transfusions of red cells and platelets. Consequently, when the number of infection-fighting white cells is low, the child is in danger of developing serious infections.

What is an ANC? (also called AGC)

The activities of families of children with leukemia revolve around the sick child's white count, specifically the absolute neutrophil count (ANC). This is sometimes called an absolute granulocyte count (AGC). The ANC (or AGC) provides an indication of the child's ability to fight infection.

When a child has blood drawn for a complete blood count (CBC), one section of the lab report will state the total white blood cell (WBC) count and a "differential." This means that each type of white blood cell will be listed as a percentage of the total. For example, if the total WBC count is 1500 mm^3, the differential might appear as in the following table:

White Blood Cell Type	Percentage of Total WBC
Segmented neutrophils (also called polys or segs)	49%
Band neutrophils (also called bands)	1%
Basophils (also called basos)	1%
Eosinophils (also called eos)	1%
Lymphocytes (also called lymphs)	38%
Monocytes (also called monos)	10%

To calculate the ANC, add the percentages of neutrophils and bands, and multiply by the total WBC. Using the example above, the ANC is 49% + 1% = 50%. 50% of 1500 (.50 × 1500) = 750. The ANC is 750.

> Erica ran a fever whenever her counts were low, but nothing ever grew in her cultures. They would hospitalize her for 48 hours as a precaution. She was never on a full dose of medicine because of her chronically low counts. She's two years off treatment now and doing great.

How to protect the child with a low ANC

Generally, an ANC over 1000 provides the child enough protective neutrophils to fight off exposure to infection due to bacteria and fungi. With an ANC this high, you can usually allow your child to attend all normal functions such as school, athletics, and parties. However, it is wise to keep close track of the pattern of the rise and fall of your child's ANC. If you know that the ANC is 1000, but is on the way down, it will affect your decision on what activities are appropriate. Each hospital has different guidelines concerning appropriate activities for children with low ANCs.

The following are parent suggestions to prevent and detect infections:

- Insist on frequent, thorough hand washing for every member of the family. Use plenty of soap and warm water, lather well, and rub all portions of the hands. Children and parents need to wash before preparing meals, before eating, after playing outdoors, and after using the bathroom.

> We always had antibacterial baby wipes in our car. We washed Justin's hands, and our own, after going to any public places such as parks,

museums, or restaurants. They can also be used to wipe off tables or high chairs at restaurants.

- Make sure that all medical personnel at the hospital or doctor's office wash their hands before touching your child.

- Keep your child's diaper area and skin creases clean and dry.

- When your child's ANC is low, make arrangements with your pediatrician to use a back entrance to the office to avoid exposure to sick kids in the waiting room. It sometimes helps to make all appointments for early morning so that your child can be seen in a room that hasn't had several sick children in it.

- Whenever your child needs a needle stick, make sure that the technician cleans your child's skin thoroughly with both betadine and alcohol.

- If your child gets a small cut, wash with soap and water, rinse with hydrogen peroxide, and cover with a Band-Aid.

- Take your child's temperature every day at the same time. When your child is ill, take his temperature every two to three hours.

- Do not take the temperature rectally (in the anus) or use rectal suppositories, as these may cause anal tears and increase the risk of infection and bleeding.

- Do not use a humidifier, as the stagnant water can become a reservoir for contamination.

- Apply sunscreen whenever your child plays outdoors. Children taking methotrexate are sun-sensitive, and a bad sunburn can easily become a site for infection.

- Your child should not be vaccinated while on chemotherapy.

- Siblings should not be vaccinated with the live polio virus (OPV). They should get the killed polio virus (IPV). Verify that your pediatrician is using the appropriate vaccine for the siblings.

> *Katy was diagnosed just a week after her younger sister Alison had been given the live polio vaccine. Because there was a small risk that Alison could infect any immunosuppressed child with polio, we were not allowed to stay on the cancer floor of the hospital.*

- If your child's ANC is low, an infected site may not become red or painful.

My daughter kept getting ear infections while on chemotherapy. They would find them during routine exams. I felt guilty because she never told me her ears were hurting. I told her doctor that I was worried because she didn't complain of pain, and he reassured me by telling me that she probably felt no pain because she didn't have enough white cells to cause swelling inside her ear.

· · · · ·

Shawn had continual ear infections while on treatment. He had two sets of tubes surgically implanted while on chemotherapy.

- Never give aspirin, Motrin, or ibuprofen for fever. They may interfere with blood clotting. If your child has a fever, call the doctor before giving any medication.

- Call the doctor if any of the following symptoms appear: fever above 101°F (38.5°C), chills, cough, shortness of breath, sore throat, severe diarrhea, bloody urine or stool, and pain or burning while urinating.

Whenever my daughter (diagnosed when one year old) was on antibiotics (frequently), she developed a vaginal yeast infection. It was very painful for her and a nightmare for me.

· · · · ·

My son's big toes became large and red from ingrown toenails while on treatment. He had several surgeries to remove the corners of each nail to prevent infection. That was several years ago, and his toes look bad but are not painful.

Two serious infections that plague children during treatment for leukemia are pneumonia and chicken pox.

Pneumonia

Pneumonia is inflammation of the lungs caused primarily by bacteria or viruses. The symptoms of pneumonia are rapid breathing, chills, fever, chest pain, cough, and bloody sputum. Children with low blood counts can rapidly develop a fatal infection, and must be treated quickly and aggressively. The following are three experiences from veteran parents whose children survived pneumonia.

My son received his high-dose methotrexate and vincristine injection just days before he was scheduled to go to the American Cancer Society's camp. His ANC was 1200 and he looked so sick, but he begged to go and I let him. It was early in his treatment and I didn't realize the pattern of his blood counts. They called me from camp on Friday to say he had a temperature of 103° and needed to go to the hospital. He was very weak and feverish; his WBC was 140, and his ANC was 0. Both lungs were full of pneumonia. I was furious at the doctor for giving him permission to go to camp and at myself for not paying closer attention to how quickly his counts dropped. I'm sure he had the pneumonia before he even went to camp. They started him on five different antibiotics, and his fever went up to 106° that night. We didn't know if he would live or die. He started to gradually improve the next morning and was completely recovered in a week.

. . . . .

At the beginning of interim maintenance, Justin developed a fever. His oncologist said to give him Tylenol and call if it didn't go down. The next day he was breathing faster and his little hands and feet were turning purple. We rushed him to the hospital, and the chest x-rays showed pneumonia in both lungs. He rapidly deteriorated over the next 48 hours, so they tried an experimental constant flow ventilator which had only been used on premature infants. It was the last-ditch effort to save his life. He gradually improved. He spent a total of five months in the hospital, four more months on a portable ventilator at home with full-time nursing care, and he breathed through his tracheostomy until he completed his treatment two years later. It was a miracle.

. . . . .

Erica complained that her back hurt for two days. Then she woke up in the night crying, and she couldn't move because it hurt her too badly. She was blazing with fever, and screamed if I touched her. Her x-ray showed that her left lung was half full of fluid. They put her on antibiotics, and within 24 hours she was on the mend.

Chicken pox

Chicken pox is a common childhood disease caused by a virus called varicella zoster. The symptoms are headache, fever, and malaise, rapidly followed by eruptions of pimple-like red bumps. The bumps typically start on the stomach, chest, or back. They rapidly develop into blister-like sores which break open, then scab over in three to five days. Any contact with the sores can spread the disease.

Chicken pox can be a fatal disease for immunosuppressed children, so extreme care must be taken to prevent exposure. Children are contagious up to 48 hours prior to breaking out. It will be necessary to educate all teachers and friends to be vigilant in reporting any outbreaks. The child can then be kept home from school or preschool until the outbreak is over.

If an immunosuppressed child is exposed to chicken pox, call the doctor immediately. If the doctor is able to administer a shot called VZIG (Varicella Zoster Immune Globin) within 72 hours of exposure, it may prevent the disease from occurring or minimize its effects.

> We knew when Jeremy was exposed, so he was able to get VZIG. He did get chicken pox, but only developed a few spots. He didn't get sick; he got bored. He spent two weeks in the hospital in isolation. We asked for a pass, and we were able to go outside for some fresh air between doses of acyclovir.

If a child develops chicken pox while on chemotherapy, the current treatment is hospitalization or, if possible, home therapy for IV administration of acyclovir, a potent antiviral medication. This drug has dramatically lowered the complication rate of chicken pox.

> Kristin broke out with chicken pox on the Fourth of July weekend. Our hospital room was the best seat in the house for watching the city fireworks. She did get covered with pox, though, from the soles of her feet to the very top of her scalp. We'd just give her gauze pads soaked in calamine lotion and let her hermetically seal herself. They kept her in the hospital for six days of IV acyclovir, then she was at home on the pump (a small computerized machine that will administer the drug in small amounts for several hours) for four more days of acyclovir. She had no complications.

A child who has already had chicken pox may develop herpes zoster (shingles). If your child develops eruptions of vesicles similar to chicken pox which are in lines (along nerves), call the doctor. The treatment for shingles is identical to that for chicken pox.

> Kristin also got a herpes zoster infection, this time on Thanksgiving. It looked like a mild case of chicken pox, limited to her upper right arm,

her upper right chest, and her right leg. They kept her overnight on IV
acyclovir and then let her go home for nine more days on the pump.

Chicken pox can be transmitted through the air or by touch. Exposure is considered to have occurred if a child is in direct contact or in a room for as little as ten minutes with an infected person. If your child has never had chicken pox, it is better to take him to beaches or parks rather than indoor play areas.

Untreated chicken pox or shingles can result in life-threatening complications including pneumonia, hepatitis, and encephalitis. Parents must make every effort to prevent exposure and be vigilant in watching for signs of the diseases while their child is on treatment.

An immunization for chicken pox has been developed which may be given to children with leukemia in the near future. Currently, there is insufficient data to evaluate its usefulness or safety in children with leukemia.

Can pets transmit diseases?

It is very unlikely that your child will be harmed from living with a household pet, but several common sense precautions are needed to protect a child with a low ANC from disease, worms, or infection:

- Make sure that the animal is vaccinated against all possible diseases.

- Have pets checked for worms as soon as possible after your child is diagnosed, and then every year thereafter (more often for puppies).

- Do not let pets eat off plates or lick your child's face.

- Keep children away from the cat litter box and any animal feces outdoors.

- Have children wash hands after playing with the pet.

- Make sure that your pet has no ticks or fleas.

- If you have a pet that bites or scratches, consider finding another home for it. On the other hand, if you have a gentle, well-loved pet, do not give it up.

I think parents should know that you should not automatically get rid of your dog because your child has a low ANC. We went through a small crisis trying to decide whether to give away our large but beloved mongrel. The doctors wouldn't really give us a straight answer, but a parent in the support group said, "DO NOT get rid of your dog. Your son will need that dog's love and company in the years ahead." She was right. The dog was a tremendous comfort to our son.

If your child wants to buy a pet while undergoing treatment for cancer, here are some suggestions:

- Do not get a puppy. All puppies bite while teething, increasing the chance that your child may contract an infection.

- Do not get a parrot or parakeet as these species can transmit psittacosis.

- Do not get a turtle or other reptile (snake, iguana) as they sometimes carry salmonella.

- Avoid buying any animal that is likely to bite or scratch.

We bought Sarah an older puppy. We were very selective about the breeder and the breed. The dog has given my little girl back to me. After she got the dog, she started to want to walk again. She started to laugh. She had reason to think beyond herself and how terrible this illness is. She had someone who needed her. Someone who was delighted to see her and made her feel special in a way no human can. It literally transformed my child.

The dog's name is Libbe, and after having Libbe for about a week, Sarah started asking when Libbe was going to die. She knew Libbe was just a baby, a puppy, but she really was asking about herself. We were able to tell her that Libbe will be around when she is a teenager and she can take Libbe with her on those big-girl sleepovers. Heck, she could take Libbe in the car for a ride, if she wanted. She beamed. It put the death and dying issue to rest.

If you have any concerns or questions about pets you already own or are thinking of purchasing, ask your oncologist for advice.

Diarrhea

Chemotherapy destroys cancer cells, as well as any cells that are produced at a rapid rate such as those that line the mouth, stomach, and intestines. This damage can cause diarrhea, ranging from mild (frequent, soft stools) to severe (copious quantities of liquid stool). Diarrhea during chemotherapy can also be caused by some antinausea drugs, antibiotics, or intestinal infections. After chemotherapy ends and immune function returns to normal, the lining of the digestive tract heals and the diarrhea ends.

The following suggestions for coping with diarrhea come from parents:

- Do not give any over-the-counter drug to your child without approval from the doctor. He may want to test your child's stool for infection prior to treating the diarrhea. Frequently recommended drugs for diarrhea are Kaopectate, Lomotil, or Immodium.

- It is very important that your child drinks plenty of liquids. This will not increase the diarrhea, but will replace the fluids lost.

  My three-year-old had stopped drinking from bottles months before her diagnosis. When she first began her intensive chemotherapy, she had uncontrollable, frequent diarrhea. Liquid would just gush out without warning. It was hard for her to drink from a cup, so one night she said in a small voice, "Mommy, would it be okay if I drank from a bottle again?" I said, "Of course, honey." It was a great comfort to her, and she took in a lot more fluids that way.

- Hot or cold liquids can increase intestinal contractions, so serve lots of room-temperature clear liquids or mild juices such as water, Gatorade, ginger ale, peach juice, or apricot juice.

- Diarrhea depletes the body's supply of potassium. Provide foods high in potassium such as bananas, oranges, baked or mashed potatoes without the skin, broccoli, halibut, mushrooms, asparagus, tomato juice, and milk (if tolerated).

- Low potassium can cause irregular heartbeats and leg cramps. If these occur, call the doctor.

- Do not serve greasy, fatty, spicy, or sweet foods.

- Do not serve roughage such as bran, fruits (dried or fresh), nuts, beans, or raw vegetables.

- Do serve bland, low-fiber foods such as bananas, white rice, noodles, applesauce, unbuttered white toast, creamed cereals, cottage cheese, fish, and chicken or turkey without the skin.

  In the middle of maintenance, my son had severe diarrhea for a week. He had large amounts of liquid stools twenty times a day. I felt so sorry for him. The doctor cultured a stool specimen, but they never identi-

fied a cause. It cleared up after a week of the BRAT diet (bananas, rice, applesauce, toast). He had a problem with diarrhea almost weekly throughout his treatment.

- Keep a record of the number of bowel movements and their volume to keep the doctor informed. Call the doctor if you notice any blood in the stool, or if your child has any signs of dehydration such as dry skin, dry mouth, sunken eyes, decreased urination, or dizziness.

- Keep the area around the anus clean and dry. Wash with warm water and mild soap after every bowel movement. Pat dry gently.

- If the anus is sore, check with the doctor before using any non-prescription medicine. She may recommend using Desitin or A&D ointment after each bowel movement.

> *While taking ARA-C my daughter had a terribly sore rectum, which was a big problem. It hurt to have bowel movements, she'd cry and have to squeeze our hands to go, then the urine would run back and burn. She was very itchy. We carried around bags with Q-tips and every known brand of rectal ointment—A&D, Preparation H, Desitin, Benadryl. Thank goodness this cleared up quickly on maintenance.*

- Call the doctor if your child has significant pain with bowel movements, especially if your child has low blood counts.

Constipation

Constipation means a decrease in the normal number of bowel movements. There are many reasons that constipation occurs on chemotherapy. Some drugs, such as vincristine, slow the movement of the stool through the intestines, resulting in constipation. Pain medication, decreased activity, decreased eating and drinking, and vomiting can all affect the normal rhythm of the intestine. When movement through the intestine slows, stools become hard and dry.

The following are parents' suggestions for preventing and helping constipation:

- To prevent constipation, encourage your child to be as physically active as possible.

- Encourage your child to drink plenty of liquid a day. Prune juice is especially helpful.

- Prepare high-fiber foods such as raw vegetables, beans, bran, graham crackers, whole wheat breads, whole grain cereals, dried fruits (especially prunes, dates, and raisins), and nuts

- Check with the doctor prior to using any medications for constipation. He may recommend a stool softener like colace. If the doctor suggests liquid ducosate, be aware that many kids don't like the taste. Metamucil or citrucel increases the volume of the stool, which stimulates the intestine. Milk of magnesia or magnesium citrate helps the stool retain fluid and remain soft.

- Do not give enemas or rectal suppositories. These can cause anal tears which can be dangerous for a child with a weakened immune system.

- When your child feels the need to have a bowel movement, sipping a warm drink can help.

> My four-year-old daughter either had diarrhea or severe constipation for the entire eight months of intensive treatment. Her bowel habits returned to normal during maintenance. When constipated, she would just sob and try to hold it in. This made her stool even harder and more painful. One time she cried, "Why is my anus round and my poop square?" We ended up just putting her in a warm bathtub, gave her warm drinks, and let her go in the bathtub.

Fatigue and weakness

Fatigue is a feeling of weariness, which is an almost universal side effect of treatment for cancer. General weakness, while different from fatigue, is caused by many of the same things, and is treated the same way. Fatigue and weakness may be constant throughout therapy or intermittent. They can be minor annoyances or totally debilitating. Many parents worry that if fatigue is present, so is the cancer, but this is not the case. Fatigue and weakness can be caused by one, or a combination, of the following things:

- Your child's body working overtime to heal tissues damaged by treatment and to rid itself of dead and dying cancer cells

- Medications to treat nausea or pain

- Mineral imbalances caused by chemotherapy, diarrhea, or vomiting

- Infection

- Emotional factors such as anxiety, fear, sadness, depression, or frustration

- Malnutrition caused by nausea, vomiting, loss of appetite, or taste aversions

- Anemia (low red cell count)

- Disruption of normal sleep patterns (common when hospitalized or when taking prednisone)

> My son is almost nineteen and just beginning his third year of maintenance for ALL. He is a quiet and studious young man, has never dated, and does not go about partying and the like. The last three months, he appears to be all right, but he is, in his own words, always "exhausted." In college and living in the dorm, he can get up in the morning at six, but if he has two classes in a row, he is quite likely to fall asleep during the second class. He's too tired to concentrate on homework for more than an hour at a time. Before diagnosis, a 50-mile bike ride was nothing to him. Even six months ago, he could ride 30 miles, although he did feel some fatigue. Now, his beloved bike rests gathering dust. It breaks my heart that my son cannot feel the exuberance of young adulthood that I experienced at his age, but I am so very thankful that the treatment for leukemia has saved his life. I hope that when he is off treatment he will finally feel good again.

The following are suggestions from parents:

- Make sure that your child gets plenty of rest. Naps or quiet times spaced throughout the day help.

> Erica took a two-and-a-half-hour nap every afternoon throughout therapy. She's four now and off treatment, but her endurance is low and she still tires easily.

- Limit visitors if your child is weak or fatigued.

> While in the hospital, my daughter was very weak. She had too many visitors, yet didn't want to hurt anyone's feelings. We worked out a signal that solved the problem. When she was too tired to continue a visit, she would place a damp washcloth on her forehead. I would then politely end the visit.

- Serve your child well-balanced meals and snacks, but don't get upset if he doesn't eat them (see next point).

- Parents and children should try to avoid physical or emotional stress.

- Encourage child to pursue hobbies or interests if able. For example, if your child is too weak to play on his athletic team, let him go to cheer the team on.

    My four-year-old daughter wanted desperately to be in the annual kid's parade in our town. She could barely stand, much less march in a parade. So I put her in a big red wagon lined with blankets, and pulled her the entire way. I think she got more cheers than the floats!

- Help your child make a prioritized list of activities. If he feels strongly that he wants to attend a certain function, and you think he may run out of energy, throw a wheelchair or stroller into the car and go.

- Encourage your child to attend a kid or teen support group, and go to the parent group yourself. Seeing that others have the same problems and talking about how you are feeling can lighten the load.

Many children breeze through the low- or average-risk protocols for leukemia without fatigue or weakness, while other children are not so lucky. The following are two typical stories.

Before Brent was diagnosed at age six, he was exceptionally well coordinated and a very fast runner. During treatment, he slowed down to about average. He played soccer and T-ball throughout, and was very competitive.

· · · · ·

Jeremy has had some major, persistent problems with weakness and loss of coordination. When he was nine years old, a year off therapy, he still could not catch a ball. When he ran, he was like a robot, and the trunk of his body stayed straight. Some kids made fun of him, and he got very frustrated with himself. He had lots of physical therapy, and now, three years off chemotherapy, his skills have improved, but he still has to work harder than the other kids. We put him into martial arts in hopes of further increasing his motor skills and his confidence.

Bed wetting

Bed wetting, although infrequent, can be a very upsetting side effect of chemotherapy. Some drugs increase thirst, while others disrupt normal sleep patterns, both of which can make bed wetting more likely. Lots of IV fluids at night are a problem for some children. When the bed wetting is caused by drugs or IVs, time will cure the problem. Once the drug or extra fluid is no longer necessary, the bed wetting will stop.

There are also psychological reasons for bed wetting during chemotherapy. The trauma of the treatment for cancer causes many children to regress to earlier behaviors such as thumb sucking, baby talk, temper tantrums, and bed wetting. Punishment for this type of bed wetting only adds to the child's trauma and rarely solves the problem. The following are veteran parents' suggestions:

- Double-sheet the bed. Put down one plastic liner with fitted and flat sheets, then put on top another plastic liner with fitted and flat sheet. During the night, simply pull off the top sheets and plastic, and there are fresh sheets below.

- Keep a pile of extra-large or beach towels next to the bed. Cover the wet spot with towels, and save the bed change for the morning.

- Give the last drink two hours before bedtime, to allow the child's bladder to totally empty right before bed.

- Change sleeping arrangements.

> Prednisone caused my child to have nightmares and frequent bed wetting. I felt if she could sleep through the night, the bed wetting might stop. I told her she could sleep with me for the month that she was on prednisone, but that after that she would move back into her own bed. It calmed her to sleep with me. The nightmares and bed wetting decreased, and she moved back into her own bed without complaint when the time came.

- Adopt an attitude that lets the child know that bed wetting is "no big deal." There should be no shaming or punishment.

- If the child is extremely distressed by his bed wetting, ask him if he wants you to set the alarm for the middle of the night in order to help him get up to go to the bathroom.

> Alex was potty-trained during consolidation. He would get major hydration with the high dose-methotrexate, but he never had a accident. We brought his potty with us to the hospital and kept it right next to his bed. If he had to go during the night he would just get out of bed and go. It worked out really well, and you can empty it in the morning.

- Give extra love and reassurance.

When my daughter started bed wetting, I didn't think it was the drugs. I thought long and hard about any additional worries that she might have, and I realized that because her dad had emotionally with-drawn from her during her illness, she might be worried that I would do the same. So I told her one night, "You know, I just realized that every day I tell you how much I love you. But I've never told you that no matter how hard life gets and no matter how mad we get at each other I will always love you. I love you now as a child, I will love you as a teenager, and I will love you when you are all grown up." She started to sob and hugged and hugged me. She has never wet the bed again.

· · · · ·

My teenaged son wet the bed whenever he was given antinausea medicine prior to high doses of chemotherapy. He was so embarrassed. I stayed with him every night at the hospital. He was so groggy that even if he woke up in time, I had to help him out of bed and support him while he stood, half asleep, to use the urinal.

· · · · ·

My son wet the bed before, during, and after the three years of his treatment for ALL. We just kept him in diapers at night. He would abso-lutely flood the bed while on prednisone. After he completed treatment, they put him on a drug called DDAVP to help cure the bed wetting.

Dental problems

Both radiation and chemotherapy can cause changes in the mouth and teeth. Awareness of the potential problems coupled with good preventive care can help keep your child more comfortable during treatment.

Some anticancer drugs and radiation can cause changes in children's ability to salivate. Plaque may build up rapidly on your child's teeth, increasing the chance for both cavities and gum infections. Take your child to the dentist for cleaning and check-up every three to four months, as long as his counts are good (ANC more than 1000, platelets more than 100,000). If your child has a central venous catheter (Hickman or Port-a-cath), he should be given antibiotics before and after each visit to the dentist. Ask your dentist to refer to the current issue of the *Pediatric Dentistry Reference Manual* to formulate a dental plan.

Get recommendations from your child's oncologist and dentist for advice on tooth care when counts are very low. Often parents are advised to use a sponge or damp gauze to gently wipe off their child's teeth after meals instead of brushing.

> My daughter had problems with thick yellow saliva during the entire time she was treated. It coated her teeth and formed a lot of plaque. I brought her to an excellent pediatric dentist every three months to have the plaque removed. She took antibiotics half an hour before treatment and then again six hours afterward. He also put sealants on all of her molars and, even though there were many weeks when her teeth could not be brushed, she never got a cavity.

Mouth and throat sores

The mouth and throat are lined with cells which divide rapidly and can be severely damaged by chemotherapy drugs. This is more common for children on very intensive protocols and those having bone marrow transplants. The sores are very painful and can prevent eating and drinking. Check your child's mouth periodically for sores, and if any are present ask advice from the oncologist. Some parent suggestions are:

- To prevent infection, the mouth needs to be kept as clean and free of bacteria as possible. After eating, have your child gently brush teeth, gums, and tongue with a soft, clean toothbrush.

- If your child is old enough, the doctor may recommend a rinse to prevent mouth sores.

> When David was told to use Peridex, I asked the doctor if we could substitute 0.63 percent stannous fluoride rinse. He said yes. As a dentist, I knew Peridex killed bacteria and lasts up to eight hours, but it tastes terrible and stains teeth. Patients did not like using it. The 0.63 percent stannous fluoride had the same bacteria killing properties and also lasts up to eight hours, but has a better taste and does not stain as badly. The fluoride also helps prevent cavities, and makes the teeth less sensitive. It comes in a variety of flavors like mint, tropical, and cinnamon. It is a prescription drug that a lot of dentists dispense.

One mixes 1/8 oz. of concentrate with warm water, making 1 oz. A measuring cup comes with the bottle. I have David swish with half the mixture for one minute (time it because it's longer than you think!). This can only be used by kids who are old enough to not accidentally swallow it. Six-year-old David has no problem taking this once a day before he goes to bed. If and when he starts developing mouth sores, he will take it morning and evening. It's important not to eat or drink for 30 minutes after rinsing. That is why David rinses before bedtime, after he has taken his meds and brushed his teeth.

- Serve bland food, meals put through the blender, or baby food.

- Use a straw with drinks or blender-processed food.

Preston got bad mouth sores every time he was on high-dose methotrexate. He could not swallow, but we were supposed to be forcing fluids to flush the drugs out. The only thing that felt good on his throat was guava nectar. It was very expensive and hard to find, and he would drink several quarts a day. Unfortunately, my daughter and husband both developed a liking for it, too. At one point we cornered the market on guava nectar at three grocery stores in our neighborhood.

- There are several prescription products available to treat mouth sores. One common product is called Magic Mouthwash, containing equal parts of Benadryl, Nystatin, Maalox, and viscous Xylocaine. Some formulations add dexamethasone. If your child has painful mouth sores, ask the oncologist for a prescription. Since large amounts of lidocaine can numb the back of the throat and cause difficulty swallowing, this medication should be used at a dose recommended by the oncologist.

Changes in taste and smell

Chemotherapy can cause changes in the taste buds, altering the brain's perception of how food tastes. Meats often taste bitter, and sweets can taste unpleasant. Even foods that children crave taste bad. The sense of smell is also impacted by chemotherapy. Smells can be heightened so that smells which other family members are unaware of can cause nausea in a child on chemotherapy.

Both the sense of smell and taste can take months to return to normal after chemotherapy ends.

Once Katy begged me to make her my special double chocolate sour cream cake. Surprisingly, it smelled really good to her as it baked. She took a big bite, spit it out all over the table, and ran back to her room sobbing. She cried for a long time. She told me later that it had tasted "bitter and horrible."

Skin and nail problems

Minor skin problems are frequent while on chemotherapy. The most common problems are rashes, redness, itching, peeling, dry skin, and acne. The following are suggestions for preventing and treating skin problems:

- Avoid hot showers or baths, as these can dry the skin.

- Use moisturizing soap such as Basic or Avena.

- Apply a water-based moisturizer after bathing.

- Avoid scratchy materials such as wool. Your child may feel more comfortable in loose, cotton clothing.

- Have your child use sunscreen with a sun protection factor of at least SPF 30.

- If your child is bald, and especially if she has had cranial radiation, insist on head coverings or sunscreen every time she goes outdoors.

- Buy your child lip gloss with sunscreen.

- If your child has chemotherapy drugs injected into the veins (rather than a central catheter), you may notice a darkening along the vein. This will fade after chemotherapy ends.

- Skin and underlying tissues can be damaged or destroyed by drugs which leak out of a vein. If your child feels a stinging or burning sensation, or you notice swelling at the IV site, call a nurse immediately.

- Rubbing cornstarch on itchy skin is often soothing.

- Call the doctor anytime your child gets a severe rash or is very itchy. Scratching rashes can cause infections, so you need to get medications to control the itching.

Chemotherapy affects the growing portion of nails located under the cuticle. After chemotherapy, you may notice a white band or ridge across the nail as it grows out. These brittle bands are sometimes elevated and feel bumpy. As the white ridge grows out toward the end of the finger, the nail may break. Keeping your child's fingernails trimmed can help prevent breakage.

Learning disabilities

Some children who have been treated for leukemia are at risk of developing learning disabilities as a consequence of their treatment. Those at highest risk are children under five years old who receive both cranial radiation and intrathecal methotrexate, children who were on a high-dose methotrexate protocol, and young children who are given significant dosages of intrathecal methotrexate. There is considerable research on the types of learning difficulties exhibited by these children. This information is covered fully in Chapter 15, *School*.

Eating problems

Most children have major nutritional problems while on chemotherapy. Chapter 14, is devoted to explaining eating problems such as anorexia (lack of appetite), food aversions, overeating, and the myriad other problems induced by chemotherapy and radiation.

There were times during my son's protocol that I felt he suffered more from the side effects of treatment than from the disease. It was emotionally painful for me to watch him go through so much. I think one of the hardest moments for me was the day he lost all his hair. Up until that point I had been living in a semi-state of denial. His bald head was more proof of our reality—he really did have cancer.

I had to learn how to accept our situation, because I needed to be strong for my child. To get through, I reminded myself every day that the treatments were necessary and that without them he would die. It was a struggle, but the unpleasant side effects soon passed and he was able to resume his normal activities. I was constantly amazed at his resilience.

CHAPTER 12

Radiation

Nothing is so strong as gentleness,
and nothing is so gentle as true strength.

—St. Francis De Sales

RADIATION IS A LIFE-SAVING THERAPY that has dramatically improved survival rates of children with high-risk leukemia. However, radiation therapy to the brain, spine, or testes can cause mild, short-term side effects, and sometimes permanent damage that may not be evident until months or years after treatment. The benefits and risks of treatment with radiation must be carefully weighed by both doctors and parents.

This chapter will help parents understand what radiation is, when and how it is used, and what side effects could develop. It will dispel myths and alleviate concerns by clearly explaining what the parent and child can expect from radiation treatment.

What is radiation?

Radiation treatment, also called irradiation or radiotherapy, is the use of high-energy x-rays to kill cancer cells. A large machine called a linear accelerator directs x-rays to the precise portion of the body needing treatment. The treatment is usually given in small doses measured in units called centigrays or rads (short for radiation-absorbed dose). Radiation is usually given every day for ten to sixteen days, excluding weekends. The daily doses allow smaller amounts of radiation to be used, lessening side effects and allowing any damaged normal cells to heal. Children do not become radioactive from these treatments.

Who needs radiation treatment?

Because of the possibility of long-term side effects from treating children with radiation, only 10 to 12 percent of children with leukemia receive radiation. Some of the children for whom radiation is prescribed are:

- Children who have leukemia blasts in their central nervous system (CNS) at diagnosis.

- Children who are determined to be at high risk of relapse in the central nervous system, for example, those with white counts above 100,000/ mm^3 at diagnosis.

- Children who have relapsed in their central nervous system or testes.

- Children who will undergo a bone marrow transplant.

Treatment for childhood leukemia is constantly evolving. Even as this book is being written, several ongoing clinical trials are evaluating alternative methods for CNS prophylaxis. Perhaps in the near future, no child with leukemia will need radiation. But for the present, although there are possible side effects, radiation to the brain provides children with certain types of high-risk leukemia or CNS leukemia the best chance to be cured.

When is radiation treatment given?

Cranial radiation is most effective if given after remission is achieved, usually at the beginning of the consolidation phase. For children who have relapsed, cranial, spinal, and/or testicular radiation is prescribed at the beginning of consolidation in the relapse protocol.

Questions to ask about radiation treatment

- Why does my child need radiation?
- What type of radiation does she need?
- What part of her body will be treated with radiation?
- What is the total dose of radiation that she will receive?
- How many treatments of radiation will be necessary?
- How much experience does this institution have in administering this type of radiation to children?
- How will she be positioned on the table?

- Will any restraints be used?

- Will anesthesia or sedation be used?

- How long will each treatment take?

- What are the possible short-term and long-term side effects?

- Could this type and dosage of radiation cause cancer later?

- What are the alternatives to radiation?

Where should your child go for radiation treatment?

To have optimal treatment, children should receive radiation therapy only at major medical centers with experience in treating children with cancer. Do not go to a local radiation center or the radiation department in your community hospital. All treatments should be supervised by physicians who are board-certified or equally experienced in radiation oncology. State-of-the-art equipment, expert personnel, and vast experience with pediatric cancers are what you should look for in choosing a center.

Radiation oncologist

A radiation oncologist is a medical doctor with years of specialized training in using radiation to treat disease. Other names for this type of specialist are radiotherapist, radiation therapist, or therapeutic radiologist. In partnership with the pediatric oncologist, the radiation oncologist develops a treatment plan tailored specifically for each individual child.

The radiation oncologist will explain to both child and parents what radiation is, how it will be administered, and any possible side effects. She will answer all questions regarding the proposed treatment. Parents will be given a consent form to review prior to signing. Take the consent form home if you need extra time to read it. Parents should not sign the consent form until they thoroughly understand all benefits, risks, and possible side effects of the radiation. The radiation oncologist will meet at least weekly with child and parents to discuss how the treatment is going and to address concerns or answer questions.

Radiation therapist

The radiation therapist is a specially trained technologist who operates the machine that delivers the dose of radiation prescribed by the radiation oncologist. This member of the medical team will give the child a tour of the radiation room, explain about the equipment, and position the child for treatment. The technologist will operate the x-ray machine, and will monitor the child via closed-circuit TV and a two-way intercom.

> When three-year-old Katy was being given the tour of the radiation room by her technologist, Brian, he was just wonderful with her. He gave her a white stuffed bear which he used to demonstrate the machine. He immobilized the bear on the table using Katy's mask (device to hold the head still during treatment), then moved the machine all around it so that she could hear the sounds made by the equipment. He then took a Polaroid picture of the bear on the table, in the mask, for Katy to take home with her.

Masks

To immobilize very young children, a mask of the youngster's face is made to hold the head perfectly still during the cranial radiation treatment. Great care should be taken to ensure that making the mask is not traumatic. This can often be accomplished by utilizing play therapy to demonstrate the procedure.

Masks are made from a lightweight, porous, mesh material. First, the technologist should explain and demonstrate the entire mask-making process to the child. The child then lies down on a table. The technologist places a sheet of the mask material in warm water to soften it. This warm mesh sheet is placed over the child's face and quickly molded to her features. The child can breathe the entire time through the mesh material but must hold still for several minutes as the mask hardens. The mask is lifted off the child's face, and the technologist cuts holes in it for the eyes, nostrils, and mouth.

> The cancer center staff had scheduled two hours for mask-making for my three-year-old daughter. I asked them to very quietly explain every step in the process. I told her that I would be holding her hand, and I promised that it would not hurt, but it would feel warm. I asked her to choose a story for me to recite as they molded the warm material to her face to make the time go faster. She picked "Curious George Goes to the Hospital." She held perfectly still; I recited the story; the staff were gentle and quick; and the entire procedure took less than twenty minutes.

· · · · ·

Shawn (two years old) needed to be sedated for his ten doses of radiation. They also made his mask while he was anesthetized.

Other immobilization devices

Different institutions use a variety of devices to immobilize children to ensure that the radiation beam is directed with precision. These are also used on adults who receive radiation. Some of the products used are custom-made plaster of paris casts, thermal plastic devices, vacuum-molded thermoplastics, and polyurethane foam forms. Custom-fitting the forms on a child who has already undergone numerous painful procedures requires skill and patience. Immobilization devices can be fitted on well-prepared, calm children or sedated children. The following are parent suggestions for preparing a child for the fitting of her immobilization device:

• Give the child a tour of the room where the fitting will take place.

• Explain in clear language each step in the process.

• Be honest in describing any discomfort the child may experience.

• For small children, fit the device onto a mannequin or stuffed animal to demonstrate the process.

• For older children or teenagers, show a video or read a booklet describing the procedure.

Seventeen-month-old Rachel was fitted with two immobilization devices. They made a mask to hold her head in position, as well as a body mold from her neck to her thighs.

The more time spent on preparation, the less time will be spent on fitting a device. If the fitting goes well, it establishes trust and good feelings that will help make the actual radiation treatments proceed smoothly.

After relapsing while on treatment, Stephan (seven years old) needed cranial and spinal radiation. I took him on a tour and explained in detail what would happen. All of his questions were answered. He would go in, have the black marks put on, and lie face down on a bed. There was a thing for his forehead to rest on, but he didn't require any other supports. He would just hold perfectly still. We kept a bucket next to the bed, because he was on high dose ARA-C, and after his radiation session, he would often need to lean over and vomit.

He was so wonderful about it. He would go up to all of the older patients who were awaiting treatment and chat. He really reached out to them, and their eyes would just sparkle.

Sedation

All infants, most preschoolers, and some school-age children require sedation or anesthesia to ensure that they will remain perfectly still during the radiation treatment. Most radiation facilities use a combination of anesthetics that are effective, yet allow the child to recover quickly so that he does not need to go to a recovery room.

Each radiation facility should give parents written instructions concerning pediatric anesthesia. Generally, the child must not eat for eight hours prior to his appointment. Clear liquids are usually allowed four hours prior to anesthesia. Children can eat and drink immediately after treatment.

The anesthetic is usually given through the child's catheter or IV while the parent is holding or comforting him. The child will go to sleep in the parent's arms, and then the parent leaves the room while the treatment takes place. The anesthesiologist will bring the child to the parent in the waiting room when the child is partly awake. Once the child is easily aroused, the child and parents can leave. The entire procedure takes from 30 to 60 minutes. Nausea and vomiting are occasional side effects of anesthesia.

> *Shawn was almost three years old when he needed his cranial radiation. He is an extremely active child, and we agreed with the medical team that he would have to be sedated. His appointment was always at 1:00 p.m., and we were told that he could have apple juice or Jell-O at 6:00 a.m. but nothing to eat or drink after that. Every single morning he would drink the juice and then throw up. At the radiation room, I would hold him while he was anesthetized, then wait in the waiting room. They would bring him out to me in 30 to 45 minutes.*

During a course of radiotherapy, the dose, drugs, and methods to sedate or anesthetize the child may need to be changed because some children develop a tolerance to certain drugs. Good communication between parents and members of the treatment team should prevent unnecessary anxiety about increased dosages or the use of a different drug. In some cases, less anesthesia is needed if the child is gently coached on ways to hold still.

*Each time my young son came in for radiation, part of the routine
was to place the hard plastic mesh mask over his face while he was
awake, just for an instant, to get him used to the idea of trying to wear it
for treatments without sedation. No pressure was ever put on him about
it, it was just mentioned as a possibility of something he could try, something that would let him keep eating and drinking all through the day,
instead of having to fast for a few hours before each sedation, which was
very hard for such a small boy who was getting sedation twice a day.*

*They left the mask on him for a tiny bit longer each time, until he
was tolerating it for several seconds, and then close to a minute. His fifth
birthday was at the exact middle of treatment, and he decided that since
he was such a big boy now, he would try to do it without sedation. I know
he was trying to please and impress all these kind people. He worked it
out quietly with a favorite technician, asked the "sleepy medicine doctor"
to wait outside the treatment room, let them screw the mask down to the
table and did the whole thing awake.*

*I've never been more proud in my life. Everyone cheered and hugged
him. He finished the rest of the treatments without sedation, sometimes
eating and drinking on his way in the door just to show off that he could!*

Radiation simulation

Prior to actually receiving any therapy, many measurements and technical x-
rays are taken to map the precise area to be treated. This preparation for
therapy is called the "simulation." The simulation will generally take longer
than any other appointment, from thirty minutes up to two hours. Because
simulation is not a treatment with high-dose radiation, parents are often
allowed to remain in the treatment room to help and comfort their child. As
discussed previously, some children will need to be sedated for the simulation.

During simulation, the radiation oncologist and technologist use a specialized x-ray machine to outline the treatment area. They will adjust the table
that the child lies on, the angle of the machine, and the width of the x-ray
beam needed to give the exact dosage in the proper place. In addition, the
oncologist or technologist will put small ink marks on the skin to pinpoint
the area to be treated. These marks should not be scrubbed in the bath or
shower. They do fade with time, so the technologist may need to add more
ink at some point in the child's treatment.

Children who wear masks during treatment will have these ink marks put on the mask, not their skin. At some institutions, children who require spinal radiation may have tiny black dots permanently tattooed on their skin. These tattoos are made by putting a drop of India ink on the skin, then pricking with a pin. They look like tiny black freckles.

After the simulation is completed, the child can go home while the radiation oncologist carefully evaluates the developed x-ray film and measurements to design the treatment field.

Description of a cranial radiation treatment

To receive cranial radiation, children are given appointments for ten weekdays, the same time each day. They usually have the weekend off. At some institutions, children go twice a day for ten days. When the parent and child arrive, they must check in at the front desk. The technologist comes out to take the child into the treatment room. Often, the parent accompanies her young child into the room. If the child requires anesthesia, it will take place in the treatment room.

For conscious children, the technologist will secure them in position with either the mask (which is screwed down to the table on either side of the head) or other device. The technologist will take measurements to verify that the child's body is perfectly positioned. Frequently, the technologist will shine a light on the area to be irradiated to ensure that the machine is properly aligned. The technologist and parents will leave the room, closing the door behind them.

At some institutions, parents are allowed to stay and watch the TV monitor and talk to their child via the speaker system. If this is the case, the parent should be careful not to distract the technologist as he administers the radiation. At other institutions, parents must wait in the waiting room. The treatment takes only five to ten minutes, and can be stopped at any time if the child experiences any difficulty. When the treatment is finished, the technologist turns off the machine and removes the immobilization device, and parents and child can go home. There is no pain at all when receiving x-ray treatment.

> I desperately wanted my three-year-old to be able to receive the radiation without anesthesia. I asked the center staff what I could do to make her comfortable. They said, "Anything, as long as you leave the room during the treatment." So I explained to my daughter that we had to find

ways for her to hold very still for a short time. I said, "It's such a short time, that if I played your Snow White tape, the treatment would be over before Snow White met the dwarves." Katy agreed that was a short time, and asked that I bring the tape for her to listen to. She also wanted a sticker (a different one every day) stuck on the machine for her to look at. I brought her pink blanket to wrap her in because the table was hard and the room cold. Each day, she chose a different comfort animal or doll to hold during treatment. So we'd arrive every day with tapes, blanket, stickers, and animals. She felt safe, and all treatments went extremely well.

• • • • •

There was something about the radiation or the anesthesia that frightened Shawn terribly. He would scream in the car all the way to the hospital. It was a scream as if he was in pain. He had nightmares while he was undergoing radiation and every night after it was over. We decided a month after radiation ended to bring a box of candy to the staff who had been so nice. Shawn asked, "Do I have to go in that room?" When I explained that it was over and he didn't need to go in the room anymore, he asked if he could go in to look at it once more. He stood for a long time and just looked and looked at the equipment. Somehow he made his peace with it, because he never had any more nightmares.

If your child is receiving spinal radiation, the back of the heart may be affected. A baseline EKG and echocardiogram should be performed prior to treatment and on a regular basis thereafter. Spinal radiation may also damage the thyroid gland, which is located behind the Adam's apple. The oncologist should evaluate the functioning of this gland if spinal radiation has been given.

Description of a testicular radiation treatment

For boys or teens with leukemic cells in the testes, radiation is included in the treatment plan. At the present time, most protocols require 2400 rads, given in 200-rad doses, once a day for twelve days. Radiation treatment is usually only given Monday to Friday, with weekends off. Treatment plans vary among protocols and institutions.

Prior to your son's radiation to the testes, the technologist or child life specialist will give a tour of the facility, describe the machines, and explain exactly how the radiation sessions will be done. Usually, only older boys require radiation to the testes, so anesthesia is rarely needed. Instead, the boy or teen will lie on the table, the technologist will support the testicles on a small piece of lead, and the penis will be taped up to keep it out of the radiation field. Each treatment will last less than five minutes, during which time the boy must hold perfectly still. As with cranial radiation, the technologist will be watching your son through a window and will be in verbal contact through a two-way intercom system.

For all sexually mature males, sperm banking should be discussed with the oncologist prior to treatment. Sperm can be kept viable for ten to fifteen years, and this may allow some teens the opportunity to become fathers later in life.

Description of a total body radiation treatment

Total body radiation (also known as total body irradiation, or TBI) is sometimes given prior to bone marrow transplantation. There are numerous protocols, each with a different treatment schedule. Two examples are: 200 rads are given twice a day for three days, or 120 rads given three times a day for four days. The treatments are usually five to six hours apart. Prior to treatment, the child will be measured by the radiation therapist using tape measures and calipers. The therapist will give the family a tour and will show the two cobalt machines on either side of the stretcher in the middle of the room.

On the first day of treatment, the child or teen will be brought to the room (at some institutions, small kids will ride a tricycle or are pulled in a wagon), and may choose to watch TV or a movie, or to listen to a tape or radio. He will lie on the stretcher between the two cobalt machines, and the therapist will position him on his side or on his back. These positions will alternate each treatment, once on the back, then on the side. It doesn't matter which side, so if a child has a sore left side, he can always lie on his right. The child can move a bit, for example, scratch his nose or cross his ankles, but cannot get off the stretcher. The therapist will remove all metal from the child or his clothing—watches, rings, zippers, clamps. Anything with tight elastic—diapers or tight socks—will be loosened or removed. Treatment time lasts from 18 to 35 minutes, depending on the size of the child or teen.

Antinausea drugs are given to prevent vomiting, and these often make the child drowsy enough to doze through the treatment. Some small or extremely active children are sedated.

> *The radiation was easy. When I wasn't sleeping, I watched TV or listened to the radio. I threw up once, but they gave me Benadryl and I never was sick again from the radiation. The room was neat, it was painted lots of bright colors and had two big blue machines on each side of me.*

Possible short-term side effects

Generally, radiation given to children with leukemia lasts less than two weeks. Many children suffer no short-term side effects at all. If side effects do occur, it is often hard to differentiate those caused by radiation and those caused by the high-dose chemotherapy that is being given at the same time. Possible short-term side effects are:

- Loss of appetite
- Nausea and vomiting
- Fatigue
- Slightly reddened or itchy skin
- Hair loss
- Low blood counts
- Changes in taste and smell
- Sleepiness (somnolence syndrome)—from cranial radiation
- Swollen parotid (salivary) glands—from TBI

Methods of coping with most of the above side effects are contained in Chapter 11, *Common Side Effects of Chemotherapy*. Somnolence syndrome is uniquely associated with cranial radiation and is characterized by drowsiness, prolonged periods of sleep (up to twenty hours a day), low-grade fever, headaches, nausea, vomiting, irritability, difficulty swallowing, and difficulty speaking. It can occur anywhere from three to twelve weeks after radiation treatment ends, and can last from a few days to several weeks.

> *Nine weeks after ending her cranial radiation, my daughter started complaining of severe headaches. She would hold her head and just sob with pain. She also vomited several times. Then she became very sleepy,*

and dozed on the couch most of the day. She developed a low fever and choked when she tried to swallow liquids or solid food. This lasted for about a week, and I was worried sick. I called her oncologist, her radiation oncologist, and her pediatrician, and they all said they didn't think that it was related to the radiation or chemotherapy. I went to the medical library and discovered somnolence syndrome.

. . . . .

Stephan (eight years old) had no side effects from the cranial and spinal radiation other than sleepiness, but he was very affected by it. First, he just started taking naps and generally slowing down. Then the naps got longer, and he was awake less. Finally, he only woke up to eat. Luckily, that part coincided with Christmas vacation so he didn't miss much school. Altogether, it lasted about six weeks.

. . . . .

Ryan (fourteen years old) had his radiation during consolidation when he was very ill from the chemotherapy. He would develop severe headaches and vomiting an hour after each radiation treatment.

. . . . .

Three weeks after her radiation ended, Rachel (eighteen months old) slept for three days. We tried to wake her to eat, but she literally would fall asleep with her face in her food. After three days, she gradually became more alert, with the whole episode lasting only a week and a half. Oddly enough, the oncology people warned me about the possibility of sleepiness, but the radiation staff insisted that it wasn't related to the radiation.

Possible long-term side effects

While short-term effects appear and subside, long-term side effects may not become apparent for months or years after treatment ends. The effects of radiation on cognitive functioning, growth, and puberty range from no late effects to severe, lifelong impacts. The possible long-term side effects of total body radiation are covered in Chapter 20.

Cognitive problems

Intrathecal and intravenous methotrexate and/or radiation to the brain can sometimes cause damage to the central nervous system. Some children develop learning disabilities which can start immediately or several years after treatment. Typically, poor performance is noted in mathematics, spatial relationships, problem solving, attention span, and concentration skills. Here are the stories of three parents:

My daughter is a year off treatment and three years past radiation and seems to have no cognitive problems at all. She is doing well in kindergarten. She reads and writes, and has taught herself to add and subtract all of the combinations up to twenty. I was worried while she was on chemotherapy that her comprehension was slow. She continually asked me to reread portions of books and didn't seem to understand without constant repetition. But that faded away after the chemotherapy ended, and now she's quick to understand stories read aloud. She does, however, have significant social problems which may be related to the radiation.

• • • • •

My son turned three years old while receiving his cranial radiation. He is now five years old and has major cognitive problems. He can't count, and so far he hasn't been able to learn the alphabet. He is in a preschool for the developmentally disabled, and the teacher feels that he has just hit a brick wall. I gave her the Candlelighters book, "Educating the Child with Cancer," and several articles. She is trying different techniques with him. He is a super kid, though, with a great attitude, and we hope for the best.

• • • • •

Rachel received 1800 rads of cranial radiation when she was seventeen months old. She's six now, in kindergarten. She has multiple cognitive problems, including problems with letter and number recognition and short-term memory. She is a child who will need extra help in school, including phonics and drilling while learning to read. It is challenging for her to sit quietly in class and listen to the teacher. After much observation, I truly think that these kids have a quirky organizational system for their brain. They seem to have a different way of inputting and outputting information. She will frequently say something completely out of the blue during a conversation that is totally unrelated to what is being discussed. My husband and I both realize that school may be a struggle for her, but we intend to get her all of the help available to persons who are traumatically brain injured. Her self-esteem is high, she is a very bright, verbal child, and we will work with each of her teachers to ensure that she gets the best education possible.

It is important to remember that doctors cannot predict which children will develop cognitive problems. Children at greatest risk for cognitive problems are those treated when less than five years of age, with those under two at the highest risk. Chapter 15, *School*, discusses in great detail the types of educational problems some children face and how to deal with them.

Problems with growth

The brain contains the hypothalamus and the pituitary gland, which control many body processes, including growth and reproduction. At the initial dosages of radiation given to most children with leukemia (1800 rads to the cranium), growth is usually not affected except in younger, female patients. Effects on growth usually begin to be seen in those children who received 2400 rads or more. If the child requires additional cranial radiation or radiation to the spine, growth can be slowed or stopped. The growth of children who receive cranial radiation or craniospinal radiation should be followed closely. Children should be measured (sitting and standing) at every follow-up visit and their growth plotted on a chart to measure velocity.

If your child is one of the rare individuals who experiences premature puberty (before the age of eight for girls and ten for boys), growth may also be affected. These children may be given daily growth hormone injections to support their growth until they reach their final height.

Children who receive total body radiation prior to bone marrow transplant also may exhibit delayed growth, especially if they had cranial and/or spinal radiation previously. These children should be under the care of a pediatric endocrinologist who is experienced in follow-up care for bone marrow transplant patients.

Early or delayed puberty

Some young children who receive radiation to the brain do not experience puberty at the appropriate age. A very small percentage of children enter precocious puberty, which means that puberty begins several years earlier than normal. This is most common in children who also have impaired growth. Conversely, puberty in some children is significantly delayed. Teenage girls who do not show signs of puberty—pubic and underarm hair, breast development—should be evaluated by a pediatric endocrinologist. Similarly, teenage boys who show no signs of puberty—growth of body hair, deepening voice—should also consult a endocrinologist.

Secondary cancers

Children who receive cranial radiation have an increased risk of malignancy (cancer) years after treatment. The risk is reported to range from 1 to 5 percent.

My eighteen-year-old daughter had AML M5 over twelve years ago and does have some late effects. She was a very early bone marrow transplant recipient (1987) so she had total body irradiation seven times. As a result of that she has ongoing endocrine problems and cataracts. She also has a reduced ejection fraction of the heart as a result of the anthracyclines. That said, you'd never pick her out of a crowd. She just graduated from high school with a perfect 4.0 GPA, is applying to university and wants to specialize in biology with the intent to go into medicine (pediatric oncology) or molecular genetics with a focus on cancer genetics. There is hope.

CHAPTER 13

Record-Keeping and Finances

*Prosperity is not without many fears
and distastes; and adversity is not
without comfort and hopes.*

—Francis Bacon

KEEPING TRACK OF THE voluminous paperwork—both medical and financial—is a trial for every parent of a child with cancer. However, it is a necessary evil, because accurate records prevent medical errors and insurance over-billings. Poor record-keeping can allow changes in lab results to go unnoticed and untreated. Poor organization of bills often results in parents being hounded by collection companies. This chapter will suggest simple systems for keeping both medical and financial records.

Keeping medical records

Think of yourself as someone with two sets of books, the hospital's and yours. If the hospital loses your child's chart or misplaces lab results, you will still have a copy. If your child's chart becomes a foot thick, you will still have your simple system that makes it easy to spot trends and retrieve dosage information. Conscientious doctors appreciate organized parents.

The following are suggested items that you should record:

- Dates and results of all lab work
- Dates of chemotherapy, drugs given, and dose
- All changes in dosages of medicine
- Any side effects from drugs
- Any fevers or illnesses
- Dates for all medical appointments and name of the doctor seen

- Dates for any procedures done
- Child's sleeping patterns, appetite, and emotions

Keeping daily records on your child's health for two or three years is hard work. But remember that your child will be seen by pediatricians, oncologists, residents, radiation therapists, lab techs, nutritionists, psychologists, and social workers. Your records will keep it all straight and help pull all information together. They will help you remember questions to ask, prevent mistakes, notice trends. They will help busy doctors remember what happened the last time your child was given a certain drug. Your records will help the entire team provide your child with the best possible care.

There are as many good ways to record the above information as there are parents. Some of the methods used by veteran parents follow.

Journal

Keeping a notebook works extremely well for people who like to write. Parents make entries every day about all pertinent medical information and often include personal information such as their own feelings or memorable things that their child has said. Journals are easy to carry back and forth to the clinic, and can be written in while waiting for appointments. They also have the advantage of having unlimited space. One disadvantage is that they can be misplaced.

In *You Don't Have To Die*, Geralyn Gaes writes of the value of keeping a journal:

> Some days my entries consisted of only a few words: "Good day. No problems." Other times I had so many notes and questions to jot down that my handwriting spilled over into the next day's space. I must confess that I probably went overboard, documenting every minute detail of Jason's life down to what he ate for each meal. If he gets over this disease, I thought, maybe this information will be useful for cancer research.
>
> I'm not so sure I was wrong. Jason went two years without a blood transfusion, unusual for a child receiving such aggressive chemotherapy. Studying my journal, one of his physicians remarked, "This kid eats more oatmeal than anybody I've ever seen." Which was true. Jason wolfed it down for breakfast, after school, and before bedtime. The doctor speculated, "Maybe that's why Jason's blood is so rich in iron and builds back up so fast."

Stephan's oncologist is kind of hard to communicate with. I learned early on to keep a journal of Stephan's appointments, drugs given, side effects, and blood counts. That way if I ever had to call the doctor I would have it right in front of me. I also recorded Stephan's temperature when his counts were low to keep track of infections.

•　•　•　•　•

Record-keeping—very important! My father came to the hospital soon after diagnosis and brought a three-ring binder and three-hole punch. I would punch lab reports, protocols, consent forms, drug information sheets, etc., and keep them in my binder. A mother at the clinic showed me her weekly calendar book, and I adopted her idea for recording blood counts and medications. Frequently the clinic's records disagreed with mine as to medications and where we were on the protocol. I was very glad that I kept good records.

Calendar

Many parents reported great success with the calendar system. They buy a new calendar each year and hang it in a convenient place such as next to the telephone. You can record counts on the calendar while talking to the nurse or lab technician on the phone and take it with you to all appointments.

Each year I purchase a new calendar with large spaces on it. I write all lab results, any symptoms or side effects, colds, fevers, and anything else that happens. I bring it with me to the clinic each visit, as it helps immensely when trying to relate some events or watch trends. I also use it like a mini-journal, recording our activities and quotes from Meagan. Now that she's off treatment, I'm superstitious enough to still bring it to our monthly checkups.

•　•　•　•　•

I wrote the counts on a calendar or on little pieces of paper which got lost. But, to be honest, I didn't keep the medical records very well. I'm upset with myself when I think of it now.

•　•　•　•　•

For a long time I was unorganized, which is very unlike the way I usually am. I found that my usual excellent memory just wasn't working well. It all seemed to run together, and I began to forget if I had given her

all of her pills. Then I began using a calendar for both counts and medica-
tions. I wrote every med on the correct days, then checked them off as I
gave them.

Blood count charts

Many hospitals supply folders containing xeroxed sheets for record-keeping. Typically, they have spaces for the date, WBCs, ANC, Hct (hematocrit), platelets, chemotherapy given, and side effects.

> *My record-keeping system was given to me by the hospital on the*
> *first day. We were given a notebook with information about the illness and*
> *treatment. Also included were charts that we could use to keep all the*
> *information about the child's blood work, progress, reactions to drugs, etc.*
> *While we were at the hospital we were able to get the information off one*
> *of the computers on our floor each afternoon. My notebook holds records*
> *and notes for three years. Perhaps I was being compulsive with my*
> *record-keeping, but it made me feel that I was part of the team working*
> *on bringing my boy back to health.*

Appendix B, *Blood Counts and What They Mean*, contains examples of actual lab sheets, and a record-keeping sheet that you can use to keep track of your child's blood counts.

Tape recorder

For parents who keep track of more information than a calendar can hold and who find writing in a journal too time consuming, using a tape recorder works well. Small machines are very inexpensive, and can be carried in a pocket.

> *I started keeping a journal in the hospital, but I was just too upset*
> *and exhausted to write in it faithfully. A good friend who was a writer by*
> *profession told me to use a tape recorder. It was a great idea and saved a*
> *lot of time. I could say everything that had happened in just a few min-*
> *utes every day. I kept a separate notebook just for blood counts so that I*
> *could check them at a glance.*

Computer

For the computer-literate, keeping all medical records on the computer is an attractive option. (Be sure to back up all information so it won't be lost if your computer crashes.) You can print out bar graphs of the blood counts in relation to chemotherapy and quickly spot trends. Some hospitals also have this information available.

> At our hospital, the summary of counts for a given child can be formatted to print out as a "trend review" with each date printed out on the left side of the page and the various values (HGB, etc.) in columns down the page. The system permits printouts from the very first blood draw if that is desired. Periodically, on slow days, I'll ask if I can have a trend review. Then I can discard the associated single printouts (much less paper that way).

Keeping financial records

You will not need a calendar or journal for financial records, just a big, well-organized file cabinet. It is essential to keep track of bills and payments. Dealing with financial records is a major headache for many parents, but keeping good records can prevent financial catastrophe.

The following are ideas on how to organize financial records:

- Set up a file cabinet just for medical records.
- Have hanging files for hospital bills, doctor bills, all other medical bills, insurance explanations of benefits (EOB), prescription receipts, tax-deductible receipts (tolls, parking, motels, meals), and correspondence.
- Whenever you open an envelope, file the contents immediately. Don't leave it on the desk or throw it in a drawer.
- Keep a notebook with a running log of all tax-deductible medical expenses, including the service, charge, bill paid, date paid, and check number.
- Don't pay a bill unless you have checked over each item listed to make sure that it is correct.
- Start new files every year.

> I bought an accordion-style file folder each year to hold everything to do with Stephan. It had a slot each for hospital bill printouts, insurance explanation of benefits, receipts for all prescriptions, all Candlelighters' newsletters, pediatrician bills, laboratory bills, and Leukemia Society information.

• • • • •

To be honest, the paper trail really gets me down. I can only deal with the stacks every few months. I open things and make sure that the insurance company is doing their part, and then I try to sort through and pay our part.

• • • • •

I started out organized, and I'm glad I did because the hospital billing was confusing and full of errors. I cleared out a file cabinet and put in folders for each type of bill and insurance papers. I filed each bill chronologically so I could always find the one I needed. I made copies of all letters sent to the insurance company and hospital billing department. I wrote on the back of each EOB any phone calls that I had to make about that bill. I wrote down the date of the call, the person's name who I spoke to, and what she said. It saved me a lot of grief.

What are deductible medical expenses?

It is estimated that families of children with cancer spend 25 percent or more of their income on items not covered by insurance. Examples of these expenses are gas, car repairs, motels, food away from home, health insurance deductibles, prescriptions, and dental work. Many of these items can be deducted on federal income tax. Often parents are too fatigued to go through stacks of bills at the end of the year to calculate their deductions. If a monthly total is kept in a notebook, then all that needs to be done at tax time is adding up the monthly totals.

Medical expenses that could be deducted for 1998 were: acupuncture, ambulance, artificial limb, artificial teeth, expenses to modify your home to provide medical care for your child, chiropractor, crutches, dental treatment, HMO fees, hearing aids, hospital services, insurance premiums, laboratory fees, special school or tutor for child with learning disabilities, lodging costs for family when child is hospitalized, meals at hospital, physician's services, medicines, nursing care, operations, osteopath, oxygen, psychiatric care, psychological care, therapy, transplants, transportation to obtain medical care, trips for medical care, wheelchair, and x-rays.

To find out what can be legally deducted for the years your child is undergoing cancer treatment, get IRS publication 502. This booklet is available at libraries and IRS offices or by calling (800) TAX-FORM ((800) 829-3676) or *http://www.irs.ustreas.gov/*.

Canadian families are able to deduct many of the same medical expenses as those living within the US. To find out what can be legally deducted in Canada for the years your child is undergoing cancer treatment, contact Revenue Canada at (800) 959-8281 and ask for IT-519R2—Medical Expense and Disability Tax Credits.

If you do keep a calendar, an easy way to keep track of tax-deductible items is to glue an envelope to the inside cover. Whenever you incur an expense that is tax deductible, put the receipt in the envelope, and file it when you get home.

Dealing with hospital billing

Unfortunately, problems with billing are the norm rather than the exception for parents of children with leukemia. Here are two typical experiences:

> Insurance was an absolute nightmare. It almost gave me a nervous breakdown. After all we go through with our children to have to deal with the messed-up hospital billing was just too much—it was the worst part of the whole experience.

> We would stack the bills up and try to go through them every two or three months. Our insurance was supposed to pay 100 percent, but the billing was so confusing that they refused to cover some things because it wasn't clear what they were being billed for. The hospital frequently double billed, especially for prescriptions. We just stopped getting our prescriptions there.

> We would call them to try to get the mess straightened out, but the billing department was just as confused as we were. They kept sending our account to collections. We did everything in our power to get it straight, but we never did.

· · · · ·

> We had two distinctly different experiences at the two institutions that we dealt with. The university hospital where my daughter received her radiation gave me a folder the first day. It included, among other things, a sheet from a financial counselor giving all the information needed for preventing and solving billing problems. I never needed to call her because the hospital billing was clear, prompt, and organized.

The children's hospital where my daughter was a frequent inpatient and clinic patient was another story altogether. They billed from three different departments, put charges from the same visit on different bills, frequently over-billed, continuously made errors, and constantly threatened to send the account to collections. I never spoke to the same billing clerk twice. It was a never-ending grind and a constant frustration.

It is impossible to prevent billing errors, but it is necessary to deal with them. Here are step-by-step suggestions on solving billing problems:

• Keep all records filed in an organized fashion.

• Check every bill from the hospital to make sure there are no charges for treatments not given or errors such as double billing.

During maintenance, my daughter went to the clinic every three months. She had identical treatments every visit—port accessed, vincristine given, physical exam, and intrathecal methotrexate given via spinal tap. Each bill was different, ranging from $329 to $740, for identical visits! There were errors on each bill, including numerous charges for IV benedryl that she never received. I would get the errors removed, then they would reappear on the next bill.

• Check to see if the hospital has financial counselors. If so, make contact early in your child's hospitalization. Counselors provide services in many areas, including help with understanding the hospital's billing system, billing insurance carriers, understanding explanations of benefits, hospital/insurance correspondence, dealing with Medicaid, working out a payment plan, designing a ledger system for tracking insurance claims, and resolving disputes.

• If you find any billing error, call the hospital immediately. Write down the date, the name of the person you talk to, and the plan of action.

I often couldn't even get through to the billing representative, I was just put on hold forever. Then I tried to discuss the problems with the director of billing, but she was never in. After about twenty phone calls, I finally said to her secretary, "You know, I have a desperately sick child here, and I have more important things to do than call your boss every day. I've been as patient and polite as I can. What else can I do?" She said, "Honey, get irate. It works every time." I told her to put me through to somebody, anybody, and I would. She connected me to the person who mediates disputes, I got irate, and we went through all the bills line by line.

- If the error is not corrected on your next bill, call and talk to the billing supervisor. Explain politely the steps you have already taken and how you would like the problem fixed.

  The hospital billing was so bad, and I had to call so often, that I developed a telephone relationship with the supervisor. I always tried to be upbeat, we laughed a lot, and it worked out. She stopped investigating every problem and would just delete the charge from the computer.

- If the problem is still not corrected, write a brief letter to the billing supervisor explaining the steps you have taken and requesting immediate action. Keep a copy of each letter that you write and all written responses.

- Every time you receive an explanation of benefits (EOB) from your insurance company, compare it to the hospital bill. Track down discrepancies.

- If you are inundated with a constant stream of bills and there are major discrepancies between the hospital charges and what is being paid for by your insurance, ask both the hospital billing department and your insurance company, in writing, to audit the account. Insist on a line-by-line explanation for each charge.

  Within five months of my daughter's diagnosis, the billing was so messed up that I despaired of ever getting it straight. When the hospital threatened to send the account to a collection agency, I took action. I wrote letters to the hospital and the insurance company demanding an audit. When both audits arrived, they were $9,000 apart. I met with our insurance representative, and she called the hospital, and we had a three-way showdown. We straightened it out that time, but every bill that I received for the duration of treatment had one or more errors, always in the hospital's favor.

  • • • • •

  Our account for last year was being audited (at my request) because there was a discrepancy in the out-of-pocket amount. My figure was way different from theirs; their records indicated that we hadn't met it, my figures said we had exceeded it by about $7,000. I had to copy all my records (more than 100 pages) and send them to the company. To make a long story short, they reprocessed the bills and sent me 43 checks—for thousands!

- If you are too tired or overwhelmed to deal with the bills, ask a family member or friend to help. He could come every other week, open and file all bills and insurance papers, make phone calls and write all necessary letters. Some friends might even enter all your records on a computer for storage.

- Don't let billing problems accumulate. Your account may end up at a collection agency, which can quickly become a nightmare.

> Our insurance was constantly months behind in paying our bills to the Children's hospital. The hospital sent our account to collections, despite my assurances that I was doing everything I could to get the insurance to pay. We were hounded on the phone constantly by the collection people, often until we were in tears. We finally just took out a second mortgage and paid off the hospital, but now I don't know if we will be reimbursed by insurance.

· · · · ·

> I had a horrible run-in with the collection agency that works for the Children's Hospital. All of our bills are current, except one from November 1997. Yesterday, a woman called me saying she is filing a subpoena against me and is having me arrested. She threatened to take away our house if that is what it takes to get this bill ($614) paid. She even tried to call my husband at work yesterday. Luckily, my brother-in-law called the company lawyer and was told that what she did was illegal. He said collection agencies have strict rules and this woman broke them all. They are not allowed to bother you at work. They can never threaten legal action. He said that medical bills cannot even go on your credit report. The attorney called the collection agency and he assured me they would never call again. He also gave me a name at the Consumer Protection Agency and if she calls here again, I am to call them (they already have the complaint on file and will take additional action if she calls again). I also filed a written complaint with the hospital. I want them to know the people they have hired are harrassing their patients. I was in tears.

Not all stories are so grim. People who are in a socialized healthcare system, some managed care systems, or on public assistance never even see bills. Many people with insurance encounter no problems throughout their child's treatment.

Our insurance paid 80 percent of everything, no questions asked and always paid us within a month. People shouldn't have to worry about finances or their insurance program at a difficult time like this.

• • • • •

We have a low income, so we are on the state plan. They give us coupons for each child, and we just hand over a coupon at each visit. I have never seen a bill.

Coping with insurance

Finding one's way through the insurance maze can be a difficult task. Understanding the benefits and claims procedures can help you get the bills paid without undue stress. The following are some steps to help prevent problems with insurance.

Understand your policy

As soon as possible after diagnosis, read your entire insurance manual. Make a list of any questions you have on terms or benefits:

- Learn who the "participating providers" are under the plan, for, in today's managed healthcare climate, there may be a limited network of providers and hefty penalties or no benefits if the patient goes outside the network.

- Find out what your deductible is.

- Find out if there is a point where coverage increases to 100 percent.

- Determine if there is a lifetime limit on benefits.

- Find out when a second opinion is required.

- Learn when you have to notify the company about hospitalizations—many firms require pre-notification except in the case of emergency.

I realized that my daughter had been treated for over four months and I had never called the insurance company. When I read the manual, I was horrified to find out that I had not pre-notified them about three scheduled hospitalizations. There was a $200 penalty for each lapse. I called in tears, and they only charged me for one mistake, not all three.

Get a copy of every form that you may need to submit, for example, claim forms for inpatient care, outpatient care, or prescriptions. You can cut down on paperwork by filling in all the subscriber information on one of each type of form (except date and signature) and then making many copies. You will have a form ready to send in with each bill.

It may be helpful to determine whether your policy has benefits for counseling. If so, find out how many visits are covered and the level of training required (sometimes only counseling by persons with an MA or PhD degree is covered). Is there a home nursing benefit? How many visits?

> We changed to a new pediatrician, and he asked me if I thought it would be easier on my son to have visiting nurses come to our home to do the chemotherapy injections and some blood work. Since he had very low counts, it made a lot of sense not to have to go out. It also lessened his fears to be able to stay at home and have the same nurse come to do the procedures. It was a pleasant surprise to find these services covered by our insurance.

Find a contact person

As soon as possible after diagnosis, call your insurance company and ask who will be handling your claims. Explain that there will be years of bills with frequent hospitalizations, and it would be helpful to always deal with the same person. Insurers may be able to offer parents a contact person for claim review or special needs. Ask the contact person to answer any questions that you have on benefits. Try to develop a cooperative relationship with your contact person because she can really make your life easier. Also, the employer may have a benefits person who can operate as a liaison with the insurer.

> My employee benefits representative was Bobbi. She was just wonderful. The hospital would send her copies of the bills at the same time as they sent mine. Since I found so many errors, she would hold the bills a week until I called to tell her that they were correct before she paid them. She was very pleasant to deal with.

Negotiate

Don't be afraid to negotiate with the insurance company over benefits. Often, your contact person may be able to redefine a service that your child needs to allow it to be covered.

Our insurance company covered 100 percent of maintenance drugs only if the patient needed them for the rest of their lives. Christine's drugs were only needed for two years but were extremely expensive. I asked my contact person for help, and she petitioned the decision-making board. They granted us an exemption and covered the entire cost of all her maintenance drugs.

· · · · ·

My husband works for a small city that contracts out health insurance. A year into our child's treatment, the contract was being renegotiated. He brought home a copy of the proposed contract, and I was horrified to see that they had halved the benefit for transplants, from $200,000 to $100,000. I called the members of the committee negotiating the contract, the union representative, the city insurance liaison, and the city attorney. I was very polite, but I told them that if my child needed a bone marrow transplant, the new contract would bankrupt us. We would lose our home and have to sell all of our belongings to pay our part of the procedure. Then I called two transplant centers, and had them fax me the estimated cost of a routine bone marrow transplant (about $220,000). I sent copies of the fax to everyone that I could think of, and followed it up with phone calls. They changed the new contract back to $200,000. One person can make a big difference.

Challenging a claim

The key to obtaining the maximum benefit from your insurance policy is to keep accurate records and to challenge any denied claims. Some tips on good record-keeping are:

- Make photocopies of everything you send to your insurance company, including claims, letters, and bills.
- Pay bills by check, and keep all of your canceled checks.
- Keep all correspondence you receive from billing companies and insurance.
- Write down the date, name of person contacted, and conversation of all phone calls concerning insurance.
- Keep accurate records of all medical expenses and claims submitted.

Policyholders have the right to appeal a claim denial by their insurance company. The following are suggested steps to contest a claim:

- Keep original documents in your files, and send photocopies to the insurance company with a letter outlining why you think the claim should be covered. Make sure you get the reply in writing.

- If the insurance company is refusing coverage because they claim the procedure is "investigational" or "experimental" and therefore not covered, contact the Childhood Cancer Ombudsman Program (listed in Appendix C, *Resource Organizations*). This organization offers a free ombudsman program to help families maximize benefits or resolve disputes.

- Contact your elected representative to the US Congress. All Senators and members of the House of Representatives have staff who help constituents with problems.

- If all of the above steps do not resolve the dispute, take your claim to small claims court, or hire an attorney skilled in insurance matters to sue the insurance company.

Above all, don't be afraid to ask questions, and be persistent!

Sources of financial assistance

Sources of financial assistance vary from state to state and town to town. To begin to track down possible sources, ask the hospital social worker for assistance. In addition, some hospitals have community outreach nurses or case workers who may point out potential sources of assistance.

Hospital policy

If you find yourself unable to pay your hospital bills, don't sell your house or let your account go to collections. Ask the social worker to set up an appointment for you with the appropriate person to discuss the hospital policy on financial assistance. Many hospitals write off a percentage of the cost of care if the patient is uninsured or underinsured. Be proactive and talk to the hospital about setting up a monthly payment plan.

SSI (Supplemental Security Income)

SSI is a federal (US) program administered by the Social Security Administration, and is an entitlement based on family income. Recipients must be blind or disabled and have a low family income and few assets. Children with cancer qualify as disabled for this program, making some of them eligible for monthly aid if the family income and assets are low enough. To find out if your child qualifies, look in the phone book under "United States Government" for "Social Security Administration." Call the nearest field office to determine if your child is eligible for SSI.

Medicaid

Medicaid is administered by state governments in the US, with the federal government providing a portion of the entitlement. Rules on eligibility vary, but families with private insurance sometimes are eligible if huge hospital bills are only partially covered. Call your local or county social service department to obtain the number for the Medicaid office in your area. If they tell you that your child is ineligible, ask if the state has an "Aged, Blind, Disabled, Medically Needy" program.

In addition to helping pay some or all hospital bills, Medicaid sometimes also pays transportation and prescription costs. Some states cover children under the age of 21 if they are hospitalized for more than 30 days, regardless of parental income. States are supposed to have Children's Medical Services programs to pay for medical treatment of physically disabled children: these programs allow a higher income level than Medicaid. Ask for a detailed list of benefits available in your state.

If you are having difficulty applying for or obtaining government benefits, contact the Childhood Cancer Ombudsman Program for free help. They have expert medical and vocational volunteers who can help you through the maze of government benefit programs.

Free medicine programs

Many drug companies have programs to provide free medicines (including chemotherapy) to needy patients. Eligibility requirements vary, but most are available to those not covered by private or public insurance programs. You can get a free copy of the Directory of Pharmaceutical Patient Assistance from the Pharmaceutical Manufacturers Association, 1100 15th St. NW, Washington D.C. 20005; *http://www.phrma.org/patients*. Their toll-free hot line for physicians is (800) PMA-INFO.

While the cost of in-hospital treatment in Canada is covered by provincial governments, families have to pay for other medications at their own expense. For those without private insurance, this usually creates an extreme financial hardship. In many instances, the Department of Social Services can help pay for medications. The qualifications vary in each province and the decision is based on financial need. Canadian parents should contact their provincial Department of Social Services for further information.

Service organizations

There are numerous service organizations that can help families in need. They provide all kinds of aid: transportation, wigs, special wheelchairs, and food. Often, all a family has to do is describe their plight, and good Samaritans appear. Some organizations that may exist in your community are: American Legion; Elks Club; fraternal organizations such as the Masons, Jaycees, Kiwanis Club, Knights of Columbus, Lions, Rotary; United Way; Veterans of Foreign Wars; and churches of all denominations. In addition, local philanthropic organizations exist in many communities. To locate them, call your local Health Department, speak to the social worker, and ask for help.

Organized fund raising

Many communities rally around a child with cancer by organizing a fund. Help is given in various ways, ranging from donation jars in local stores to an organized drive using all of the local media. There are many pitfalls to avoid in fund raising, and great care must be exercised to protect the privacy of the sick child as much as possible. If you are contemplating starting a fund, read Sheila Peterson's *A Special Way to Care* (listed in Appendix D, *Books and Online Sites*). This guide gives detailed, step-by-step advice on determining the needs of the family, finding benefits, using publicity, generating community support, and managing the fund.

If your child is on or seeking Social Security or Medicaid eligibility, funds must be held in a special needs trust and paid directly to providers. If the family receives the money, or the child's Social Security number is used to open the bank account, the child can lose both Social Security and Medicaid.

We were making inquiries into hospice care, feeling it was time to explore that option. I found out that the only pediatric hospice provider in the state of Georgia was not on the preferred provider list. They would pay for benefits, but at a reduced rate; not a good thing since the lifetime maximum for hospice care was $7,500. With these benefits, we would get 78 days of hospice care. I felt like my only options were reduced pediatric care or full benefits using adult services. I wrote a letter of appeal stating that medically and ethically, neither of these were good choices. Well, we got a better outcome than I asked for. Not only will they cover the pediatric provider, but they have waived the lifetime maximum.

CHAPTER 14

Nutrition

Let your food be your medicine
and your medicine be your food.

—Hippocrates (fifth century B.C.)

THE EATING HABITS OF CHILDREN WITH LEUKEMIA go haywire. Parents know that eating the right types of food will help their child heal faster, feel better, and continue to grow. Moreover, cancer treatment itself increases the need for balanced nutrition. The child's body works hard to repair the damage to healthy cells caused by chemotherapy, and to break down and excrete the cancer cells killed by treatment. Just metabolizing the numerous chemotherapy drugs given stresses children's systems.

Despite knowing that children need to eat nutritious meals, the reality is that sick children often do not want to eat. This chapter discusses eating problems, explains good nutrition, suggests ways to pack extra calories into small servings, and offers tips on how to make food more appealing to children.

Treatment side effects and eating

Eating is tremendously impacted by most types of chemotherapy. Listed below are several common side effects of treatment which conspire to prevent good eating. Other common side effects, including nausea, vomiting, diarrhea, constipation, and mouth and throat sores, are covered in detail in Chapter 11, *Common Side Effects of Chemotherapy*.

Loss of appetite

Anorexia, or loss of appetite, is one of the most common problems associated with the treatment of cancer. Children suffering from nausea and vomiting, diarrhea or constipation, altered sense of smell and taste, mouth sores, and other unpleasant side effects understandably do not feel hungry. Loss of appetite is most pronounced during the intensive periods of treatment, such as induction, consolidation, or delayed intensification. If your child loses more than 10 to 15 percent of her body weight, she may need to be fed intravenously or by tube. Sometimes this can be avoided by parents learning how to increase calories in small amounts of food.

> *My son looked like a skeleton several months into his protocol for high-risk ALL. I used to dress him in "camouflage" clothes—several layers thick. This kept him warm and prevented stares.*

In addition to simple loss of appetite, your child may experience a side effect of chemotherapy called early filling. This means that the child has a sense of being full after only a few bites of food. If the child is suffering from early filling and only eats when hungry, she may begin losing weight and become malnourished. This chapter provides dozens of creative ways to encourage your child to eat more.

Increased appetite and weight gain

When children are given high doses of steroids such as prednisone or dexamethasone, they develop voracious appetites. They are hungry all the time, develop food obsessions, and frequently wake parents up during the night begging for another meal.

> *Early in her treatment when Carrie Beth was taking dexamethasone, she would start hitting me in the face in the middle of the night demanding food. I learned to have a bag of snacks and a bottle sitting next to the bed, so I could just hand them over and go back to sleep.*

Most parents become very concerned as their child consumes huge quantities of food and gains weight. A moon face with chubby cheeks and a rotund belly are classic features of a child on high-dose steroids. Much of the extra weight is fluid which steroids cause the body to retain. Avoid foods with increased salt that can contribute to fluid retention and high blood pressure. There are two important points for parents to remember about treatment with steroids: when the steroids stop, the extra fluid is excreted and weight drops, and the child's appetite usually goes from voracious to poor.

Do not put your child on a diet when he is taking steroids. Instead, try to make the most of this brief time of good appetite to encourage consumption of a variety of nutritious foods. A well-balanced diet now will help your child withstand the rigors of treatment ahead.

If you are concerned about the weight gain, consult your child's oncologist. If the fluid retention is extreme, the doctor may have you restrict your child's salt intake, and in some cases children are given drugs called diuretics to rid the body of excess fluid.

Lactose intolerance

Lactose intolerance is when the body can't absorb the sugar (lactose) contained in milk and other dairy products. Both antibiotics and chemotherapy can cause lactose intolerance in some individuals. The part of children's intestines that breaks down lactose stops functioning properly resulting in gas, abdominal pain, bloating, cramping, and diarrhea. If your child develops this problem, it is important to talk to a nutritionist to learn about low-lactose diets and alternate sources of protein. The following are suggestions for parents of lactose-intolerant children:

- Adding enzyme tablets or drops to dairy products makes them digestible for some children. Some of these are over-the-counter additives, while others require a prescription. Discuss these additives with the oncologist prior to using.

- Replace milk with cheese, nonfat yogurt, buttermilk, or sour cream.

- Replace milk with acidophilus milk or soy milk, which are easier to digest.

- Remember that milk is a common ingredient in other foods, even bread. Read ingredient lists carefully.

- If no dairy products are tolerated, supply calcium by serving canned salmon, sardines, or calcium-fortified fruit juices. Consult your child's oncologist and nutritionist about calcium supplements.

- Always be sure that products are pasteurized, not raw.

Diet and Nutrition and *Eating Hints* are free booklets from the National Cancer Institute, (800) 4-CANCER. They both contain recipes and suggestions for lactose-restricted diets.

Altered taste and smell

One common reason why children do not eat is because food has no taste or tastes bad. If the problem is food having no taste, try serving highly seasoned food (e.g., Italian, Mexican, or curried foods). If foods taste bitter or metallic, avoid using metal pots, pans, and utensils. Serve the child's food with plastic knives, forks, and spoons. Replace red meat with tofu, chicken or turkey, eggs, and dairy products.

Some children's taste returns to normal when maintenance starts, some after treatment ends, and for a few children, it takes years before some foods taste pleasant again.

What is a balanced diet?

A good diet includes sufficient calories to ensure a normal rate of growth, fuels the body's efforts to repair and replace damaged normal cells, and provides the energy the body needs to break down the various chemotherapy drugs given and excrete their by-products. Research has shown that a well-nourished body will:

- Tolerate more treatment
- Tend to have fewer side effects
- Maintain weight
- Recover faster from treatment

When the body becomes malnourished, body fat and muscle decrease. This leads to:

- Weakness, lack of energy, weight loss
- Decreased ability to digest food
- Limited ability to heal and fight infection

To keep your child's body well-nourished, foods from all of the five basic food groups are needed. The five groups are breads and cereals, fruits, vegetables, dairy products, and meats and meat substitutes. The groups and recommended daily servings are shown in Figure 14-1.

Below are examples of foods contained in each group, with a small child's serving size in parentheses beside each food. Consult a nutritionist to determine the serving size appropriate for your child.

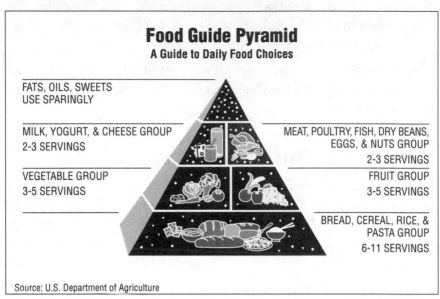

Food Guide Pyramid
A Guide to Daily Food Choices

FATS, OILS, SWEETS
USE SPARINGLY

MILK, YOGURT, & CHEESE GROUP
2-3 SERVINGS

MEAT, POULTRY, FISH, DRY BEANS,
EGGS, & NUTS GROUP
2-3 SERVINGS

VEGETABLE GROUP
3-5 SERVINGS

FRUIT GROUP
3-5 SERVINGS

BREAD, CEREAL, RICE, &
PASTA GROUP
6-11 SERVINGS

Source: U.S. Department of Agriculture

Figure 14-1. Food guide pyramid

Meat and meat substitutes *(two or three servings per day)*

Meat (1 ounce)	Eggs (1)
Fish (1 ounce)	Peanut butter (2 tbsp.)
Poultry (1 ounce)	Dried beans, cooked (1/2 cup)
Cheese (1 ounce)	Dried peas, cooked (1/2 cup)

These foods provide protein, which helps build and maintain body tissues, supply energy, and help form enzymes, hormones, and antibodies. Some typical one-ounce servings of meat and meat substitutes are: a meatball one inch in diameter, a one-inch cube of meat, one slice of bologna, a one-inch cube of cheese, or one slice of processed cheese. As you can see, two to three meatballs a day provide all the protein needed by a school-aged child.

Dairy products *(two or three servings per day)*

Milk (1/2 cup)	Tofu (1/2 cup)
Cheese (1 ounce)	Custard (1/2 cup)
Ice cream (1/2 cup)	Yogurt (1/2 cup)

These foods provide calcium, vitamin D, and protein.

Breads and cereals (six to eleven servings per day)

Bread (1/2 slice)

Oatmeal (1/2 cup)

Cream of wheat (1/2 cup)

Graham crackers (1 square)

Rice (1/2 cup)

Dry cereal (1/2 cup)

Granola (1/2 cup)

Cooked pasta (1/2 cup)

Saltines (3 squares)

Potatoes (1 baked)

These foods supply vitamins, minerals, fiber, and carbohydrates. Try to use only products made with whole wheat flour and limited sugar to get more nutrients per serving. One sandwich made with two slices of bread provides four servings of this food group.

Fruits (two to four servings per day)

Fresh fruit (1 medium piece)

Canned fruit (1/4 cup)

Dried fruits (1/4 cup)

Fruit juice (1/4 cup)

Fruits provide many vitamins, minerals, and fiber. Add dried fruits to cookie and muffin recipes. Fruits can be camouflaged by puréeing them with ice cream in the blender to make a tasty milkshake.

Vegetables (three to five servings per day)

Raw vegetables (1/4 cup)

Cooked vegetables (1/4 cup)

Vegetables, like fruit, are excellent sources of vitamins, minerals, and fiber. If your child does not want vegetables, they can be grated or puréed and added to soups or spaghetti sauce. If you own a juicer, add a vegetable to fruits being juiced.

Fats (several servings a day)

Butter or margarine

Mayonnaise

Peanut butter (or nuts)

Meat fat (in gravy)

Ice cream

Cheese

Whipped cream

Avocado

Olives

Chocolate

Although the food pyramid calls for fats to be used sparingly, higher consumption of fats is needed for children being treated for cancer. Experiment to find the fats that your child enjoys eating, and serve them frequently.

Are vitamin supplements necessary?

Yes, vitamin supplements are usually necessary. The nutritional needs of kids with cancer are higher than other children's, yet kids on treatment eat less food. Most children with cancer are unable or unwilling to eat the variety of foods necessary for good health. In addition, damage to children's digestive systems from chemotherapy alters the body's ability to absorb the nutrients contained in the food they do manage to eat.

Vitamin supplementation should only be done in consultation with your child's oncologist. Oversupplementation of some vitamins, folic acid for example, can make your child's chemotherapy less effective. But providing other vitamins can make the difference between a child with dull hair, no energy, and dry peeling skin to one with stronger hair, clear skin, and a better attitude. Vitamin supplements should be individually tailored for your child in consultation with the oncologist and nutritionist.

> *Halfway through maintenance, my daughter just looked awful. Her new hair began to thin out and break easily and her skin felt papery. I had been giving her a multivitamin and mineral tablet every day because her appetite was so poor, but it didn't seem to be enough. I talked to her doctor, then began to give her more of the antioxidant vitamins: betacarotene, E, and C. I bought the C in powder form, which effervesced when mixed with juice. She really liked her "bubble drinks." The betacarotene and E she swallowed along with the rest of her pills. Within a few weeks her hair stopped falling out, her skin stopped peeling, and she felt better.*

· · · · ·

> *I gave my teenaged daughter supplements of vitamins and some minerals. I also increased her vitamin intake by using the juicer every day. She always drank a big glass of fruit or vegetable juice, and I really think it helped her do as well as she has.*

Making eating fun and nutritious

In some homes, mealtimes turn into battlegrounds, with worried parents resorting to threats or bribery to get their child to eat. After such scenes, parents, the ill child, and siblings are exhausted, and nutritious food still has not been consumed. The next several sections are full of methods used successfully by many veteran parents to make mealtimes both fun and nutritious.

How to make food more appealing

Many children are finicky eaters at the best of times. Cancer and its treatment can make eating especially difficult. Here are some general suggestions to make eating more enjoyable for your child:

- Give small portions throughout the day rather than three large meals. Feed your child whenever she is hungry.

- Remember that your child knows best which foods he can tolerate.

    In the beginning of treatment, we decided that my son had to eat what the rest of the family was having. If he didn't eat that, he got no more food. He usually just didn't eat. Some mornings, I had trouble waking him up. He was limp and would have his eyes rolled back in his head. He was tested and diagnosed with hypoglycemia (low blood sugar). The doctor told us to make sure he ate something right before bed, even if it was ice cream or cookies and milk. Since he has been off chemotherapy, he has not had any problems.

- Explain clearly to your child the importance of eating a balanced diet.

- Make mealtimes pleasant and leisurely.

- Rearrange eating schedules to serve the main meal at the time of day when your child feels best. If she wakes up feeling well most days, make a high-protein, high-calorie breakfast.

- Praise and encourage eating well.

- Don't punish the child for not eating.

- Set a good example by eating a large variety of nutritious foods.

- Have nutritious snacks available at all times. Carry them in the car, to all appointments, and packed in knapsacks for school.

- Serve fluids between meals rather than with meals to keep your child from feeling full after only a few bites of food.

- Limit the amount of less desirable foods in the house. Potato chips, corn chips, soda pop, and sweets with large amounts of sugar may fill your child up with empty calories.

- If your child is interested, include him in making a grocery list, shopping for favorite foods, and food preparation.

Make mealtime fun

Here are some suggestions on how to make mealtime more fun:

- Try to take the emphasis off eating food because it's good for you and focus instead on setting a mood of enjoying each other's company while sharing a meal. Encourage good conversation, tell stories and jokes, perhaps light some candles.

- Make one night a week "restaurant night." Use a nice tablecloth, candles, allow the children to order from a menu, and pretend the family is out for a night on the town.

- Since any change in setting can encourage eating, consider having a picnic on the floor occasionally. Order pizza or other takeout, spread a tablecloth on the floor, and have an in-home picnic. Some parents even send lunch out to the treehouse for a lark.

> *My son enjoyed eating in different places around the house and seemed to eat more when he was having fun. I sometimes fed the kids on their own picnic table outdoors in good weather, and at the same picnic table in the garage during the winter. They were thrilled to wear their coats and hats to eat. Occasionally I would let them eat off TV trays while watching a favorite program or tape.*

- Some families have theme meals, such as Mexican, Hawaiian, Chinese. They use decorations, wear costumes, and cook foods with exotic spices.

- Some children seem to eat better if food is attractively arranged on the plate or is decorated in humorous ways. Preschoolers enjoy putting a smiling face on a casserole using strips of cheese, nuts, or raisins. Sandwiches can be cut into funny shapes using knives or cookie cutters.

> *My daughter liked to have food decorated. For example, we would make pancakes look like a clown face by using blueberries for eyes, strawberry for a nose, orange slices for ears, etc. She also enjoyed eating brightly colored food, so we would add a drop of food coloring to applesauce, yogurt, or whatever appealed to her.*

How to serve more protein

Since many children cannot tolerate eating meat while on chemotherapy, here are some suggestions for increasing protein consumption:

- Add one cup of dried milk powder to a quart of whole milk, then blend and chill. Use this extra-strength milk for drinking and cooking.

- Use extra-strength milk (above), whole milk, evaporated milk, or cream instead of water to make hot cereal, cocoa, soup, gravy, custards, or puddings.

- Add powdered milk to casseroles, meat loaf, cream soups, custards, and puddings.

- Add chopped meat to scrambled eggs, soups, and vegetables.

- Add chopped, hard-cooked eggs to soups, salads, sauces, and casseroles.

- Add grated cheese to pizza, vegetables, salads, sauces, omelets, mashed potatoes, meat loaf, and casseroles.

- Serve bagels, English muffins, hamburgers, or hot dogs with a slice of cheese melted on top.

- Spread peanut butter on toast, crackers, and sandwiches. Dip fruit or raw vegetables into peanut butter for a quick snack.

- Spread peanut butter or cream cheese onto celery sticks or carrots.

- Serve nuts for snacks, and mix nuts into salads and soups.

- Serve yogurt and granola bars for extra protein. Top pie, Jell-O, pudding, or fruit with ice cream or whipped cream.

- Use dried beans and peas to make soups, dips, and casseroles.

- Use tofu (bean curd) in stir-fried vegetable dishes.

- Add wheat germ to hamburgers, meat loaf, breads, muffins, pancakes, waffles, vegetables, and as a topping for casseroles.

Guidelines for boosting calories

Parents need to alter their perceptions of what constitutes healthy food when they are struggling to feed a child on chemotherapy. Many parents have ingrained habits of low-fat cooking and food preparation. That habit must be replaced by methods to constantly find ways to add calories to their child's food:

- Add butter or margarine to hot cereal, eggs, pasta, rice, cooked vegetables, mashed potatoes, and soups.

- Use melted butter as a dip for raw vegetables and cooked seafood such as shrimp, crab, and lobster.

- Use sour cream to top meats, baked potatoes, and soups.

- Use mayonnaise instead of salad dressing on salads, sandwiches, and hard-cooked eggs.

- Add mayonnaise or sour cream when making hamburgers or meat loaf.

- Use cream instead of milk over cereal, puddings, Jell-O, and fruit.

- Make milkshakes, puddings, and custards with cream instead of milk.

- Serve your child whole milk to drink instead of 2 percent milk.

- Sauté vegetables in butter.

- Serve bread hot so it will absorb more butter.

- Spread bagels, muffins, or crackers with cream cheese and jelly or honey.

- Make hot chocolate with cream, and add marshmallows.

- Add granola to cookie, bread, and muffin batters. Sprinkle granola on ice cream, pudding, and yogurt.

- Serve meat and vegetables with sauces made with cream and pan drippings.

- Combine cooked vegetables with dried fruit.

- Add dried fruits to recipes for cookies, breads, muffins.

- Add honey to cereal, milkshakes, yogurt.

- Glaze chicken with honey when cooking.

Nutritious snacks

Try to get into the habit of always bringing a bag of nutritious snacks whenever you leave home with your child. This allows you to feed her whenever she is hungry and avoids stopping for non-nutritious junk food. Here are some examples of healthful snacks:

- Apples or applesauce
- Baby foods

- Burritos made from beans or meat
- Buttered popcorn
- Celery sticks stuffed with cheese or peanut butter
- Cookies made with wheat germ, oatmeal, granola, fruits, nuts
- Cereal
- Cheese
- Cheesecake
- Chocolate milk
- Cottage cheese
- Crackers with cheese, peanut butter, tuna salad
- Custards made with extra eggs and cream
- Dips made with cheese, avocado, butter, beans, or sour cream
- Dried fruit such as apples, raisins, apricots, or prunes
- Fresh fruit
- Granola mixed with dried fruit and nuts
- Hard-cooked and deviled eggs
- Ice cream made with real cream
- Juice made from 100 percent fruit
- Milkshakes made with whole milk or cream
- Muffins
- Nuts
- Peanut butter on crackers or whole wheat bread
- Pizza
- Puddings
- Sandwiches with real mayonnaise or butter
- Vegetables such as carrot sticks or broccoli florets
- Yogurt, regular or frozen

Ask for help

It is very helpful to consult the hospital nutritionist to obtain more information and ideas on how to add more protein and calories to your child's diet.

> I had two quite different experiences with hospital nutritionists. At the children's hospital, I couldn't get the doctors concerned about my daughter's dramatic weight loss. She was so weak she couldn't stand, and her muscles seemed to be wasting away. I finally asked the receptionist to please send in a nutritionist. A very young woman came in and talked to me about the major food groups. I felt my cheeks begin to flush, and my eyes glistened as I said, "I know what she is supposed to eat, I need to know how I can make her want to eat." I must have sounded a bit crazy, because she just handed me a booklet and backed out the door.

> The next week when my daughter began her radiation, the radiation nurse took one look at her and called the nutritionist right down. This nutritionist was very warm and caring. She helped me to understand that I needed to think fat, protein, and calories, and she gave me lots of practical suggestions on how to boost calories. I think that she probably saved my daughter from tube feedings.

Another resource is the American Institute for Cancer Research Nutrition Hot Line, (800) 843-8114, Monday through Friday, 9:00 a.m. to 5:00 p.m. EST. A registered nutritionist will answer your questions about your child's nutrition.

What kids really eat

The previous part of the chapter listed ideas for increasing calories and making food more appealing. What follows are accounts of what several kids really ate while on chemotherapy. You'll notice how varied the list is, so experiment to see what your child finds palatable. Remember also that children's tastes and aversions change as time passes while on treatment.

> Judd craved chicken chow mein and fried rice takeout from a Chinese restaurant. He also loved SpaghettiOs and hot dogs.

> • • • • •

> I let Preston eat whatever tasted good to him, which was usually lots of potatoes and eggs. He liked spicy food (especially Mexican) while on prednisone.

· · · · ·

Katy typically only ate one food for days or weeks at a stretch. One time, she ate pesto sauce (made from olive oil, garlic, Parmesan cheese, and basil leaves) on pasta every meal for weeks. She also went through a spicy barbecue sauce phase, in which she wouldn't eat any food unless it was completely immersed in sauce. She ate no fruits, vegetables (except potatoes), or meat for the entire period of treatment. She ate mostly cereal and beans when she was feeling well, and mostly puréed baby food when she was really sick.

· · · · ·

In the beginning when Meagan lost so much weight, we snuck Poly-cose (a powdered nutritional supplement) into everything. She finally got stuck on cans of mixed nuts. They are high calorie and were instrumental in putting back on the weight. She also craved capers and would eat them by the tablespoonful.

· · · · ·

All Brent asks for are "peanut butter and jelly sandwiches, cut in fours, no crusts, with Fritos." The only fruit he has eaten for three years is an occasional banana, and he eats no vegetables. He always ate everything before his diagnosis at age six.

· · · · ·

The doctor told me to keep Kim on a low-salt, low-folic-acid diet. She wouldn't eat anything, so he eventually said he didn't care what she ate, as long as she ate. She liked SpaghettiOs, Chick-fil-A nuggets, Chick-fil-A soup, and McDonald's sausage and pancakes.

· · · · ·

All that Carl ate was dry cereal, dry waffles, oatmeal, and bacon. He ate no other meat or vegetables throughout treatment, but did drink milk. I thought that he would never be healthy, but he's fifteen now (diagnosed when two), eats little junk food, never gets sick, and looks great.

· · · · ·

While on prednisone I felt like I could never get out of the kitchen because Shawn ate nonstop. The rest of the time he ate almost nothing. He survived on bagels, dry cereal, french fries, popcorn, and burritos.

· · · · ·

Stephan's appetite went back to normal on maintenance. But after he relapsed and had cranial and spinal radiation, things have never been the same. He only wants junk food such as hot dogs and chicken nuggets. Most meats make him sick, and he's having problems with smells making food unappetizing.

· · · · ·

John (fourteen months old) craved creamed corn and pork and beans. I would just sit him on a potty chair at the table and let him eat, and it would go in one end and out the other. When on prednisone, he would sit at the table almost all day. He also drank a gallon of apple juice a day. He rarely eats meat to this day (two years off treatment).

· · · · ·

On prednisone, Rachel ate only hot dogs, bologna, scrambled eggs with cheese, and potato chips. She would eat until she literally threw up. Now, two years off treatment, she is gradually expanding her repertoire. She only drinks milk (no water, juice, or soda), eats no sweets, and prefers all salty foods. I really have no idea whether it is learned behavior or is a result of the cancer treatment.

· · · · ·

I guess Carrie Beth is the exception that proves the rule. She is on maintenance and has an excellent appetite. She eats fruits, vegetables, and lots of meat.

Parent advice

Several veteran parents whose children have completed therapy offer the following suggestions on how to handle the inevitable eating problems of children on therapy:

- Doctors sometimes reassure parents by saying, "His appetite will return to normal on maintenance." Don't be surprised if this does not happen.

- Let the child control what type of food and how much he wants. In the beginning, any food is good food.

- Buy a juicer, and use it every day. This was the only way we got any fruits or vegetables into our daughter. Make apple juice and sneak in a carrot. Sometimes we would make the juice, then blend it in the blender with ice cubes to make an iced drink, which we would serve with a straw.

- I solved my daughter's salt cravings by buying sea salt and letting her dip french fries in it once a week. For some reason, that satisfied her and stopped her from begging for regular table salt at every meal.

- Try not to worry about your child's future eating habits. During treatment, you just have to let go of normal requirements and feed him whatever he wants, whenever he is hungry.

- When your child is on prednisone, don't try to restrict his food intake. It can be hard to watch these rotund little ones just shovel the food in, but once they get off the prednisone, they stop eating and quickly lose the weight. Then you have the opposite problem: how to get them to eat anything!

- Try to work around their taste problems. For example, my son wouldn't drink milk, so I made his oatmeal and cream of wheat with milk instead of water.

- If you only keep good food in the house, and don't buy junk food, your child will eat more nutritious food.

- Take good care of yourself by eating well. We are all under tremendous stress and need good nutrition. I gave my daughter healthy foods and glasses of juiced fresh fruits and vegetables while I was living on lattés (a coffee drink). I now have breast cancer and wish that I had eaten well during my daughter's treatment.

- There is reason for hope. My daughter ate almost nothing while on treatment. After treatment ended, she ate more food but still no variety. She didn't turn the corner until a year off treatment, but now she is gradually trying new foods, including fruits and vegetables again. I'm glad I never made an issue of it.

Commercial nutritional supplements

Many children cannot tolerate solid food or can only eat small amounts each day. Liquid supplements can help provide the necessary calories. The following is a sampling of the variety of supplements that can be purchased at pharmacies or grocery stores. If you are unable to locate a particular brand, your pharmacist may be able to order it for you:

- Sustacal. Lactose-free liquid. Flavors are chocolate, vanilla, eggnog, and strawberry. Also comes in a high-protein or extra-fiber formula. 240 calories and 15 grams protein per 8 oz. can (Mead Johnson).

- **Sustacal Pudding**. Like Sustacal in pudding form. Flavors are chocolate, vanilla, and butterscotch. 240 calories and 6.8 grams protein per 5 oz. can (Mead Johnson).

- **Sustacal HC**. Concentrated liquid. Flavors are vanilla, chocolate, strawberry, eggnog. 360 calories and 14 grams protein per 8 oz. can (Mead Johnson).

- **Ensure**. Lactose-free liquid. Flavors are chocolate, vanilla, black walnut, coffee, butter pecan, banana, and strawberry. Other formulas are high protein or extra fiber. 250 calories and 9 grams protein per 8 oz. can (Ross Laboratories).

- **Ensure Plus**. Concentrated liquid. 355 calories and 13 grams protein per 8 oz. can (Ross Laboratories).

- **Isocal**. Lactose-free liquid. Vanilla. 250 calories and 8 grams protein per 8 oz. can (Mead Johnson).

- **Enrich**. Liquid with fiber. Lactose free. 260 calories and 9 grams protein per 8 oz. can (Ross Laboratories).

- **Instant Breakfast**. Powder, which is added to milk. Variety of flavors. When mixed with 8 oz. whole milk, provides 280 calories and 15 grams protein (Carnation Co.).

- **Citrotein**. Powder, which is added to water or juice. Orange flavor. 127 calories and 8 grams protein per 1/4 cup (Doyle Pharmaceutical).

- **Polycose**. Liquid or powder. Adds carbohydrates for extra calories. Add to milk, juice, gravy, soups. One tablespoon adds 30 calories.

Feeding by tube and IV

Tube feedings or TPN are a necessity for some children with leukemia. These types of feedings do not represent a failure on the part of parents or children to "eat properly." Although feeding by tube and IV may require additional hospitalization, parents need to understand the benefits clearly. If a child with cancer becomes malnourished, events are set in motion that can have grim consequences. As appetite and weight decrease, the child's ability to repair cellular damage caused by treatment is impaired. The child becomes progressively weaker and resistance to infection decreases. Infections and weakness may require interruptions in treatment. This scenario needs to be prevented. Most protocols require tube or IV feeding after a certain percentage of body weight is lost. There are two types of supplemental feeding.

Total parenteral nutrition (TPN)

Total parenteral nutrition, also known as hyperalimentation, is a form of intravenous feeding used to prevent malnutrition in those children who cannot eat or eat enough to meet basic nutritional needs. Some of the many reasons why your child may require TPN are severe mouth and throat sores which prevent swallowing, severe nausea, vomiting, and diarrhea, or a loss of more than 10 percent of body weight. TPN ensures that the child receives all of the protein, carbohydrates, fats, vitamins, and minerals she needs. The TPN is administered through the central or IV line, but children receiving TPN can also eat solids and drink fluids.

Enteral nutrition

If a child requires supplemental feeding and the bowel and intestines are still functioning well, enteral nutrition may be recommended. Enteral nutrition is feeding via a tube placed through the nose, mouth, or directly into the stomach through the abdominal wall. Nutritionally complete liquid formulas are fed through the tube. The appropriate formula will be decided by the oncologist and nutritionist. Infrequent side effects of enteral nutrition are irritated throat, nausea, or constipation.

One parent shared her thoughts on her son's chemotherapy-induced eating problems with these words:

> I feel good nutrition is very important to good health, but the reality of the situation with our child was that he hated anything nutritious when he was on chemotherapy. I could doctor it up, add the best toppings, make it look terrific, season it just right, and it would still be rejected. So I decided since my son wasn't allowed to make any decisions in regards to the pills, treatments, tests, or hospital stays, he wouldn't be forced to eat everything nutritious if he didn't want to. Whether this was a right or wrong decision, I don't know. I just know that I served him a lot of processed foods during those years and he's a healthy and happy boy ten years later. After he was finished with chemotherapy, however, we did require that he eat healthier foods.

CHAPTER 15

School

Most of us had two feelings at the same time:
wanting to go back to school and
being scared of going back.

—Eleven children with cancer
There Is a Rainbow
Behind Every Dark Cloud

CHILDREN WITH CANCER often experience disruptions in their education due to repeated hospitalizations, side effects from chemotherapy, or generally not feeling well enough to fully participate in daily school life. As their health improves and treatment allows, returning to school can be either a relief or a challenge for children with cancer.

For many children, school is a refuge from the world of hospitals and procedures, a place for fun, friendship, and learning. Because school is the defining structure of every child's daily life, returning to school signals normalcy; indeed, expectations of school attendance impart a clear and reassuring message that there is a future. Other children, especially teens, may dread returning to school because of temporary or permanent changes to their appearance or concerns that prolonged absences may have changed their social standing with their friends. Additionally, school can become a major source of frustration for those children who develop learning disabilities as a result of treatment. These learning differences, if handled in an insensitive or uninformed manner, can affect a child's confidence and self-esteem.

The issues of educating children with cancer are complex, but most can be successfully managed through planning and good communication. In this chapter, many veteran parents share advice and experiences to help you meet the educational needs of your child.

Keeping the school informed about treatment

Communicating with the school often does not enter a parent's mind during the nightmarish days after diagnosis. Keeping the school informed, however, lays the foundation for the months or years of collaboration as the child goes through the rigors of treatment for cancer. Parents need to forge a strong alliance with the school professionals to ensure that their child, who may be emotionally and/or physically fragile, continues to be welcomed and nurtured at school. As soon as possible, parents should notify the principal in writing of the child's diagnosis and hospitalization. Otherwise, "perfect participation" policies are sometimes used to lower the child's grades.

The first step in ensuring a good relationship is choosing an advocate to be the liaison among hospital, family, and school. The advocate will work to keep information flowing between the hospital and school, and will help pave the way for a successful school reentry for the sick child. Often the advocate is the hospital social worker, but it can also be a hospital or school nurse, psychologist, principal, or other motivated individual. The most important qualifications for this role are good communication skills, knowledge of educational programs and procedures, comfort in dealing with school issues, and organizational skills. It must be someone you trust to fairly act on your child's behalf.

The advocate should locate a contact person at the school (or hospital) and should provide frequent updates about the child's medical condition, treatment, emotional state, and tentative reentry date. The advocate should encourage questions, and address staff concerns about having a seriously ill child in school. Privacy laws prohibit these exchanges unless parents first sign a release form authorizing the school and hospital to share information. These forms are available at schools.

> We had absolutely no problem keeping the school informed, as we lived directly behind it. The teacher would frequently stop by on her way home to drop off homework assignments and cards or messages from Stephan's classmates. The school nurse, psychologist, and teacher were at my beck and call. Whenever I felt that we needed to talk, I'd call and they would set up a meeting within 24 hours. I gave them the Candlelighters' book Educating the Child with Cancer and they even attended a Candlelighters meeting. They have been wonderful.

Keeping teacher and classmates involved

While your child is hospitalized, it is vital to his well-being to stay connected with his teacher and classmates. Children go to school for instruction, developing communication skills, and increasing socialization skills with peers. Even when instruction is not possible, the other skills can continue to grow.

The teacher should be getting updates through the advocate, but the parent can help by calling the teacher periodically and bringing notes or taped messages to the classroom. The following are suggestions for keeping the teacher and classmates involved:

- Give the teacher a copy of *Educating the Child with Cancer* (listed in Appendix D, *Books and Online Sites*).

- Have the pediatric oncology nurse or social worker come to class to give a presentation about what is happening to their classmate and how he will look and feel when he returns. This should include a question and answer session to clear up misconceptions and allay fears. All children, especially teenagers, should be involved in deciding what information should be given to classmates.

- Take pictures of your child on treatment (some families fill a photo album) and share it with her class.

- Encourage classmates to keep in touch by sending notes, calling on the phone, sending class pictures, or making a banner.

Call the American Cancer Society, (800) ACS-2345, to ask for a comprehensive listing of the printed materials and outreach programs available for teachers and parents. Canadians can obtain information through the Canadian Cancer Society's Cancer Information Service, (888) 939-3333.

> Communication was the key. I wrote weekly updates and made copies for each teacher, put their names on it and delivered it to school. I learned that a single copy of a letter didn't get passed around to everyone (Joel was in high school). Some classes used a tape recorder; they all kept a record of what he'd missed and his math teacher got together with the librarian and arranged to videotape his math classes. They did so much on the board, on overheads, and with discussion in that class that an audio-

tape would not have helped. All teachers were willing to meet with him after or before school to essentially reteach the concepts that he had missed.

I also told his teachers it was okay to discuss Joel, his leukemia, and his treatment with the other kids in the class. They would never have done it without my okay. I tried to phrase things in my updates in a way that the kids would understand what was going on. I knew that in the absence of information, there would be rumors flying. This might not work for everyone, but it served us well.

Keeping up with schoolwork

Whenever your child is able, keeping up with schoolwork should be a priority. Learning can continue despite school absences. Parents should communicate with the teacher to keep abreast of the subjects being covered in school. Often, the teacher will send assignments and materials home with siblings, or arrangements can be made for pick-up.

Public schools are required to provide a free education to all children. To keep up in school, the parents need to request special education eligibility so that the child can qualify for an itinerant teacher. Without an individual education plan (IEP) or 504 plan in place, the child is entitled to nothing except what the school voluntarily provides, and this is not enforceable. (IEP and 504 plans are discussed later in this chapter.)

Joanne Holt, a high school Director of Special Education, suggests:

If children are having difficulty remaining interested in school work due to fatigue and not feeling well, it may be useful to consider alternative learning activities. In such circumstances, a parent and child might identify an area of special interest or curiosity (e.g., dinosaurs, space, animals, nature, the Wild West, etc.). Children may find it more interesting to develop reading skills, learn math concepts, develop writing skills, and learn research and study principles in the context of a high-interest area while still learning and maintaining the concepts being introduced in school. Play is a significant part of such activities and can often spark imaginative activities. It is important that the school be aware of and supportive of such an approach; most often they are and, in fact, may be valuable resources for ideas and activities. The goal is to encourage confidence and prepare the child for the least disruptive reentry to school routines.

Siblings need help, too

The diagnosis of cancer catastrophically affects all members of the family. Siblings can be overlooked in the early months when the parents are spending most of their time caring for the ill child at the hospital, clinic, or in the home. Many siblings keep their feelings bottled up inside to prevent placing additional burdens on their distraught parents. Often, the place where siblings act out the most is at school. It is very common for siblings to withdraw or become disruptive in the classroom, cry easily, become frustrated, fall behind in classwork, bring home failing grades, cut classes, become rebellious toward authority, or have fistfights with classmates.

Send a letter to the principal about each sibling. Ask the principle to alert teachers, counselors, and nurses about the situation.

> Lindsey was in kindergarten when Jesse was first diagnosed. Because we heard nothing from the kindergarten teacher, we assumed that things were going well. At the end of the year, the teacher told us that Lindsey frequently spent part of each day hiding under her desk. When I asked why we had never been told, the teacher said she thought that we already had enough to worry about dealing with Jesse's illness and treatment. She was wrong to make decisions for us, but I wish we had been more attentive. Lindsey needed help.

If possible, try to include the siblings' teachers in all conferences at school. If your child has several different teachers (middle or high school) ask the principal to send a school representative. Teachers need to be aware of the stresses facing the family, and understand that feelings may bubble to the surface in their classroom. It is essential that parents advocate for the healthy child's emotional and educational needs as well as their sick child's. Chapter 16, *Siblings*, deals exclusively with the problems, feelings, and burdens of the siblings, and contains suggestions for coping.

Returning to school

Although it is normal that parents don't think about school during the early efforts to save their child's life, hospital personnel should reinforce the importance of an early return to school. Going to school helps children regain a sense of normalcy and provides a lifeline of hope for the future.

Preparation is the key to a successful reentry to school. The parent should ask the physician or primary nurse to prepare a letter for the school staff containing the following information:

- The student's health status and its probable affect on attendance.

- Whether she will attend full or half days.

- Whether he can attend unrestricted general physical education classes, general P.E. with restrictions (e.g., no running), or support a request for adaptive physical education for disabled children.

- How much recess is allowed, if any.

- A description of any changes in her physical appearance (e.g., will she bring a wig?).

- Her feelings about returning to school.

- Any anticipated behavioral changes resulting from medication or treatment.

- The possible effect of medications on her academic performance.

- If any medications or other health services need to be given at school.

- Reminder to never give any medication, especially aspirin, which can cause uncontrollable bleeding, without parental permission.

- Dietary restrictions.

- Any special considerations such as extra snacks, rest periods, or extra time to get from class to class, use of the nearest restroom (even if teachers') and the need to go to the restroom without permission. Depending on the age of the child and her knowledge about her situation, how much weight to give to her requests.

- Concerns about exposure to communicable disease.

- List of signs and symptoms requiring parent notification, e.g., fever, nausea, pain, swelling, bruising, or nosebleeds. In the case of divorce, which parent to notify, or notify first.

- Any uniform changes (e.g., scarf or hat).

- Stress that the teacher's job is to teach, and the parent and nurse will take care of all medical issues.

Once faculty have had a chance to read the letter, request an IEP meeting that includes faculty, administrators, school nurse, school counselor or psychologist, and special education personnel. At this meeting, answer any questions about the information contained in the letter, pass out booklets on children with cancer in the classroom, formulate a communicable disease notification strategy (if necessary), discuss the ongoing need for appropriate discipline, and do your best to establish a rapport with the entire staff. Take this opportunity to express appreciation for the school's help and your hopes for a close collaboration in the future to create a supportive climate for your child.

> *I still feel unbelievable gratitude when I think of the school principal and my daughter's kindergarten teacher that first year. The principal's eyes filled with tears when I told her what was happening, and she said, "You tell us what you need and I'll move the earth to get it for you." She hand-picked a wonderful teacher for her, made sure that a chicken pox notification plan was in place, and kept in touch with me for feedback. She recently retired, and I sent her a glowing letter which I copied to the school superintendent and school board. Words can't express how wonderful they were.*

· · · · ·

> *Jeremy's kindergarten teacher was the pits. He was on chemotherapy, and she told Jeremy not to wash his hands, as it took too long. I was disappointed that even after the nurse came to class and gave a presentation, the kids still teased my son. They would say things like, "You've got Jeremy germs, you are going to catch cancer" and "You can't get rid of cancer, you always die." During his kindergarten year, Jeremy needed to have heart surgery. I called the teacher to let her know, but he did not hear from anyone in his class, not one card or phone call even from the teacher. She didn't even tell the class why Jeremy was absent.*

The following are additional parent suggestions on how to prevent problems through preparation and communication:

- Keep the school informed and involved from the beginning. This fosters a spirit that "we're all in this together."

- Reassure the staff that even if the child looks frail, he really needs to be in school.

The school librarian had a bed set up in the library for ailing students to use. I found out that sometimes Preston would spend the whole day there, because he was just too exhausted to attend class. It was very important to him and his sense of well-being to be at school. He would just drag himself in there in order to be with the other kids. Fortunately, all of his classmates were always nice to him.

· · · · ·

There was a beanbag chair in the back of Brent's class, and he just curled up in it and went to sleep when he needed to.

- Reassure them that the child poses no health threat to anyone.

- Bring the pediatric oncology nurse back into the class to talk about cancer and answer questions whenever necessary. This should also be done at the beginning of each new year to prepare the new classmates.

- Ask the school to bend some rules and policies if you think it will help your youngster. For example, wearing a hat can sometimes eliminate teasing.

My sixteen-year-old son was allowed to leave each textbook in his various classrooms. This prevented him from having to carry a heavy backpack all day. They also let him out of class a few minutes early because he was slower moving from room to room.

- For elementary school children, enlist the aid of the hospital advocate or school counselor to help select the teacher for the upcoming year. Although this violates the policy at some schools (and you have no legal right to it), you can ask nicely that the policy be modified for your child.

Because my son has had such a hard third-grade year, I have really researched the fourth-grade teachers. I sat in and observed three teachers. I sent a letter to the principal, outlining the issues, and requested a specific teacher. The principal called me and was very upset. He said, "You can't just request who you want. What would happen if all the parents did that? You'll have to give me three choices just like everybody else." I said, "My son has had three years of chemotherapy, has a seizure disorder, behavior problems, and learning disabilities. Can you think of a child who has greater need for special consideration?" My husband and I then requested a meeting with him, and at the meeting he finally agreed to honor our teacher request.

- Prepare both teacher(s) and student for the upcoming year.

> *I asked for a spring conference with the teacher selected for the next fall and explained what my child was going through, what his learning style was, and what type of classroom situation seemed to work best. Then, I brought my son in to meet the teacher several times, and let him explore the classroom where he would be the next year. This helped my son and the future teacher adjust to one another.*

- Get help from school counselors to talk about grades, classes, and other issues of what goes on in school. A mental health therapist can talk with your child about emotions and the child's life both inside and beyond school.

> *My daughter went to a psychotherapist for the years of treatment. It provided a safe haven for frank discussions of what was happening, and also provided a place to practice social skills, which was a big problem for her at school.*

- Recognize that children's response to treatment varies.

> *Chemotherapy can really zap some kids, leaving them a pale, tired version of themselves. Other children can have chemo and still have lots of energy to participate in school. Some children have always gotten every little bug they are exposed to—others are never sick.*

> *We were some of the lucky ones. Robby continued to attend school, do karate, and play baseball. Had minimal hospitalizations and rarely even had a cold. Cancer was pretty much just a reason he had to go to the doctor every once in a while. We didn't dwell on it, but we also didn't deny it. He still had to make his bed every morning and do his homework and behave in an acceptable manner.*

- Realize that teachers and other school staff can be frightened, biased, overwhelmed, and discouraged by a child with a life-threatening illness in their classroom. Accurate information and words of appreciation can provide much needed support.

Avoiding communicable diseases

The dangers of communicable diseases to immunosuppressed children are discussed in Chapter 11, *Common Side Effects of Chemotherapy*. To prevent exposure, parents need to work closely with the school to develop a chicken pox, shingles, and measles outbreak plan if the school does not already have a disease notification plan in place. Parents need to be notified immediately if their child has been exposed to chicken pox so that the child can receive the varicella zoster immune globulin (VZIG) injection within 72 hours of exposure.

There are several methods used to ensure prompt reporting of outbreaks. Some parents notify all the classmates' parents by letter to ask for help. If the parent has a good rapport with the teacher, she can have the teacher report any cases.

> *My daughter's preschool was very concerned and organized about the chicken pox reporting. They noted on each child's folder whether he or she had already contracted chicken pox. They told each parent individually about the dangers to Katy, and then frequently reminded everyone in the monthly newsletters. The parents were absolutely great, and we always had time to keep her out of school until there were no new cases. With the help of these parents, teachers, our neighbors, and friends, Katy dodged exposure for almost three years. She caught chicken pox seven months after treatment ended and had a perfectly normal case.*

· · · · ·

> *My son was diagnosed at age fourteen. He was starting ninth grade, the last year of junior high. He missed about a third of that year. He was able to keep up thanks to some terrific teachers and a very cooperative administration, not to mention being a really motivated kid. He hated missing school and would go even when he didn't feel very good, just to say he'd been to school that day, even if only for two periods. Our oncologists gave him the okay to be in school, saying that infection in kids his age was usually from bacteria they were already carrying around, so other kids, providing they weren't sick, were not a big threat.*

Other parents enlist the help of the office workers who answer the phone calls from parents of absent children.

> *We asked the two ladies in the office to write down the illness of any child in Mrs. Williams's class. That way the teacher could check daily and call me if any of the kids in her class came down with chicken pox.*

What about preschoolers?

A large proportion of children diagnosed with cancer are preschoolers. Parents face the dilemma of continuing preschool through treatment, risking exposure to all the usual childhood viruses and diseases, or holding their child out, which denies them the opportunity for social growth and development. The decision is a purely personal one made after considering such issues as:

- Has the child already had chicken pox?
- Is the child already enrolled and comfortable in a preschool program?
- Are social needs being met by siblings and/or neighbors?
- Is preschool an option given medical considerations?

> Elizabeth was in preschool at the time of her diagnosis. The manager did a wonderful job of integrating her back into the fold. All of the other children at the school were taught what was happening to Elizabeth and what would be happening (such as hair loss). They learned that they had to be gentle with her when playing. The manager was a former home health nurse, so I was very confident that she would be able to take care of my daughter in the event of an emergency. She was already familiar with central lines and side effects from chemotherapy. She was a gem!

The terminally ill child and school

In the sad event that the child's health continues to deteriorate and all possible treatments have been exhausted, it is time for the students and staff to discuss ways to be supportive during his final days. Classmates need timely information about their ill classmate, so that they can deal with his declining health and prepare for his death. The possibility of death from cancer should have been sensitively raised in the initial class presentation prior to the student's return to school, but additional information is needed if the student's health declines. The following are suggestions on how to prepare for the death of a classmate:

- The entire school staff needs to be in continuous communication with parents and hospital. They need to be reassured that death will not suddenly occur at school, that the child will either die at home or in the hospital.

- Staff needs to be aware that participation at school is vital to a sick child's well-being. They should welcome and support the child's need to attend school as long as possible.

- Staff can design flexible programs for the ill student, for example, part-time school attendance and/or part-time home tutoring (if appropriate) for a child too weak to attend school all day.

  Jody was lucky because he went to a private school, and there were only sixteen children in his class. Whenever he could come to school, they made him welcome. Because children worked at their own pace, he never had the feeling that he was getting behind in his classwork. He really felt like he belonged there. Sometimes he could only manage to stay an hour, but he loved to go. Toward the end when he was in a wheelchair, the kids would fight over whose turn it was to push him. The teacher was wonderful, and the kids really helped him and supported him until the end.

- Staff can designate a "safe person" and "safe haven" in the school building so that the student can retreat if physically or emotionally overwhelmed.

- The hospital advocate should meet with school personnel and the student's class to answer questions about the student's health status and to address fears and misconceptions about death.

- It is helpful to provide reading materials on death and dying for the ill child's classmates, siblings' classmates, teachers, and staff.

- Extraordinary efforts should be made to keep in touch once the child can no longer attend school. Cards, banners, tapes, telephone calls, or conference calls (on the principal's speaker phone) from the entire class are good ways to share thoughts and best wishes.

- Visits to the hospital or child's home should be made, if appropriate. If the child is too sick to entertain visitors, the class could come wave at the front window and drop off cards or gifts.

- The class can send a book of jokes, a Walkman and tapes, or a basket of small gifts to the hospital.

- The class can decorate the family's front door, mailbox, and yard when the child is returning home from the hospital.

All of the above activities encourage empathy and concern in classmates, as well as help them adjust to the decline and imminent death of their friend.

When the child dies, a memorial service at school gives students a chance to grieve. School counselors or psychologists should talk to the classmates to allow them to express their feelings.

Parents appreciate receiving stories or poems about their departed child from classmates, and other children attending the funeral also supports the grieving family.

Identifying cognitive late effects

State-of-the-art treatment for childhood cancer has increasingly resulted in greater numbers of long-term survivors, but not without cost. Some survivors suffer neurotoxic effects, which cause changes in their learning style as well as social behavior. These differences in school may be treatment related, may have been preexisting and aggravated by treatment, or may be caused by prolonged absences from school and friends.

It is important that parents and educators remain vigilant for potential learning problems to allow for quick intervention. The signs of possible learning disabilities are problems with:

- Handwriting.
- Spelling.
- Reading or reading comprehension, especially compound sentences.
- Understanding math concepts, remembering math facts, comprehending math symbols, sequencing, and working with columns and graphs.
- Difficulty in using calculators or computers.
- Auditory or visual language processing. These children have trouble with vocabulary, blending sounds, and syntax.
- Attention deficits. Some children become either inattentive or hyperactive or both. These behaviors are indicative of neurologically based deficits in attention, which can cause children to be more impulsive and distractible than their peers.
- Short-term memory and information retrieval.
- Planning and organizational skills.
- Social maturity and social skills.

You should also suspect learning difficulties if:

- Your child was an A student prior to cancer, and she is working just as hard and getting Cs.

- Your child takes three hours to do homework that used to take one hour.

- Your child reads a story and then has trouble explaining the plot.

- Your child frequently comes home frustrated from school, saying he just doesn't understand things as well as the other kids.

- Your child's teacher complains that she "just doesn't pay attention" or "just needs to work harder."

If any of the above situations are occurring, take action to begin the evaluation process before your child's self-esteem plummets. It is often hard to take this first step because children affected by radiation and/or chemotherapy can reason well and think clearly and may be above average academically in several areas. They may fall behind their classmates, however, on tasks that require fast processing skills, short-term memory, sequential operations, and organizational ability (especially visual). Once identified, these differences can be addressed by strategies such as resource services in memory enhancement, eliminating timed tests, improving organizational skills, and providing extra help in mathematics, spelling, reading, and speech.

> *When she entered adolescence, my daughter became very angry about her learning disabilities. She used to be gifted, and now does very well, but it is a struggle for her. We honestly explained that the choices were life with the possibility of some academic problems versus death, and we chose life.*

Your legal rights (United States)

The cornerstone of all federal special education legislation in the United States is Public Law 94-142, the Individuals with Disabilities Education Act (IDEA). The major provisions of this legislation are the following:

- All children, regardless of disability, are entitled to a free and appropriate public education and necessary related services. Schools are required to provide an individually designed instructional program for every eligible child. An amendment to 94-142, called Public Law 99-457, requires early intervention programs for at-risk infants and toddlers.

- Children will receive fair testing to determine if they need special education services.

- Children with disabilities will be educated in the least restrictive environment, usually with children who are not disabled.

- The decisions of the school system can be challenged by parents, with disputes being resolved by an impartial third party.

- Parents of children with disabilities participate in the planning and decision making for their child's special education.

Of course, each school district has different interpretations of the requirements of the law, and implementation varies, so you should contact the school superintendent, director of special education, or special education advisory committee to obtain a copy of the school system's procedures for special education ("Notice of Parents' Rights"). Depending on the district, this document may range from two to several hundred pages. Also write to your state Superintendent of Public Instruction to obtain a copy of the state rules governing special education. To get the address, ask the school principal, a reference librarian, or refer to the resource section of *Negotiating the Special Education Maze* listed in Appendix D.

Children on and off treatment may also be eligible for services and accommodations under the federal Rehabilitation Act (Section 504). Section 504 applies when the child does not meet the eligibility requirements for specially designed instruction, but still needs accommodations to perform successfully in school. For example, a child undergoing chemotherapy might need some special accommodations to address health needs (e.g., use of separate bathroom when neutropenic, different behavior management for prednisone days, water bottle on the desk, different medication administration policies, reduced homework during periods of frequent illness, waiving regular attendance/tardy policies and procedures). A child off therapy with cognitive impairments that do not meet the IDEA requirements might need to have accommodations that eliminate timed tests or provide more time to finish written assignments.

> Robbie was diagnosed in January of his kindergarten year. He returned to kindergarten the same day he got out of the hospital. His teacher was wonderful. She moved the desks around in the classroom so that if Robby got tired, she would go get his cot and put it in the center of the classroom so he could lay down and still listen. If a child had a cold, she would move him/her to the other side of the classroom. The kids

washed their hands at least four times a day. The teacher's aide would sit in the rocking chair holding Robby if he was sad (prednisone days). Also on prednisone days, Robby was allowed to have his lunch box, which weighed at least ten pounds a day, at his desk and he could eat all day.

Your legal rights (Canada)

The Canadian special education process is very similar to that used in the US. Provincial guidelines are set down by the national Ministry of Education and governed by the Education Act, but most decisions are made at the regional, district, or school level. Evaluations are done by a team that may include a school district psychologist, a behavior specialist, a special education teacher, other school or district personnel, and in some cases a parent, although the latter is not required by law as it is in the US.

Children between the ages of 6 and 22 may qualify for special education assistance under the Designated Disabled Program (DDP), the Special Needs Program (SNP), or the Targeted Behavior Program (TBP), depending on the evaluation.

A full range of placement options is available for Canadian students, from home-based instruction to full inclusion. Students from rural or poorly served areas may receive funding to attend a day program outside of their home area.

Referral for services

You will need to be an advocate for your child as he goes through the several steps necessary to determine the best possible education available to him. The steps that will be taken are referral, evaluation, eligibility, developing an individual education plan (IEP), annual review, and triennial assessment.

> *My son had problems as soon as he entered kindergarten while on treatment. He couldn't hold a pencil, and he developed difficulties with math and reading. By second grade, I was asking the school for extra help, and they tested him. They did an IEP, and gave him special attention in small remedial groups. The school system also provided weekly physical therapy, which really helped him.*

Parents or teachers can make a referral by writing the school principal, requesting special education testing. Some school districts automatically will set up an IEP for any child who has had cranial radiation as part of his therapy, while other school districts are extremely reluctant even to evaluate struggling children for possible learning disabilities. Therefore, it is best for the parent or physician to send a written request to the principal, stating that the child is "health impaired" due to treatment for cancer, list his problems, and request assessments and an IEP meeting.

Once the referral is made, an evaluation is necessary to find out if the school district agrees that the child needs additional help, and if so, what types of help would be most beneficial. Usually a multidisciplinary team consisting of at least the teacher, school nurse, district psychologist, speech and language therapist, resource specialist, medical advocate (whoever is serving as the hospital liaison with the school), and social worker meet to administer and evaluate the testing. Parents should always request that the ADA/504 coordinator be present at the IEP meeting. Schools call the teams that write 504 plans either Child Study Teams or Student Study Teams (it's the same thing, just different names). Areas usually included in the evaluation process are educational, medical, social, psychological, and others.

Some survivors of childhood cancer require neuropsychological testing, which is best administered by psychologists experienced in testing pediatric patients. Most large children's hospitals have such personnel, but it sometimes takes very assertive parents to get the school system to use these experts. Your written consent is required prior to your child's evaluation, and you have the right to obtain an independent evaluation if you believe that the school's evaluation is biased or flawed in any way. However, you are responsible for this cost unless the district agrees or you follow the notice procedures.

After the evaluation, a conference is held to discuss the results and reach conclusions about what actions will be necessary in the future. Make sure that in all written correspondence with the school, you clearly express a wish to be present at all meetings and discussions concerning your child's special education needs. You know him best, and you and your spouse have the right to be there.

Parents need to be aware that children of very high intelligence unfortunately can fall into a gap where services will not be offered. This is because they may continue to perform "adequately," according to the school district standards (e.g., achievement scores within two grade levels of the child's age). Gifted children may receive good enough grades (As, Bs, Cs) even though their potential is that of an A+ student. These assertions may be unlawful if the child meets other eligibility requirements. This discrepancy can frustrate them significantly. In this case, parents should be strong advocates, and continue to seek special services through the school or private tutoring if they can afford to pay out of pocket for it.

Individual education plan (IEP)

The individual education plan describes the special education program and any other related services specifically designed to meet the individual needs of your child with learning differences. It is developed as a collaboration between parents and professional educators to determine what the student will be taught, and how and when the school will teach it. Students with disabilities need to learn the same things as other students: reading, writing, mathematics, history, and other preparation for college or vocational training. The difference is that, with an IEP in place, many specialized services, such as small classes, home schooling (usually five hours per week), speech therapy, physical therapy, counseling, and instruction by special education teachers, are used.

> Initially, the school was reluctant to test Gina because they thought she was too young (six years old). But she had been getting occupational therapy at the hospital for two years, and I wanted the school to take over. I brought in articles from Candlelighters Childhood Cancer Foundation, and spoke to the teacher, principal, nurse, and counselor. She had a dynamite teacher who really listened, and she helped get permission to have Gina tested. Her tests showed her to be very strong in some areas, and very weak in others. Together, we put together an IEP which we have updated every spring. Originally, she received weekly occupational therapy and daily help from the special education teacher. She's now in fourth grade and is doing so well that she no longer needs occupational therapy, and she only gets extra help during study hall. They even recommended her for the student council, which has been a tremendous boost for her self-confidence.

The IEP has five parts:

1. **A description of the child.** Includes present level of social, behavioral, and physical functioning, academic performance, learning style, and medical history.

2. **Goals and objectives.** Lists skills and behaviors that your child can be expected to master in a specific period of time. These should not be

vague like "John will learn to cooperate," but rather, "John will prepare and present an oral book report with two regular education students by May 1." Each goal should answer the following questions: Who? What? How? Where? When? How often? When will the service start and end?

3. **Related services.** There are many specialized services that might be mandated by the IEP which will be provided at no cost to the family. These can include hearing or speech therapy, health services, occupational therapy, parent counseling and training, physical therapy, and transportation. For these services, the IEP should list the frequency and duration, e.g., "Jane will receive physical therapy from 9:00 to 10:00 a.m. on Tuesday and Thursday from September until December, when her needs will be reevaluated."

4. **Placement.** Describes the least restrictive setting in which the above goals and objectives can be met. For example, one student would be in the regular classroom all day with an aide present, while another might leave the classroom for part of each day to receive specialized instruction in the resource room or physical therapy. The IEP should state the percent of time the child will be in the regular education program and the frequency and duration of any special services.

5. **Evaluating the IEP.** At least once a year, and more frequently if requested by a parent or teacher, a meeting is held to review the progress towards meeting the short- and long-term goals and objectives of the IEP. Some states have limits on the number of IEP meetings per year.

It is best to create a positive relationship with the school so that you are able to work together to promote your child's well-being. If, for whatever reason, communication deteriorates and you feel that your child's IEP is inadequate or not being followed, there are several facts that you need to know:

• Changes to the IEP cannot be made without parental consent.

• If parents disagree about the content of the IEP, they can withdraw consent and request (in writing) a meeting to draft a new IEP or they can consent only to portions of the IEP with which they agree.

• Parents can request to have the disagreement settled by an independent mediator and hearing officer.

This year (third grade) has been a nightmare. My son has an IEP that focuses on problems with short-term memory, concentration, writ-

ing, and reading comprehension. The teacher, even though she is special-ed qualified, has been rigid and used lots of timed tests. She told me in one conference that she thought my son's behavior problems were because he was "spoiled." We asked her at the beginning of the year to please send a note home with my son if he has a seizure, and she has never done it. She even questions him when he tells her that he had a seizure at recess. I began communicating directly with the principal, and I finally received a written notice that he had a seizure. I learned that the IEP is only as valuable as the teacher who is applying it.

The IEP in Canada is almost identical to those used in the US. In Canada, the IEP is updated yearly, or more frequently if needed. A formal review is required every three years. In Canada, if disputes arise between the school or the district and the parents, there is a School Division Decision Review process available to resolve them. The concept known as due process in the US is usually referred to as fundamental justice in Canada.

Services for infants and preschoolers

US federal law also mandates early intervention services for disabled infants and toddlers, and in some cases, children at risk of having developmental delays. Infants, toddlers, or preschoolers with cancer may be eligible for these services in order to avoid developmental delays caused by cancer treatments. These services are administered either by the school system or the state health department. You can find out which agency to contact by asking the hospital social worker or by calling the special education director for your school district.

The law requires services not only for the infant or preschooler, but for the family as well. Therefore, instead of an IEP, an Individualized Family Service Plan (IFSP) is developed. This plan includes:

1. Description of child's physical, cognitive, language, speech, psychosocial, and other developmental levels

2. Goals and objectives for family and child

3. Description, frequency, and delivery of services needed, such as:

   - Speech, occupational, and physical therapy

   - Health and medical services

- Family training and counseling

4. A caseworker who locates and coordinates all necessary services

5. Steps to support transition to other programs and services

> We have had an excellent experience with the school district through-out preschool and now in kindergarten. We went to them with the first neuropsychiatric results, which were dismal. They retested him, and suggested a special developmental preschool and occupational therapy. Both helped him enormously. He had an IEP done, and now has a full-time aide in kindergarten. He is getting the help he needs.

Record-keeping

Other than medical record-keeping, no records are more important to keep than those concerning your child's special education. Many parents recommend that you keep a yearly file that includes the name of the teacher, principal, and district psychologist, copy of the IEP, all test results, all correspondence, a current copy of the local and state regulations, and all of your child's report cards. You should also include in the file a list of the medications taken by your child during the year. Do not throw these records out—give them to your child when she reaches eighteen, as they can be crucial for college testing and accommodations.

The thought of this may seem overwhelming, but try to think of it this way: appropriate schooling is what will enable your child to overcome the cancer experience and become a productive adult. And your child needs your help to secure that future.

On accepting disabilities

Many of the disabilities of survivors of childhood cancer are invisible. To help children and teens reach their true potential, changes in intellectual functioning and social skills must be diagnosed early and addressed. Students whose style of learning has changed as a result of treatment need their parents and teachers to explore the many excellent methods to enhance their ability to learn.

It is also important to remember that higher cognitive functioning often remains intact, it is just getting the information in ("processing") that is impaired. Children who were gifted usually remain so; children with average abilities retain them. Their performance may be slower; they may require extra instruction in memory enhancement and organizational skills, but they can still achieve to their potential. There are thousands of survivors in their late teens and twenties who are successfully attending college, or who have graduated and are pursuing professional careers. A disabled survivor of Wilms tumor who is now an expert on disability law wrote:

> These children are not going to have their rights protected, or be eligible (presuming they are eligible) for various services, benefits, programs, and affirmative action unless they say they are disabled. As far as the civil rights laws are concerned, they will be considered disabled from diagnosis till death, even if they are as healthy as the average person. Furthermore, the limited civil rights protection that applies to their parents, siblings, spouses, and partners won't apply unless they say they are disabled.

> I do not think that there is anything shameful or stigmatizing about saying you are disabled. I think the efforts some parents have gone to so they can avoid this word are similar to the old days, when black children wore their hair like white children, and other families changed their last names and stopped speaking their native tongues for fear of "not fitting in." I think if disability is correctly explained to children, they will understand and accept. When I was a child, I was told I wasn't disabled (that was for people who were deaf, retarded, or in a wheelchair), I was merely "very sick" most of the time. It is better to make the effort to teach and have the children enjoy friendships with both nondisabled and disabled children. Otherwise, you end up with adults who feel isolated from even their own siblings.

Armed with the information from this chapter, and material from Appendix D, you will be prepared to effectively work with the school to ensure the very best education possible for your child, the survivor.

The following passage was written by Brigit Tuxen and is reprinted from Candlelighters Youth Newsletter, Fall 1994, Vol. XVI No. 4.

> My diagnosis of high-risk ALL gave me a 50 percent chance of survival. Cranial radiation and three years of blood tests, IV, chemotherapy, bone marrows, and spinal taps were my prescription. A positive outlook

pushed me through the bad times. Somehow I understood that all the hurt was for a good reason, and that it would make me well.

Call it a miracle, luck, or determination to live—I survived! But I would soon realize that I would never be like all the other kids. The radiation which destroyed cancer cells also harmed some of my brain cells. For the past five years, I have had slight difficulty with math and science courses at school, but, with the help of a tutor, I've managed to pull through challenging honors classes with As and Bs. However, I am often the last to finish class assignments or tests. It is very frustrating and often embarrassing. The SAT has become my ultimate challenge. Despite this minor disability, I continue to set high standards for myself. I feel extremely lucky to have beaten this disease, and I want to do anything I can to help those who are fighting cancer or some other hardship.

CHAPTER 16

Siblings

Why was his hair falling out? Why was he
going to the hospital all the time? Why was he
getting bone marrows all the time? It never
occurred to me that he might die. What was
happening? I didn't get to go to the hospital to
see him. What was leukemia? Why was he
getting so many presents???

—Chet Stevens
Straight from the Siblings:
Another Look at the Rainbow

CHILDHOOD CANCER TOUCHES all members of the family, with especially long-lasting effects on siblings. The diagnosis creates an array of conflicting emotions in siblings; not only are the siblings concerned about their ill brother or sister, but they usually resent the turmoil that the family has been thrown into. They feel jealous of the gifts and attention showered on the sick child, yet feel guilty for having these emotions. The days, months, and years after diagnosis can be difficult indeed, for the sibling of a child with leukemia.

Of all the topics covered in this book, parents expressed the most regret and guilt over how they handled the pain and worry of their "healthy" children. They will share with you their experiences, in the hope that it will help you find the time to listen to and love the frequently overlooked brothers and sisters.

Emotional responses of the siblings

Brothers and sisters are shaken to the very core by leukemia in the family. Their parents, the leaders of the family clan, sometimes have no time, and little energy, to focus on the siblings. During this major crisis for the siblings—this time when their beings are flooded with anger and concern, jealousy and love, when they are in conflict as never before—they often have no one to turn to for help. If you recognize these strong, ever-changing emotions of siblings as normal, not pathological, you will be better able to help your child talk about and cope with his overpowering feelings.

Although the time after diagnosis is emotionally potent, stress levels associated with life-threatening illnesses tend to decrease over time. Siblings also tend to have good psychological outcomes. In many cases, siblings report the experience as life changing in many positive ways.

Concern for sick brother or sister

Children really worry about their sick brother or sister. It is hard for them to watch someone they love be hurt by needles, sickened by medicines, lose weight, and be bald. It is hard to feel so healthy and full of energy when the brother or sister has to stay indoors because of weakness or low blood counts. The siblings may also be old enough to understand that death is a possibility. There are plenty of reasons for concern.

> *Christine's younger sister has really developed the nurturing side of her personality as a result of the leukemia. She frequently puts her arm around her sister, comforts her with soothing words or touches, and seems to feel her pain.*

. . . . .

> *I'm the mother of three children. Logan was nineteen months old when diagnosed. It was very hard on all of us. Kathryn (she was five and a half at time of diagnosis) felt that she had to take so much on herself. She was there with us the entire time Logan was in the hospital. She had a cot right next to Logan's bed and only she and I were the ones that could take care of "our Logan." She is a doll.*

> *She used to love to visit the other kids on the hospital floor and entertain them. She hated to go home. She would get so involved with the other kids and didn't want to leave them. She actually got very close to two little girls that lost the battle, so here she was at six, dealing with the loss of two friends.*

Fear

It is very common for young siblings of children with cancer to think that the disease is contagious, that they can "catch it." Many also worry that one or both parents may get cancer. The diagnosis of cancer changes all of the children's view that the world is a safe place. They feel vulnerable, and they are afraid. Depending on their age, siblings worry that their brother or sister may get sicker or may die. Some siblings develop symptoms of illness in an attempt to regain attention from the parents.

Fears of things other than cancer may emerge: fear of being hit by a car, fear of dogs, fear of strangers. Many fears can be quieted by accurate and age-appropriate explanations from the parents or medical staff.

> My three-year-old daughter vacillated between fear of catching cancer ("I don't ever want those pokes") to wishing she was ill so that she would get the gifts and attention ("I want to get sick and go to the hospital with Mommy"). She developed many fears and had frequent nightmares. We did lots of medical play which seemed to help her. I let her direct the action, using puppets or dolls, and I discovered that she thought there was lots of violence during her sister's treatments. She continues to ask questions, and we are still explaining things to her, four years later.

Jealousy

Despite feeling concern for the ill brother or sister, almost all siblings also feel jealous. Presents and cards flood in for the sick child, Mom and Dad stay at the hospital with the sick child, and most conversations revolve around the sick child. When the siblings go out to play, the neighbors ask about the sick child. At school, teachers are concerned about the sick child. Is it any wonder that they feel jealous?

The siblings' lives are in turmoil, and, being human, they feel a need to blame someone. It's natural for them to think that if their brother didn't get sick, life would be back to normal.

> Our nine-year-old son seemed to be dealing with things so well until one evening as I was tucking him in he confided that he had tried to break his leg at school by jumping out of the swing. He began to cry and told me he doesn't want his brother to be sick anymore; that he needs some attention, too. As parents, we were always so concerned with our sick child that we didn't realize how much our healthy child was suffering, too.

Guilt

Young children are egocentric; they feel that the world revolves around them. It is logical to them to feel that since their sister has cancer, they caused it. They may have said in anger, "I hope you get sick and die," and then their sister got sick.

It is vital that this notion be dispelled right after diagnosis. Children really need to be told, many times, that cancer just happens, and no one in the family caused it. They need to understand that just because you think something or say something, it doesn't make it happen.

Beyond feeling guilt for causing the cancer, virtually every sibling feels guilt for their normal responses to cancer like anger and jealousy. They think, "How can I feel this way about my brother when he's so sick?" Assure them that the many conflicting feelings they are experiencing are normal and expected. As a parent, share some of your conflicting feelings (anger at the behavior of a child on prednisone, guilt about being angry).

Some children even feel guilt for being healthy! They think, "Why should I feel great when she's so frail and sick?"

Abandonment

If parental attention revolves around the sick child, siblings may feel isolated and resentful. Even when parents make a conscious effort not to be so preoccupied with the ill child, siblings sometimes still perceive that they are not getting their fair share of attention and may feel rejected.

> One day when my four-year-old son was in day care, we had to unexpectedly bring Erica in for emergency surgery on a septic hip. (It turned out to be a life-threatening surgery, and she ended up staying in for weeks.) I called the day care and said that I couldn't pick up Daniel by closing time and the teacher said, "No problem, I live right across the street and I'll take him home for dinner." We went to get Daniel that evening, and he was very withdrawn. Later, he exclaimed, "All the mommies came. Then teacher turned out the lights, and you didn't come to get me." Then he burst into tears. In hindsight, one of us should have gone to bring him to the hospital to just sit with us. It was tense there, but at least he would have been with us, included as part of the family.

Sadness

Siblings have many very good reasons to be sad. They miss their parents and the time they used to spend together. They miss the life they used to have, the one they were comfortable with. They worry that their brother or sister may die. Some children show their sadness by crying often; others withdraw and become depressed. Often children confide in relatives or friends that they think their parents don't love them anymore.

> When Jeremy was very sick and hospitalized, we sent his older brother Jason to his grandparents for long periods of time. We thought that he understood the reasons, but a year after Jeremy finished treatment, Jason (nine years old) said, "Of course, I know that you love Jeremy more than me anyway. You were always sending me away so that you could spend time with him." It just broke my heart that every time he made that long drive over the mountains with his grandparents, he was thinking that he was being sent away.

· · · · ·

> Months after his four-year-old sister's treatment ended, my six-year-old son confided to his grandmother that his parents loved her more than him. He still has never told his father or me, but he does sometimes ask if his sister is going to die. When I say no, he looks sort of disappointed.

Anger

Children's lives are disrupted by the diagnosis of a sister or brother with cancer, and it can make siblings very angry. Questions such as "Why did this happen to us?" or "Why can't things be the way they used to be?" are common. Children's anger may be directed at their sick brother, their parents, relatives, friends, or doctor. Children's anger may have a variety of causes, for instance, being left with baby-sitters so often, unequal application of family rules, or additional responsibilities at home. Because each member of the family may have frayed nerves, explosions of temper can occur.

> As we were driving home from school one day, Annie was talking, and I was only half listening. All of a sudden I realized that she was yelling at me. She screamed, "See, this is what I mean. You never listen, your mind is always on Preston." I pulled the car over, stopped, and said, "You're right. I was thinking about Preston." I told her that from now on I would try to give her my full attention. I realized that I would really have to make an effort to focus on what she was saying and not be so distracted. This conversation helped to clear the air for a while. I tried to take her out frequently for coffee or ice cream to just sit, listen, and concentrate on what she was saying.

Worry about what happens at the hospital

Children have vivid imaginations, and when they are fueled by disrupted households and whispered conversations between teary parents, children can imagine truly horrible things. Seeing how their ill sister looks upon returning from a hospital stay can reinforce their fears that awful things happen at the clinic or hospital. Age-appropriate, verbal explanations can help children be more realistic in what they think happens at the hospital, but nothing is as powerful as a visit. Of course the effectiveness of a visit depends on your child's age and temperament, but many parents said bringing the siblings along helped everyone. The sibling gained an accurate understanding of hospital procedures, the sick child is comforted by the presence of the sibling, and the parent gets to spend time with both (or more) children.

> My son is only in kindergarten. He has separation anxiety worse than a six-month-old. He doesn't want to go to bed alone. The last time Karissa had the flu, I thought he was going to die of worrying so much. He cried himself to sleep every night and woke up crying. He was so worried. He hasn't gotten much better since she has started feeling better, either. He doesn't even want to go near the hospital with his sister.

Another method to minimize worry is to read age-appropriate books together. Many children's hospitals have coloring books for preschoolers that explain hospital procedures with pictures and clear language. School-age children benefit from reading *You and Leukemia: A Day at a Time* with a parent (see Appendix D, *Books and Online Sites*). Adolescents might be helped by seeing videos on the subject or joining a sibling support group.

Veteran parents suggested that another way to reduce siblings' worries is to allow even the youngest children to help the family in some way. As long as children have clear explanations of the situation, and concrete jobs to do that will benefit the family, they tend to rise to the occasion. Make them feel that they are a necessary and integral part of the family's effort to face leukemia together.

Concern about parents

Exhausted parents are sometimes not aware of the strong feelings of their healthy children. They sometimes assume that children understand that they are loved, and would be getting the same attention if they were the one who had cancer. But siblings frequently do not share their powerful feelings of anger, jealousy, or worry because they love their parents and do not want to place additional burdens on them. It is all too common to hear siblings say, "I have to be the strong one. I don't want to cause my parents any more pain." But burdens are lighter if shared, and parents need to try to encourage all of their children to talk about how they are feeling.

Sibling experiences

Simply understanding the depth of the pain and fears of your healthy children eases their path. Being available to listen, to say, "I hear how painful this is for you," or "You sound scared. I am, too," makes siblings feel that they are still valued members of the family; that even though their brother or sister is absorbing the lion's share of parents' time and care, they are still cherished. Even if parents do not have large amounts of time to spend with them, siblings need to hear that what they feel matters. If parents understand that these overwhelming emotions are normal, expected, healthy, they can provide solace.

In the hope that telling their stories will illuminate the difficulties faced by the siblings, brothers and sisters of children with leukemia shared the following.

Silent hurting heart

Dayna Erickson is thirteen years old. One of Dayna's brothers died of a brain tumor, and her other brother is in remission from ALL. This poem was published in *Bereavement* magazine.

> *"Oh, nothing's wrong," she smiled,*
> *grinning from ear to ear.*
> *The frown that just was on her face*
> *just seemed to disappear.*
>
> *But deep down where secrets are kept,*
> *the pain began to swell.*
> *All the hurt inside of her*
> *just seemed to stay and dwell.*
>
> *All the pain in her heart*
> *was too much for her to take.*
> *Pretending everything's OK*
> *is much too hard to fake.*

She'd duck into the bathrooms
and hide inside the stalls
Because no one could see her tears,
behind those dirty walls.

She was sick and tired of losing
and things never turning out right.
She had no hope left in her.
She was ready to give up the fight.

But she wiped away the teardrops,
put a smile back on her face,
pulled herself together and
walked out of that place.

Life went on and things got better.
She thought that was a start.
But still, no one could see inside
her silent hurting heart.

Alana's story

Alana Friedman (eleven years old) remembers how family life changed when her sister, Laura, had cancer.

My sister was in fifth grade, and had been sick for the last week or so. Laura always seemed to be my hero, although we got into arguments, all siblings get into fights, so I didn't worry. I didn't know what was about to happen, but neither did anyone else.

I don't quite remember how my parents told me she had cancer, but I do remember a lot of tears.

As time progressed my life changed. I lived with my best friend and her parents, Catherine and Bill, but that changed too. Kelsie (my friend) and I got into a lot of arguments, but we still do. I don't know if that is why my grandmother and grandfather moved up to live in our house so that they could take care of me. Living with them was different. My grandmother had different expectations of me than my mother did.

My parents would each take turns staying at the hospital. Some nights I would live with my mom, grammy, and grandpy; and the next it would be with my dad and them.

Of course going through this dilemma I felt left out. Here I was living with my grandparents, and my sister got to live with our parents. She got lots of flowers, cards, and gifts and all I got was the feeling of love from my relatives. I know that love is better than material things, but when you are six years old, you don't think so.

Things stayed the same for a long time. Then my sister went into remission and started living at home. I had to get used to my parents again and missed my grandparents.

My sister was spoiled at home too. They bought her a waterbed, so she wouldn't get cold. What did I get? A heating blanket; a used heating blanket.

A few months after she came home, her remission ended. She went back to live in the hospital, and my grandparents moved up to live with me.

Things went downhill from there. My life was turned around again. My sister went into a coma, and didn't really have much of a chance of coming out of it. Soon it would be her best friend's birthday, and Laura had to miss it. She was taken to heaven that day. Taken out of her misery and leaving us with a feeling of shock.

The day my sister died I had no idea what was happening. Kelsie's mom took care of me and everything was going great. To me, that is, but when her mom took me back home, I remember my dad at the door talking to her. I headed in the other direction, but my father stopped me. My dad went into my parents' bedroom with me, and there I found my mom, lying on the bed helplessly, and to this day I still remember what she said to me, "It's over." Those words didn't make a lot of sense to me, I didn't know if the earth was going to explode. And then those two words sunk into my heart and I knew: my sister had died.

Having a sister with leukemia

Alison Leake (six years old) describes the experience of having a sister with leukemia:

I think having a sister with leukemia is not fun. My mom paid more attention to Kathryn my sister. I had to stay with Daddy! Mommy picked Kathryn up and not me! I wanted my sister's PJs. Guess what? I did not get them! Although my mommy wanted to stay with me she did not want to leave my sister alone. Sometimes I felt like I was going to throw up. But now it has been five years since she has stopped having medicine and she is completely better. To celebrate that my sister and me were such good sports when my sister had leukemia we are going to Disneyland.

Siblings: The "forgotten children" in childhood cancer

Allison Ellis (twenty years old), now a graduate of Smith College and counselor at a camp for children with childhood cancer and their siblings, discusses how siblings of cancer patients can become "forgotten children":

> *I remember walking into my sister's room one morning and seeing large clumps of blond hair on her pillow. "Mommy, why is Lisa's hair falling out?" I asked.*
>
> *"She's sick," was the only reply possible from my mother; she had no time for lengthy explanations to a three-year-old. So I was left to solve the mystery for myself. I went with Lisa and my mother several times a week to the hospital where Lisa would get finger "pokies" and sometimes "bone marrows" (which I thought of as "bone arrows" because the procedure entailed being punctured in the back by a large needle). Lisa would always cry afterward—the kind of childhood cry that seems to go on for hours at a deafening pitch. She lost all of her hair, so she wore bonnets that my grandmother made for her until her hair grew back. Sometimes she would get sick and throw up, and sometimes she stayed overnight at the hospital. I remember not understanding at all what was happening to my sister and not receiving any explanations. I remember the toys, gifts, and candy that were given in surplus to Lisa in a futile attempt to ease her pain. I felt jealous, neglected, and isolated because of Lisa's illness and the subsequent attention that was given to her and taken from me. I spent a lot of time with baby-sitters and television and less with my parents and the relatives who visited only to see Lisa. It seemed as though she was the only one people cared about. In this, I was the typical sibling of a victim of childhood cancer.*
>
> *Lisa was diagnosed with leukemia in 1973 when she was just two years old and I was three. It was not expected that Lisa would live; in fact, all diagnoses of leukemia before 1970 were terminal. My parents*

were told not to talk about the disease with anyone; a child dying of cancer was just too frightening. Lisa underwent radiation therapy as well as chemotherapy to rid her body of the cancer-causing cells.

Yet, the result of this trauma was that I, as a sibling, received no attention relative to the rest of my family, and I felt extremely left out. I remember having a baby-sitter who stayed with me and my newborn baby sister during Lisa's treatment who seemed to understand how I was feeling. She would say, "Allison, I bet you're feeling a little bit left out with all the fuss over your sisters." (The youngest was given a lot of attention because everyone pays attention to newborn babies.)

I would always utter a modest, "Yeah, I guess so" while really thinking, "Yes, nobody pays attention to me. All I do is watch Sesame Street and watch Lisa play with her new toys that she got because she is sick and she won't share them with me. You bet I feel left out!"

I remember going places with my mother and being totally ignored by the people we would meet. People would say to my mother, "How is your daughter?" I would always say, "Fine," but they were never referring to me.

"Not you," they would say, "The other one," rendering my health and condition completely unimportant. I felt like a nonentity.

I began to taunt my sister, and we would fight frequently over sharing toys or clothes, which for the most part could be attributed to normal sibling rivalries, yet a lot of my hostilities ran deeper than a few pulled hairs. Lisa was the favored member of the family, and she received deferential and preferential treatment. When she came home crying after school, which was frequently the case in the first few years after her treatment was completed, she was always met with solace and understanding, whereas if I was ever upset, I was left to work things out for myself.

Today I understand better why I had the feelings that I did regarding my sister's cancer. For many years I resented her for something she had no control over and was angry at my parents for treating her differently than me. I now realize that no parent is superhuman and that they were doing what they thought was best under the unfortunate circumstances. Yet I know there are certain things I cannot change, such as being the first born. Whereas cancer made my sister vulnerable and my parents more protective, being the sibling of a cancer patient made me more independent. I was forced to find other sources of comfort at an early age, which usually meant that it had to come from within myself. Being at camp made me realize that I wasn't the only one who had experienced such a difficult role, however, and that there are many others who have been affected by childhood cancer much more deeply than me.

In conclusion, I wish to offer some advice. Siblings: please tell your parents in any way you can how you are feeling. Remember that you are not alone and you need not be forgotten, but try to understand where your parents are coming from. Parents: listen to your children. Recognize that siblings have different needs from cancer patients and try to even out attention-giving. Don't be surprised if your sibling child is angry at you. Professionals and neighbors: sometimes you are the only hope for a neglected sibling, yet you also have the potential to make things worse. Don't forget the sibling.

My brother's a legend

To Erin Hall (eighteen years old), her brother has become a "legend" by surviving childhood cancer.

I'm really proud of my brother Judson for handling everything so well. During those years there were times when I was jealous of him, not only for the attention he received, but for his courage as well. This little boy was going through so much and I still cowered at getting my finger pricked. As I look back, I wonder if I would have been able to make it through, not only physically, but emotionally as well.

According to some people a person needs to be dead in order to be a legend, or to have been famous, or well liked. A legend to me though, is someone who has accomplished something incredible, enduring many hardships and pains, and still comes out of it smiling.

Judd is a legend to me because he didn't give up in a time that he might have. He is a legend because he survived an illness that many do not. Now I look at him after being in remission for almost five years, and I hope that someday if I am ever faced with a challenge like his, I will have the same strength and courage he had.

My brother has leukemia

Eight-year-old Amanda Moodie experienced many ups and downs when her brother had cancer.

> Sometimes having a brother with leukemia is fun, like when my family goes on the Fantasy Flight to the North Pole, and going to the special summer camp, and getting special privileges at Disney World.
>
> But other times, it can be really hard, especially when William gets put in the hospital. Right now, he can't leave his room in the hospital, and the doctors wear masks when they come in. I HATE seeing that. And he stays in for very long periods of time. The first time, he was there for almost three weeks! It comes so suddenly. He has stayed out for five months, then BAM! He's back in. And the worst of it is, people are always pitying us. "Poor little boy." "Poor William." I guess they like pitying us.
>
> So, leukemia has ups and downs like everything else, but to me it's mostly downs.

For brothers and sisters

Ellen Zimmerman discusses the impact that her cancer had on her siblings. (Reprinted with permission from *Candlelighters Youth Newsletter,* Summer 1994, Vol. XVI No. 3.)

> I am the first of four children and the only girl. When I was diagnosed with ALL at the age of fourteen, it affected all our lives. My brother Wes was thirteen, Matthew was four, and Erik was two. They and my parents were my support system.
>
> When I was first diagnosed and in the hospital, Dr. Plunkett asked if I wanted anyone besides my parents present when he gave us the diagnosis. I told him I wanted Wes with me. Wes is only fourteen months younger than I am, and we have always been very close. He took it all in, and we all decided that we would face this thing, and beat it, as a family. Then he and I sent our parents off so we could have some private time together.
>
> Wes was my support at school and at home. He stuck up for me and kept an eye on me. I lost some of my "friends" after I was diagnosed because of my illness and their fear of it. Wes was always there for me.

That's not to say we didn't have our fights. Poor Wes—I could hit him,
but he couldn't hurt me physically because of my low blood counts. Some-
times I took advantage of that.

Matt and Erik were also a great source of comfort and support. They
would accompany my mom and me to treatments and hold my hand
when I got stuck. If one of them wasn't with me when I went in, the nurses
would ask me where they were. These little boys made it easier for me to
be brave.

I hope my brothers know how much I appreciate, too, the extra time
they gave me with our parents during my illness. My parents were very
good about splitting time between me and my brothers. If one was with
me at treatment or the hospital, then the other was spending time with the
boys. Family and friends were also a big help.

I've been out of treatment for ten years now. I teach second grade
and spend a week of my summer as a counselor at a camp for kids with
cancer. I am the proud sister of three Eagle Scouts. Wes is married now
and lives in another state. I realize how much he meant to me during that
trying time and how much he means to me now.

If you are a sibling to someone with cancer and wonder if you make
a difference to your sick brother or sister, I would like to tell you that you
make a very big difference.

When my brother got cancer

Annie Walls (fifteen years old) relates a positive outcome to her and her
brother's battle with childhood cancer.

One experience in my life that was in no way comfortable for my
family or myself and caused me a lot of confusion and grief was when my
brother had leukemia. Along with the disruption of this event, it also
caused me to grow tremendously as a person. The Thanksgiving of my
third-grade year, Preston, my brother, became very ill and was diagnosed
a few weeks later with having cancer.

This event helped me to grow to become a better person in many
ways. When my brother had very little hair or was puffed out from cer-
tain drugs I learned to respect people's differences and to stick up for them

when they're made fun of. Also, when Preston was in the hospital I was taught to deal with a great amount of jealousy that I had. He received many gifts, cards, flowers, candy, games, and so many other material things that I envied. Most of all though, he received all the attention and care of my mother, father, relatives, and friends. This is what I was jealous of the most. As I look back now, I can't believe that I was that insensitive and self-centered to be mad at my brother at a time like that.

The thing that made this a "graced" experience was the fact that it enabled me to be very close to my brother as we grew up. My brother and I are now good friends and are able to talk and share our experiences with each other. I don't think that we would have this same relationship if he never had leukemia and I think that has been a very positive outcome. Another thing that has been a positive outcome of this event is the people I've been able to meet. Through all the support groups, camps, and events for children with cancer and their siblings, I have met some people with more courage and more heart than anyone could imagine. In no way am I saying that I'm glad my brother had cancer, but I will say I'm very glad with some of the outcomes from it.

My sister had cancer

Eleven-year-old Jeff Pasowicz explains what happened when "My Sister Had Cancer." (Reprinted from CCCF Canada CONTACT newsletter Vol. XVI No. 2 Spring 1994.)

My sister Jamie got cancer when she was twenty-three months old. I was eight, and my two other sisters were six and four.

My sisters and I were scared that my sister was going to die. We weren't able to go to public places and also weren't allowed to have friends in my house. We missed a lot of school when there was chicken pox in our school. I got teased in school sometimes because my sister had no hair. Once an older kid called my sister a freak. My mom was sad most of the time. It was very hard.

We are all pleased that Jamie is doing well, and our lives are getting back to normal. It was an experience I'll never forget, and I hope it has made me a stronger person.

From a sibling

Fifteen-year-old Sara McDonnall won first prize in the 1995 Candlelighters Creative Arts Contest with her essay, "From a Sibling."

Childhood cancer—a topic most teens don't think much about. I know I didn't until it invaded our home.

Childhood cancer totally disrupts lives, not only of the patient, but also of those closest to him/her, including the siblings. First, I was numbed with unbelieving shock. "This can't be happening to me and my family." Along with this came a whole dictionary full of incomprehensible words and a total restructuring of our (up to that time) fairly normal life-style.

One day in July 1988, I was waiting for my parents to pick me up from summer camp and anticipating the start of our family vacation to Canada. When they arrived, they informed me that my older brother Danny was very sick, and we wouldn't be taking that trip after all. The following day the call came that confirmed the diagnosis. Instead of packing for vacation, we packed our bags and headed for Children's Hospital in Denver, 200 miles away, where Danny was scheduled for surgery and chemotherapy.

I developed my own disease (perhaps from fear I would "catch" what Danny had), with symptoms similar to my brother's:

Sympathy pains. I asked, "Why him?" when he came home from the hospital, exhausted from throwing up a life-saving drug for three days.

Fear. "How much sicker is Danny going to get before he gets well? He is going to get well, isn't he?"

Resentment. My parents seemed so worried about him all the time. They didn't seem to have time for me anymore.

Confusion. Why couldn't Danny and I wrestle around like we used to? Why couldn't I slug him when he made me mad?

Jealousy. I felt insignificant when I was holding down the fort at home.

The parts I hated the most were: not understanding what was being done to him; answering endless worried phone calls; and hearing the answers to my own questions when my parents talked to other people.

I was helped to sort out these feelings and identify with other siblings when I attended a program held just for teens who had siblings with cancer. We got together, tried to learn how to cross-country ski, and talked about our siblings and ourselves.

Perhaps you remember this story: "US [speed skating] star Dan Jansen, 22, carrying a winning time into the back straightaway of the 1000 meter race, inexplicably fell. Two days earlier, after receiving word that his older sister, Jane, had died of leukemia, Dan crashed in the 500 meter" (Life Magazine). Having a sibling with cancer can immobilize even an Olympic athlete. Dan was expected to bring home two gold medals, but cancer in a sibling intervened. He became, instead, the most famous cancer sibling of all time. He shared his grief before a television audience of two billion people. Dan later went on to win the World Cup in Norway and Germany, and capture the gold at the Olympics. He is the first to tell you the real champions can be found in the oncology wards of children's hospitals across our nation, and the siblings who are fighting the battle right along beside them.

Siblings: Having our say

Naomi Chesler gives advice to parents and siblings of those with childhood cancer.

Twelve young people aged 7 to 29 met at the 25th Anniversary Candlelighters Conference to talk about what it is like having a sibling with cancer in the family. We talked about our families, our anger, jealousy, worries, and fears, and thought about what we wanted to tell others about our experiences. In fact, we made lists of things we wanted other people to know: one for parents, one for other children or young adults in our position, and one for the child who has been diagnosed with cancer.

Some parts of these lists reflect anger and bitterness, but that was not the overriding feeling in the session. I hope it isn't the only message you take away. If nothing else, the issues raised here may provide you with a good starting point for discussions in your own family.

To parents:

- *We know you are burdened and trying to be fair. But try harder.*

- *Give us equal time.*

- *Be tough on disciplining the child with cancer. No free rides.*

- *Put yourself in our shoes once in a while.*

- *If you are away from home a lot, at least call and tell us, "I love you."*

- *Tell us what is going on. Don't just sit us in front of a video (about cancer); talk with us about it.*

- *Keep special time with us like lunch once a week or something. Time for just us. And if you can't be with us, find someone who can.*

- *When you talk to family members, say how everyone is doing— what we are doing is important, too.*

- *Ask how we are feeling. Don't assume you know.*

To siblings of newly diagnosed kids:

- *Keep a diary if you don't want to talk to your parents.*

- *Expect to not get as much attention.*

- *Expect that your parents are going to be extra cautious about what your brother/sister does, who he/she hangs out with, etc.*

- *Hang in there. You're all you've got for now.*

- *Don't feel like you have to think about the illness all the time.*

- *Be understanding of your parents and stay involved.*

- *Tell someone how you are feeling—don't bottle it up.*

- *Go to the hospital to visit when you can.*

- *Make as many friends as possible at school.*

To our siblings who struggled or are struggling with cancer:

- *The world does not revolve around you.*

- *Stop feeling sorry for yourself.*

- *Not everything is related to cancer. Stop using that as an excuse for everything.*

- *I'm jealous of you sometimes, but I'm not mad. I know it sometimes seems like I'm mad, but I'm not.*

- *Don't take advantage of all the extra attention you get.*

- *Tell mom and dad to pay attention to me sometimes, too.*

- *Now that you are feeling better, where's the gratitude for all those chores that I did?*

- *I really admire your strength and courage. I wouldn't have gotten through your illness without you.*

Helping siblings cope

The following are the experiences and advice from several families on things that help brothers and sisters cope:

- Make sure that you explain leukemia and its treatment to the siblings in terms that they understand. Create a climate of openness, so that they can ask questions and know that they will get answers. If you don't know the answer to a question, write it on your list to ask the doctor at the next appointment, or ask your child if he would like to go to the appointment with you and ask the question himself.

   We drew a lot of pictures of red cells, white cells, and platelets. We showed each doing its job: red cells carrying oxygen around, white cells gobbling up cold germs as well as leukemia blasts, and platelets clumping up to form scabs. Drawing opened the floodgates of questions, and I was always amazed at how each child understood some things so clearly, and really was confused and frightened by other things.

   $\cdot \quad \cdot \quad \cdot \quad \cdot \quad \cdot$

   We always, always explained everything that was happening to Brent's older brother Zac (eight years old). He never asked questions, but always listened intently. He would say, "Okay. I understand. Everything's all right." We tried to get him to talk about it, but through all these years, he just never has. So we just kept explaining things at a level that he could understand, and he has done very well through the whole ordeal. The times that he seemed sad, we would take him out of school, and let him stay at the Ronald McDonald House for a few days, and that seemed to help him.

- Make sure that all the children clearly understand that cancer is not contagious. They cannot catch it, nor can their ill brother give it to anyone else. Impress upon them that nothing the parents or brothers and sisters did caused the cancer.

- Bring home a picture of the brother or sister in the hospital, and carry a tape recorder back and forth to relay songs and messages.

- It is very hard for mothers and babies or toddlers to be separated. Some families leave out family photo albums for the caregiver to show the toddler whenever she gets sad.

My daughter was eighteen months old when her three-year-old sister was diagnosed. Each member of the family flew in to stay at the house for two-week shifts, so she had a lot of caregivers. A friend of mine gave her a big key chain which held eight pictures. We put a picture of each member of the family (including pets) on her key chain, and she carried it around whenever we were away. It seemed to comfort her.

- Try to spend time individually with each sibling.

We began a tradition during chemotherapy that really helped each member of our family. Every Saturday each parent would take one child for a two-hour special time. We scheduled it ahead of time to allow excitement and anticipation to grow. Each child picked what to do on their special day—such as going to the park, eating lunch at a restaurant, riding bikes. We tried to put aside our worries, have fun, and really listen.

· · · · ·

Kim's hospitalizations were very hard on five-year-old Kelly. My parents kept Kelly during the week, so this helped a lot. Dennis would pick her up after work. I remember being at the hospital all week long, then Dennis would come on the weekends, and I would go home and do things with Kelly. We would go out to eat or rollerskating, etc. I really missed her, and it was just so hard on everyone. I remember being so tired, but I feel that you need to spend time with all of your children because they need you also.

- If people only comment on the sick child, try to bring the conversation back to include the sibling. For example, if someone exclaims, "Oh look how good Lisa looks," you could say, "Yes, and Martha has an attractive new haircut, too. Don't you like it?"

- Share your feelings about the illness and its impact on the family. Say, "I'm sad that I have to bring your sister to the hospital a lot. I miss you when I'm gone." This allows the sibling an opportunity to tell you how she is feeling. Try to make the illness a family project by expressing how the family will stick together to beat it.

> *I never kept my feelings secret from Shawn's two older brothers (five and seven years old). If I was scared, I talked about it. Once when we thought he was relapsing, my stomach was so knotted up that I could barely walk. Kevin said, "Mom, I'm really worried about Shawn." I told him that I was, too, and then we both just hugged and cried together. They really opened up when we didn't hide our feelings.*

- Include siblings in decision-making, such as giving choices on how extra chores will be done or devising a schedule for parent time with the healthy children.

> *We always gave the boys choices about where they would stay when Shawn had to be in the hospital. I felt like it gave them a sense of control to choose baby-sitters. They usually stayed at a close neighbor's house where there were younger children. It allowed them to ride the same bus to school and play with their neighborhood friends. Their lives were not too disrupted. They also really pitched in and helped with the younger kids. I think it helped them to help others.*

- Allow siblings to be involved in the medical aspects of their brother's illness, if they wish it. Often the reality of clinic visits and overnight stays are easier than what siblings imagine. Many siblings are a true comfort when they hold their brother's hand during spinal taps or bone marrows.

> *Just yesterday, Spencer (who screamed and shrieked at the blood draw for the BMT typing, and didn't match) out of the blue said "Mom, I wish I could have donated my marrow to Travis." And he's five! He also donated money to plant a tree in Israel today at Sunday school and asked us to write that it was "In honor of God and my brother, Travis." Oh man, we can never forget how this experience is seared in the memory of our*

children who don't have cancer. I am convinced that for Spencer, too, we will be seeing effects of this entire experience in many ways, long into the future.

- Give lots of hugs and kisses.

    We assumed everything was fine with Erin because she had her grandma, who adored her, staying with her. We made a conscious decision to spend lots of time with her and include her in everything. But we realized later that she felt very left out. My advice is to give triple the affection that you think they need, including lots of physical affection such as hugs and kisses. For years, Erin felt jealous. She thought her brother got more of everything: material things, time with parents, opportunities to do things she was not allowed to do. She finally worked it out while she was in college.

- Be sure to alert teachers of siblings about the tremendous stress at home. Many children respond to the worries about cancer by developing behavior or academic problems at school. Teachers should be vigilant for the warning signals, and provide extra support or tutoring for the stressed child or teen. Continue to communicate frequently with the teachers of the siblings to make sure you are aware of any developing problems.

- Expect your other children to have some behavior problems as part of living with cancer in the family. This is a "normal," not pathological, response.

    When my four-year-old healthy child screams and sobs over a minor skinned knee, she gets as much sympathy as my child with leukemia does during a bone marrow aspiration. I put a bandage on the knee, rock her, sing a song, and get her an ice pack. The injuries are not equal, but the needs of each child are. They both need to be loved and cared for; they both need to know that mom will help, regardless of the severity of the problem. I even let the sibling use EMLA for routine shots. My pediatrician laughs at me, but I just tell him, "Sibs need perks, too."

- The child with cancer receives many toys and gifts, resulting in hurt feelings or jealousy in the siblings. Provide gifts and tokens of appreciation to the siblings for helping out during hard times, and encourage your sick child to share.

- Encourage a close relationship between an adult relative or neighbor and your other children. Having a "someone special" when the parents are frequently absent can help prevent problems and help your child to feel cared for and loved.

- Take advantage of any workshops, support groups, or camps for siblings. These can be of tremendous value for siblings, providing fun and friendships with others who truly understand their feelings.

Positive outcomes for the siblings

After stating all of the above potential troubles that your children might experience, it is important to note that many siblings evade the negative possibilities and exhibit great warmth and active caretaking while their brother or sister is being treated for leukemia. Their empathy and compassion seem to grow with the crisis. Some brothers and sisters of children with cancer feel that they have benefited from the stressful experience in many ways, such as: increased knowledge about disease, increased empathy for the sick or disabled, increased sense of responsibility, enhanced self-esteem, greater maturity and coping ability, and increased family closeness. Many of these siblings mature into adults interested in the caring professions, such as medicine, social work, or teaching. Character can grow from confronting personal crisis, and many parents speak of the siblings with admiration and pride.

I don't think it matters how old the siblings are—it's a reality that the healthy ones will not get their fair share for a while. From what I've been able to observe in my own and other families, the siblings do eventually take it in stride and even seem to benefit from the opportunity to learn compassion, selflessness, and responsibility. As they get older, they even take comfort in the realization that, had they been the sick one, they would have received all the necessary attention, and that their parent(s) can cope (somehow) with whatever comes around. Libby added to her observations that she noted carefully how I reacted to Casey's illness at first (fell apart!), but that the next day I could gather my strength and do what had to be done. She likes to think she would also react similarly should the occasion arise (although, at her age, every blip in her universe is a catastrophe).

CHAPTER 17

Feelings, Communication, and Behavior

When I approach a child, he inspires in me
two sentiments: tenderness for what he is,
and respect for what he may become.

—Louis Pasteur

UNDER THE BEST OF CIRCUMSTANCES, child rearing is a daunting task. When parenting is complicated by an overwhelming crisis such as leukemia, communication within the family may suffer. Prior to the diagnosis, children know the family rules and understand the limits for their behavior. Afterwards, normal family life is disrupted, and all sorts of confusing and distressing feelings appear. Parenting must change in response to the frequently shifting needs of the ill child and affected siblings.

This chapter examines some emotional and behavioral changes in both children and parents, and presents suggestions on how to maintain effective communication and appropriate behavior within the family.

Feelings

Chapter 1, *Diagnosis*, provides an extensive list of feelings that parents may experience after the diagnosis of leukemia in their child. It is important to remember that children, both siblings and the ill child, are also overwhelmed by strong feelings, and they generally have fewer coping skills than adults. At varying times and to varying degrees, children and teens may feel fearful, angry, resentful, powerless, violated, lonely, weird, inferior, incompetent, betrayed. Children have to learn strategies to deal with these strong feelings to prevent "acting out" behaviors (behavioral problems) or "acting in" behaviors (depression, withdrawal). Good communication is the first step toward helping your family identify how child behavior and family functioning is being impacted and how family members may work with each other and with professionals to restore order and a nurturing climate.

Communication

Communicating with your child or teen is the foundation for trust. Children need to know from the very beginning that you will answer questions truthfully and take the time to talk about feelings.

Preventing isolation

For your ill child and his brothers and sisters to feel secure, they must always know that they can depend on you to tell them the truth, be it good news or bad. This reduces isolation and a sense of disconnection within the family.

> We were always very honest. We felt that if she couldn't trust us to tell her the truth how scary that would be. I've seen a few incidents in the clinic of people with totally different styles who don't tell their kids the truth. I ran into the bathroom at the clinic crying after overhearing a mother who had deceived her child into coming to the clinic. Then he found out he needed a back poke and completely lost it. It makes me cringe. Children just have to be prepared. If they can't trust their parents, who can they trust?

Listening

Just trying to get through each day consumes most parents' time, attention, and energy. Consequently, one of the greatest gifts parents can give their children is time—a special time when they really focus on what children are saying; when they listen to not only the words, but the feelings that generate them.

> After my relapse at age thirteen, the chemotherapy was much more difficult to tolerate. My appearance changed dramatically due to hair loss and rapid weight gain from prednisone. The L-asparaginase made my legs stiff and sore so that it was difficult to walk. After a two-month absence, when I returned to school, the treatment I received from the other students was unbearable. I finally refused to go to school. I felt so strongly about not going to school that once, on the way there, I jumped out of the car at an intersection. This helped mom and dad make the deci-

sion to send me to a private school. The kids and staff at the new school knew my situation and were very compassionate. The decision to change schools was one of the best things my parents ever did for me.

• • • • •

When my daughter was seven, three years after her treatment ended, I realized how important it was to keep listening. She was complaining about a hangnail and I told her that I would cut it for her. She started to yell that I would hurt her. I asked her, "When have I ever hurt you?" and she said, "In the hospital." I sat down with her in my arms, rocked her, and explained what had happened in the hospital during her treatment, why we had to bring her, and how we felt about it. I told her that I cried along with her when she was hurt by procedures. I asked her to tell me her feelings about being there. We cleared the air that day, and I expect we will need to talk about it many more times in the future. Then she held out her hand so that I could cut off her hangnail.

Talking

If you are not in the habit of talking to your children about how you are feeling, it is hard to start in a crisis. But now, more than ever, it's important to try. Parents can provide an opening for discussion by simply stating how much they miss their other children, for example, "I really miss you when I have to take your sister to the hospital. I'll call you every night just so I can hear your voice," or, "Sometimes I really get mad at the cancer. I wish the family didn't have to be separated so much." It is also helpful to tell your child with leukemia how the illness is affecting her siblings, for example, "It is very hard for Jim to stay at home with a baby-sitter when I bring you to the hospital. Let's try to think of something nice to do for him." These statements not only reassure children of your continued love for them and distress about being separated from them, but creates an opportunity for them to share with you how they feel about what is happening to the family.

My daughter, diagnosed when one year old and now entering fifth grade, has three older siblings, so we have been through many developmental stages as far as communication goes. I try to answer their questions honestly, but only tell them what I think they can understand without overwhelming them with information. I remember one of my boys, soon after my daughter's diagnosis, asked me if she was going to die, and I said "no" emphatically. I regretted it immediately, and realized that I would have to deal with my fears about the possibility of her dying, then go back and tell him the truth. So, later, I told him that I hadn't given an accurate answer because I was scared; that we didn't know if she was going to die, we hoped not, but we would have to wait and see.

I have found that as their understanding deepens, they come back with more questions, needing more detailed answers. So, my motto is, be honest, but don't scare them. If you say everything is okay, but you are crying, they know something is wrong, and that they can't trust you for the truth.

Common behavioral changes of children

Discipline under the best of circumstances can be difficult. But when one child has leukemia, parents are stressed, siblings are angry, and the situation may become unmanageable. The first step is to decide whether the ill child is going to be treated as if she only has a few months to live, or as if she will survive and need to learn strategies for how to self-regulate difficult emotions. Step two is to examine your own behavior to see if you are modeling the conduct that you expect from your children. Step three is to develop a consistent response to the angry or destructive child to help the child develop social and emotional competence.

Barbara Sourkes, an experienced child psychologist, wrote in her book *Armfuls of Time: The Psychological Experience of the Child with a Life-Threatening Illness*:

> *While loss of control extends over emotional issues, and ultimately over life itself, its emergence is most vivid in the child's day-to-day experience of the illness, in the barrage of intrusive, uncomfortable, or painful procedures that he or she must endure. The child strives desperately to regain a measure of control, often expressed through resistant, noncompliant behavior or aggressive outbursts. Too often, the source of the anger —the loss of control—goes unrecognized by parents and caregivers. However, once its meaning is acknowledged, an explicit distinction may be drawn for the child between what he or she can or cannot dictate. In order to maximize the child's sense of control, the environment can be structured to allow for as much choice as is feasible. Even options that*

appear small or inconsequential serve as an antidote to loss, and their impact is often reflected in dramatic improvements in behavior.

In the following sections, parents share how they handled various behaviors of their ill child.

Anger

Parents respond to the diagnosis of leukemia with anger, and so do children. Not only is the child angry at the disease, but also at the parents for bringing her in to be hurt, at having to take medicine that makes her feel terrible, at losing her hair, at losing her friends, and on and on. Children with cancer have good reasons to be angry.

> I think that much anger can be avoided by giving choices and letting kids have some control. Parents need to clearly explain that there are some things that simply have to be done (spinal taps) but that the child or teen is in control of positions, people present, music, even timing. For example, if your teen gets bad headaches after spinals, help him negotiate the date and time when the spinal will be done so that sports or social life will not be impacted.

• • • • •

> Justin has extreme bursts of anger sometimes. I don't know if it's related to the leukemia, or if it's just personality or normal development. He starts yelling, and I feel like I have a Tasmanian devil loose in my house. But I just use time-outs ("You go sit on your bed until you are over this") or loss of privileges ("You do this now or you won't be able to watch a movie later").

• • • • •

> We have a case of the halo or the horns. Our son is either very defiant or an absolute angel. He argues about every single thing. I really think that it is because he has had so little control in his life. I have very clear rules, am very firm, and put my foot down. But I also try to choose my battles wisely, so that we can have good times, too. My husband reminds me when I get aggravated that if he wasn't this type of tough kid, he wouldn't have made it through so many setbacks. Then I am just glad to still have him with us.

Tantrums

Healthy children have tantrums when they are overwhelmed by strong feelings, and so do children with leukemia. In some cases, tantrums can be predicted by parents paying close attention to what triggers the outburst. This knowledge helps parents prevent tantrums by avoiding situations that create overload for their child. In other cases, there is no warning of the impending tantrum.

> *We never knew what would set off three-year-old Rachel, and to tell the truth, she didn't know what the problem was herself. She was very verbal and aware in many ways, but she had no idea what was bothering her and causing the anger. I would just hold her with her blanket, hug her, and rock until she calmed down. Later she would say, "I was out of control," but she still didn't know why.*

Withdrawal

Some children withdraw rather than blow up in anger. Like denial, withdrawal can be temporarily helpful as a way to come to grips with strong feelings. However, too much withdrawal is not good for children. It can also be a sign of the kind of depression which some children suffer. Parents or counselors need to find ways to gently allow withdrawn children to express how they are feeling.

> *My daughter became very depressed and withdrawn as treatment continued. She started to talk only about a fantasy world that she created in her imagination. She seemed to be less and less in the real world. She didn't ever talk to her therapist about her feelings, but they did lots of art work together. At the beginning, she only drew pictures of herself with her body filling the whole page. After EMLA became available, and she was less terrified of being hurt, she began to draw her body more normal sized. As she got better, she began to draw the family again. When she drew a beautiful sun shining on the family, I cried. She just couldn't talk about it, but she worked so much out through her art.*

Comfort objects

Many parents worry when, after diagnosis, children regress to using a special comfort object. Many young children ask to return to using a bottle, or cling to a favorite toy or blanket. It is reasonable to allow your child to use whatever he can to find comfort against the terrible realities of treatment. The behaviors usually stop either when the child starts feeling better or when treatment ends.

> *My daughter was a hair twirler. Whenever she was nervous, she would twirl a bit of her hair around her finger. As her hair fell out, she kept grabbing at her head to find a wisp to curl. I told her that she could twirl mine until hers grew back. She spent a lot of time next to me or in my lap with her hand in my hair. It was annoying for me sometimes, but it had a great calming effect on her. When hers grew back, I would gently remind her that she had her own hair to twirl. She also went back to a bottle although we did limit the bottle use to home or hospital. Both behaviors, hair twirling and drinking from a bottle, disappeared within six months of the end of treatment, when she was six years old.*

· · · · ·

> *My son was a blanket baby. I remember getting so much advice about how to take the blanket away from him, when actually I was not at all concerned. He eventually cuddled it less and less, and it finally was packed into my memory box—until he was diagnosed with leukemia. He was fifteen, and he actually asked me to bring it to the hospital. In tears, I dragged that pitiful looking, raggedy blanket to the hospital.*

Talking about death

Part of effective parenting is allowing children to talk about topics that make us uncomfortable. In our culture, the subject of death has become taboo. A diagnosis of cancer forces both parents and children to acknowledge that death is a very real possibility. Even children as young as three years old think about death and what it means.

> *Eighteen months into treatment, five-year-old Katy said, "Mommy, sometimes I think about my spirit leaving my body. I think my spirit is here (gesturing to the back of her head) and my body is here (pointing to her belly button). I just wanted you to know that I think about it sometimes."*

· · · · ·

> *After my first relapse at age thirteen, my parents always kept the focus on the future. On the way to every procedure, we would plan the*

wonderful things that we were going to do afterwards. They never discussed death. But when I asked if leukemia could kill people, my father was honest and he told me, "Yes, some kids die." I appreciated him being straight with me, and I went right back to being optimistic.

After my third relapse, my nurse said something to me about death and dying. I clearly remember my reaction. I told her, "I know kids die from this, but I'm not going to!"

Trusting your child

There is a fine line between providing adequate protection for our children or teens and becoming overly controlling due to worry about the disease. You might ask yourself, "If she didn't have cancer, would I let her do this?"

Early one summer morning, twelve-year-old Preston and I left the hospital after a week-long stay for his high-dose methotrexate infusion. He had been heavily sedated, and was groggy and shaky on his feet. My husband and daughter were getting ready to go on a boat trip, and I felt Preston was too sick to go. We sadly saw them off, then returned to the car. Preston said, "Mom, I really need to go fishing. I know you don't understand, but I really need to do this."

It made me very uncomfortable, but we went home to get his equipment. We then drove up to the mountains to a very deserted spot on the river, and Preston said that he needed to be out of my sight. So I watched him put on his waders, walk into the swift river and disappear around a bend upstream. I went out into the river and sat on a rock. I waited for two hours before Preston came back. He said, "That's what I needed; I feel much better now."

Coping well

Some children, due to both temperament and the environments in which they have lived, are blessed with good coping abilities. They understand what is required, and they do it. Many more develop emotional competence from facing and coping with the difficulties of cancer. Many parents expressed great admiration for their child's strength and grace in the face of adversity.

Stephan has not had any behavior problems while being treated for his initial diagnosis (age five) or his relapse (age seven). He has never complained about going to the hospital and views the medical staff as his friends. He has never argued or fought about painful treatments. Unlike many of the parents in the support group, we've never had to deal with any emotional issues. We are fortunate that he has that confident personality. He just says, "We've got to do it, so let's just get it done."

Common behavioral changes of parents

It's impossible to talk about children's behavior without discussing parental behavior. Children's development does not occur in a vacuum, but rather in the context of their family. At different times during their child's treatment, parents may be under enormous physical, emotional, financial, and existential stress. The crisis can cause them to behave in ways of which they are not always proud.

Some of the problem behaviors mentioned by veteran parents follow.

Dishonesty

As stated earlier, children feel safe when their parents are honest with them. If the parents start to keep secrets from the child or "protect" her from bad news, the child feels isolated and fearful. She thinks, "If mom and dad won't tell me, it must be really bad," or, "Mom won't talk about it. I guess there's nobody that I can tell about how scared I am."

Denial is a type of "unconscious" dishonesty. This occurs when parents say things to children such as, "Everything will be just fine," or, "It won't hurt a bit." This type of pretending just increases the distance between child and parent, leaving children with no support. However horrible the truth, it seldom is as terrifying to a child as a half-truth upon which his imagination builds.

Depression

Feeling sad or depressed may occur in parents of children with cancer. If you are consistently experiencing any of the following symptoms, it would probably be helpful to get professional help: changes in sleeping patterns (sleeping too much, waking up frequently during the night, early morning awakening), appetite disturbances (eating too little or too much), loss of sex drive, fatigue, panic attacks, inability to experience pleasure, feelings of sadness and despair, poor concentration, social withdrawal, feelings of worthlessness, suicidal thoughts, or drug or alcohol abuse. Depression is very common and very treatable, and should be dealt with early.

> Find a counselor you click with. Stick with that person until you truly feel some peace about your experiences and strength for dealing with the ongoing stress of treatment or whatever else might come up. I regret that I toughed it out and didn't recognize the depression I was experiencing for such a long time. I think finding sources of support in a variety of ways at the earliest moment possible can greatly mitigate long-term difficulties in coping.

Losing your temper excessively

All parents lose their temper sometimes. They lose their tempers with spouses, healthy children, pets, even strangers. But it is especially painful when the target of the anger is a very sick child. Abuse of spouses and children increases at times when either or both spouses feel incompetent and powerless. If you find yourself unable to control your temper, seek professional counseling.

> I had my share of temper tantrums. The worst was when he was having his radiation. I tried to make him eat because it would be so many hours before he could have any more food. He always threw up all over himself and me, several times, every morning. It seemed like we changed clothing at least three times before we even got out of the house each day. I remember one day just screaming at him, "Can't you even learn how to throw up? Can't you just bend over to barf?" I really flunked mother of the year that day. I can't believe that I was screaming at this sick little kid, who I love so much.

· · · · ·

> In the beginning, my two-year-old daughter was incredibly angry. She would have massive temper tantrums, and I would just hold her and tell her that I wouldn't let her hurt anybody. I would continue to hold her until she changed from angry to sad. When she was on the dexamethasone, she would either be hugging me or pinching, biting, or sucking my neck. It drove me crazy. Now, on maintenance, she's not having as many

fits, but she still pushes her sisters off swings or the trampoline. She has a general lack of control. Sometimes, when I can't stand it anymore, I swat her on the bottom, and then I feel really bad.

· · · · ·

I had always taught my children that feeling anger was okay, but we had to make good choices about what to do with it. Hitting other people or breaking things was a bad choice; hitting pillows, running around outside, or listening to music were good choices. But, as with everything else, they learned the most from watching how I handled my anger, and during the hard months of treatment my temper was short. When I found myself thinking of hitting them, I'd say, in a very loud voice, "I'm afraid I'm going to hurt somebody so I'm going in my room for a time-out." If my husband was home, I'd take a warm shower to calm down; if he wasn't, I'd just sit on the bed and take as many deep breaths as it took to stop feeling homicidal.

Unequal application of household rules

You will guarantee family problems if the ill child enjoys favored status while the siblings must do extra chores. Granted, it is hard to know when is the right time to insist that your ill child must resume making his bed or setting the table, but it must be done. Siblings need to know from the very beginning that any child in the family, if sick, will be excused from chores, but will have do them again as soon as he is physically able.

I spoiled my sick daughter and tried to enforce the rules for my son. That didn't work, so I gave up on him and spoiled them both. He was really acting out at school. What he needed was structure and more attention, but what he got was more and more things. They both ended up thinking the whole world revolved around them, and it was my fault.

Overindulgence of the ill child

Overindulgence is a very common behavior of parents of children with cancer.

I bought my daughter everything that I saw that was pretty and lovely. I kept thinking that if she died she would die happy because she'd be surrounded by all these beautiful things. Even when I couldn't really afford it, I kept buying. I realize now that I was doing it to make me feel better, not her. She needed cuddling and loving, not clothes and dolls.

• • • • •

Four days into Selah's diagnosis, we were doing anything to keep her happy. Our sweet little four-year-old had turned into a demon child in that short time. Luckily, my very dear friend took me outside into the hallway, pushed me against the wall, and demanded to know exactly what I was doing. I just looked at her and said "I have no idea." I just didn't want my daughter to die and that was my only focus. She then told me I was giving my daughter no boundaries, no behavior expectations, and she had no respect for anyone who walked into the room. She was so right and I couldn't see it for fear that Selah would die. Through my tears and our hugs, she assured me that the way we were going, if she didn't die from leukemia, we were going to want to kill her because of the monster we were creating. I am still so grateful that she wasn't afraid to tell me what I needed to hear.

One aspect of overindulgence that is quite common is the parent's reluctance to teach the sick child life skills. After years of dealing with a physically weak and sometimes emotionally demanding child, parents may forget to expect age-appropriate skills.

I realized that I had formed a habit of treating my child as if she was still young and sick. I was still treating her like a three-year-old, and she was seven. One day, when I was pouring her juice, I thought, "Why am I doing this? She's seven. She needs to learn to make her own sandwiches and pour her own drinks. She needs to be encouraged to grow up." Boy, it has been hard. But I've stuck to my guns, and made other extended family members do it, too. I want her to grow up to be an independent adult, not a demanding, overgrown kid.

Overprotection of sick child

For a child to feel normal, he needs to be treated as if he is normal. Ask the doctor what changes in physical activity are necessary for safety, and do not impose any additional restrictions that go beyond this on your child. Let the child be involved in sports or neighborhood play, and even though it is hard, stop yourself from constant reminders to be careful.

Not spending enough time with the sibling(s)

While acknowledging that there are only so many hours in a day, the parents interviewed for this book felt the most guilt about the effect of the leukemia on the siblings. They wished that they had asked family and friends to stay with the sick child more often, allowing them to use more of their precious time with the siblings. Many expressed pain that they didn't know how severely affected the sibs had been.

> We didn't have problems with our child with cancer, but his brother (six years old) really suffered. He would get the flu and sob all night. He would scream that he would have to go to the hospital and that he would die. He also had behavior problems at school. I ended up quitting work because my son with leukemia was having trouble making it through the entire school day, and his brother needed some loving attention. Many of the sibling problems cleared up with lots of one-on-one attention.

Using substance abuse to cope

Some parents find themselves turning to alcohol or drugs to help them cope. Not only illegal drugs are abused; overuse of over-the-counter sleeping pills or other medications also occurs. If you find yourself drinking so that your behavior is affected or using drugs to get through the day or night, seek professional help.

Coping

Many parents find unexpected reserves of strength and are able to ask for help from their friends and family when they need it. They realize that different needs arise when there is a great stress to the family, and they alter their expectations and parenting accordingly. These families usually had strong and effective communication prior to the illness, and pull together as a unit to deal with it.

The majority of families, however, have periods of calmness and other times when nerves are frayed and tempers short. But usually families survive intact and are often strengthened by the years of dealing with cancer.

Improving communication and discipline

Parents suggest the following ways to keep the family on a more even keel:

- Make sure that the family rules are clearly understood by all of the children. Stressed children feel safe in homes that are very structured with regular, predictable routines.

After yet another rage by my daughter with leukemia, we held a family meeting to clarify the rules and consequences for breaking them. We asked the kids (both preschoolers) to dictate a list of what they thought the rules were. The following was the result, and we posted copies of the list all over the house (which created much merriment among our friends):

1. No peeing on rug

2. No jumping on bed

3. No hitting or pinching

4. No name calling

5. No breaking things

6. No writing on walls

If they broke a rule, we would gently lead them to the list and remind them of the house rules. It really helped.

- Have all caretakers consistently enforce the family rules.

We kept the same household rules. I was determined that we needed to start with the expectation that Rachel was going to survive. I never wanted her to be treated like a "poor little sick kid" because I was afraid she would become one. We had to be careful about baby-sitters because we didn't want anyone to feel sorry for her or treat her differently. I do feel that we avoided many long-term behavior problems by adopting this attitude early.

- Give all the kids some power by offering choices and letting them completely control some aspects of their lives, as appropriate.

For a few months we ignored Shawn's two brothers as we struggled to get a handle on the situation. We just shuttled them around with no consideration for their feelings. When we realized how unfair we were being, we made a list of places to stay, and let them choose each time we had to go off to the hospital. We worked it out together, and things went much smoother.

. . . . .

My bald, angry, four-year-old daughter asked me for some scissors one day. I asked what she was going to do, and she said cut off all her Barbies' hair. I told her those were her dolls and she could cut off their hair if she chose. I asked her to consider leaving one or two with hair, because when she had long hair again, she might want dolls that looked like her then, too. But I said it was up to her. She cut most completely off, and left some intact. It really seemed to make her feel better.

- Take control of the incoming gifts. Too many gifts make the ill child worry excessively ("If I'm getting all of these great presents, things must be really bad") and makes the siblings jealous. Be specific if you want people not to bring gifts, or if you want gifts for each child, not just the sick one.

- Recognize that some problems are caused solely by the drugs (see the prednisone section of Chapter 10, *Chemotherapy*). It helps to remember that these children are not naturally defiant or destructive. They are feeling sick, powerless, and altered by massive doses of toxic drugs, and parents need to try to help by sympathizing, yet setting limits. Remember, when they get off the drugs, their real personalities will return.

- Even though many oncologists tell parents that during the maintenance phase of treatment life will return to "normal," it usually does not. It is better than the intensive parts of treatment, but often, emotional and behavioral difficulties arise when the child regains his strength during maintenance. Be glad if your child's difficulties subside during maintenance, but expect them not to.

- If your child likes to draw, paint, knit, do collages, or other artwork, encourage it. Art is both soothing and therapeutic, and it allows the child a positive outlet for feelings and creativity. Making something beautiful really helps raise children's spirits.

When Jody was in the laminar airflow (isolation) room for weeks after his bone marrow transplant, he passed the time by doing many collages. I kept him well-supplied with all sorts of materials, and he created beautiful things.

- If your child does artwork or writing, recognize that powerful emotions may surface for both child and parents.

  At my daughter's preschool, once a week each child would tell the teacher a story, which the teacher wrote down for the child to take home. Most of my daughter's stories were like this: "There was a rhinoceros. He lived in the jungle. Then he went in the pool. Then he decided to take a walk. And then he ate some strawberries. Then he visited his friend." But the week before or after a painful procedure, she would dictate frightening stories (and this from a kid who wasn't allowed to watch TV). Two examples are: "Once there were some bees and they stung someone and this someone was allergic to them and then they got hurt by some monkeybars and the monkeybars had needles on them and the lightning came and hit the bees," and, "Once upon a time there were six stars and they twinkled at night and then the sun started to come up. And then they had a serious problem. They shot their heads and they had blood dripping down."

- Allow your child to be totally in charge of his art. Do not make suggestions or criticize (e.g., "stay inside the lines" or "skies need to be blue not orange"). Rather, encourage them and praise their efforts. Display the artwork in your home. Listen carefully if your child offers an explanation of the art, but do not pry if it is private. Above all, do not interpret it yourself or disagree with your child on what the art represents. Being supportive will allow your child to explore ways to soothe himself and clarify strong feelings.

  Jody was continually making "projects." We kept him supplied with a fishing box full of materials, and he glued and taped and constructed all sorts of sculptures. He did beautiful drawings full of color, and every person he drew always had hands shaped like hearts. If we asked him what he was making, he always answered, "I'll show you when I'm done."

- Come up with acceptable ways for your child to physically release anger. Some options are: ride a bike, run around the house, swing, play basketball or soccer, pound nails into wood, mold clay, punch pillows, yell, take a shower or bath, or draw angry pictures. In addition, teach your child to use words to express his anger, for example, "It makes me furious when you do that" or "I am so mad I feel like hitting you." Releasing anger physically and expressing anger verbally are both valuable life skills to master.

> Shawn was very, very angry many times. We had clear rules that it was okay to be angry, but he couldn't hit people. We bought a punching bag which he really pounded sometimes. Play-Doh helped, too. We had a machine to make Play-Doh shapes which took a lot of effort. He would hit it, pound it, push it, roll it. Then he would press it through the machine and keep turning that handle. It seemed to really help him with his aggression.

- Treat the ill child as normally as possible.

> When Justin was in the hospital, I could never stand to see him in those little hospital gowns. I asked if we could dress him in his own outfits, and they said yes. So even when he was in the ICU with all the tubes coming out of his body, we dressed him every day in something cute. It just felt better to see him in his clothes. Several months later my mother said that she had really admired us for doing that because we were sending the message to Justin that everything was going to be okay. That even though he couldn't breathe on his own, he was still going to get up every day and get dressed. Now I think it probably did communicate to him that things were going to be normal again.

- Get professional help whenever you are concerned or run out of ideas on how to handle emotional problems. Mental health care professionals (see Chapter 9, *Sources of Support*) have spent years learning how to help resolve these kinds of problems, so let them help you.

> My daughter and I both went to a wonderful therapist throughout most of her treatment for ALL. My daughter was a very sensitive, easily overwhelmed child, who withdrew more and more into a world of fantasy as cancer treatment progressed. The therapist was skilled at drawing out her feelings through art work and play. She also helped me with very specific suggestions on parenting. For instance, when I told the therapist that my daughter thought that treatment would never end (a reasonable assumption for a preschooler), she suggested that I put two jars on my daughter's desk. One was labeled "ALL DONE," and the other was labeled "TO DO." We put a rock for every procedure and treatment already completed in the ALL DONE jar, and one rock for every one yet to do in the TO DO jar. (Only recommended if the child is more than halfway through treatment.) Then, each time that we came home, my

daughter would move a rock into the ALL DONE jar. It gave her a concrete way to visualize the approach of the end of treatment. She could see the dwindling number of pebbles left. On the last day of treatment, when she moved the last pebble over and the TO DO jar was empty, I cried, but she danced.

- Most emotional problems that children develop as a result of treatment for cancer can be resolved by professional counseling. However, some children may also need medications to get them through particularly rough times.

My daughter was doing really well throughout treatment until a combination of events occurred that was more than she could handle. Her grandmother died from cancer during the summer, one of her friends with cancer died on December 27, then another friend relapsed for the second time. She was fine during the day, but at night she constantly woke up stressed and upset. She had dreams about trapdoors, witches brewing potions to give to little children, and saw people coming into her room to take her away. She would wake up smelling smoke. She was awake three or four hours in the middle of the night, every night. Her doctor put her on sleeping pills and antianxiety medications, and the social worker came out to the house twice a month.

- Teach children relaxation or visualization skills to help them cope better with strong feelings (see Appendix D, *Books and Online Sites*, for books on such skills).

- Have reasonable expectations. If you are expecting a sick four-year-old to act like a healthy six-year-old, or a teenager to act like an adult, you are setting your child up to fail.

It seemed like we spent most of the years of treatment waiting to see a doctor who was running hours behind schedule. Since my child had trouble sitting still and was always hungry, I came well prepared. I always carried a large bag containing an assortment of things to eat and drink, toys to play with, coloring books and markers, books to read aloud, and Play-Doh. He stayed occupied and we avoided many problems. I saw too many parents in the waiting room expecting their bored children to sit still and be quiet for long periods of time.

- As often as possible, try to end the day on a positive note. If your child is being disruptive, or if your feelings toward your child are very negative, here is an exercise that can end the day in a pleasant way. At bedtime, parent and child each tell one another something they did that day that made them proud of themselves, something they like about themselves, and something they are looking forward to the next day. Then a hug and a sincere "I love you" bring the day to a calm and loving close.

Checklist for parenting stressed children

A group of veteran parents compiled the following checklist to help you parent your stressed child:

- Model the type of behavior you desire. If you talk respectfully and take time-outs when angry, you are teaching your children to do so. If you scream and hit, that is how your children will handle their anger.

- Seek professional help for any behaviors that trouble you.

- Teach your children to talk about their feelings.

- Listen to your children with understanding and empathy.

- Be honest and admit your mistakes.

- Help your children examine why they are behaving as they are.

- Distinguish between feelings (always okay) and acting on strong feelings in destructive or hurtful ways (not okay).

- Have clear rules and consequences for violations.

- Teach children to recognize when they are losing control.

- Discuss acceptable outlets for anger.

- Give frequent reassurances of your love.

- Provide plenty of hugs and physical affection.

- Notice and compliment your child for good behavior.

- Recognize that the disturbing behaviors result from stress, pain, and drugs.

- Remember that with lots of structure, love, and time the problems will become more manageable.

Children Learn What They Live

If a child lives with criticism, he learns to condemn.
If a child lives with hostility, he learns to fight.
If a child lives with ridicule, he learns to be shy.
If a child lives with shame, he learns to feel guilty.
If a child lives with tolerance, he learns to be patient.
If a child lives with encouragement, he learns confidence.
If a child lives with praise, he learns to appreciate.
If a child lives with fairness, he learns justice.
If a child lives with security, he learns to have faith.
If a child lives with approval, he learns to like himself.
If a child lives with acceptance and friendship,
He learns to find love in the world.

—Dorothy Law Nolte

CHAPTER 18

End of Treatment and Beyond

The best formula for longevity:
Have a chronic disease, and cure it.

—Oliver Wendell Holmes

THE LAST DAY OF TREATMENT is a time for both celebration and fear. Most families are thrilled that the days of pills and procedures have ended, but some fear a future without drugs to keep the disease away. Concerns about relapse are an almost universal parental response, but for the majority of families, the months and years roll by without recurrence of leukemia. Many children and teens quickly return to excellent physical and mental health, while others have lingering or permanent effects from the treatment. This chapter covers the emotional and physical aspects of ending treatment, as well as medical follow-up and possible long-term side effects.

Emotional issues

Many parents describe ending treatment as almost as wrenching an experience as diagnosis. Families begin to experience the gamut of emotions—from elation to terror—months before the final day.

> *I had a lot of anticipatory worry—it started about six months before ending treatment. By the last day of treatment I had been worrying for months, so it was just a relief to quit.*

· · · · ·

> *I expected to feel a profound sense of relief when treatment ended. The six months prior to ending treatment I felt almost euphoric. But when she was finally finished, I began to be unexpectedly fearful. I just started to worry. I didn't really relax until she was a year off treatment. Now*

weeks go by without me thinking of relapse, although I still think of the years of leukemia treatment frequently.

• • • • •

The last day was traumatic. It just wasn't a celebration because it felt exactly like every other day that we had to drive for hours, wait for hours, then have painful treatments. When it was over, he was just as physically exhausted and emotionally drained as on other clinic days. I just felt numb. But then, over time, there was a gradual awakening that it was really over.

• • • • •

We were thrilled when treatment ended. I knew many people who felt that celebrating would jinx them; they just didn't feel safe. Well, I felt that we had won a big battle—getting through treatment—and we were going to celebrate that. If, heaven forbid, in the future we had another battle to fight, we'd deal with it. But on the last day of treatment, we were delighted.

Parents should anticipate that after years spent watching their child go through the rigors of treatment, they will have lost the feeling of a "normal" life. They may experience relapse scares, and they may need to call the doctor to describe the symptoms and be reassured.

Several months after my son ended treatment, I was driving down the street, and I started to worry that he seemed excessively tired lately. I started to feel my throat constricting, and tears sprang to my eyes. I had to pull over because I literally couldn't breathe. I had to force myself to calm down, breathe slowly, and realize that I was just having a normal attack of being petrified that he would relapse.

• • • • •

We live in a cool climate, but went back east during a summer heat wave to visit relatives. My daughter was a year off treatment and doing extremely well. After a few days of 100-degree weather, she started waking up in a bed soaked with sweat. I was terrified because she had done that at diagnosis. All of those horrible feelings washed over me, and I had to stand in the shower and sob. I called my doctor who was 3,000 miles away, and listed all the normal things: good appetite, good color, good energy level, no behavior problems, no bruising, but my voice shook when I described the sweats in an air-conditioned house. He reassured me that it was almost certainly the hot weather. He said if I was too worried to enjoy my visit, he would arrange for her to get a CBC, but otherwise, just bring her by when we got back. I relaxed, didn't get the CBC, and the night sweats stopped when we got home.

With diagnosis came the awareness that life can be cruel and unpredictable. Many parents feel safe during treatment and feel that therapy is keeping the cancer away. The end of treatment leaves some parents and children feeling exposed and vulnerable. When treatment ends, parents must find a way to live with uncertainty, to find a balance between hope and reasonable worry.

The first few weeks after Casey ended treatment, I was not worried at all. The sense of relief was so great! Finally our lives weren't controlled by the disease and fevers and meds. Only once a month are we bothered by doctor office visits. It is so nice.

I remember about one month after treatment ended Casey ran a high fever. As I bathed him I told him wasn't it nice we didn't have to rush off to the hospital, he could have a fever like a normal kid! We had decided to have his port taken out in August just for that simple reason— he can run a fever and we don't have to rule out infection in the port.

Now, as his counts start to rebound, my fear is growing. Up until now there was evidence that his body still retained the drugs—now he is on his own. I'm a nervous wreck. Every bruise stands out like a neon sign. I worry on his tired days. My paranoia is not healthy and I'm working hard to reduce it. In the meantime, I've taken a step back, relying on the survival skills learned in the early days of treatment. Today he is well and I have no control over tomorrow, so I try to relish the good health that he enjoys today. No energy I put into worrying will affect the outcome in the long run. So much easier said than done, isn't it?

Last day of treatment

Although individual cases vary, generally on the last day of treatment a child in remission from leukemia has a diagnostic spinal tap, a bone marrow aspiration, a complete blood count and chemistry screen, a thorough physical exam, and a discussion with the oncologist. The oncologist should review the treatment, outline the schedule for blood tests and exams for the future, and sensitively inform the family of the potential for long-term side effects. After the procedures, the family will usually wait to hear the preliminary report on the bone marrow aspiration, as true relief does not come until they hear that no leukemic blasts are present.

One group of parents presented to physicians at a major children's hospital the following list of suggestions for the last day of treatment:

- Schedule enough time to have a conversation.
- Bring a sense of closure to the active phase of treatment.
- Express happiness that all has gone well.
- Be realistic but hopeful about the future.
- Praise the child for handling a very difficult time in her life with grace (or courage, or whatever word is appropriate).
- Praise the parents for all of their hard work.
- Allow time for the parents to give the physician feedback and thanks.
- Give a certificate of accomplishment to the child.
- Be aware that families are relieved but fearful of the future.

Our last day of treatment was horrible. The fellow was angry at me because I had arranged to have my daughter sedated. The fellow was signing the necessary forms muttering over and over, "This is ridiculous." When I asked her what was bothering her, she said that she was going on a business trip, which I was delaying, and her son had chicken pox and she was worried about it. She said another doctor was going to do the procedures because she was in a hurry. When I asked if I should wait for the results of the bone marrow, she said, "End-of-treatment bone marrows are at the bottom of the pathologist's priority list, emergencies come first, he'll get to it when he can, and the report won't be written for days." I thought that she was being heartless, but I didn't want to fight in front of my daughter. So I went across the hall and asked the director of the clinic if she would please call me that afternoon with the results of the bone marrow. She replied, "Absolutely." She called, told me it was clear, and we felt jubilant and relieved.

· · · · ·

The nurses at our clinic really made a big deal on the last day of treatment. They brought out a cake and balloons, and sang "Going off Chemo" to the tune of "Happy Birthday to You." They made Gina a banner and bought her a present. I sat in a corner and cried, because I was scared to death of the future. A nurse came over, hugged me, and said, "This must be so hard, we're taking away your security blanket." She was exactly right.

Catheter removal

Children usually cannot wait for the catheter to be removed, as it symbolizes that treatment has truly ended. Physicians differ a great deal on when is the best time to remove the catheter. Some recommend removal when the child starts maintenance. Others remove it when the child is sedated for the last bone marrow aspiration, while some doctors advise waiting until several weeks or months have passed. Ask the doctor for her reasons for her recommendation, and discuss it fully if you or your child have strong feelings about the timing.

Removal of the external catheter (Hickman or Broviac) is usually an outpatient procedure, although it may also be done under general anesthesia by the surgeon or radiologist who inserted it. The child is given a mild sedative, then the oncologist pulls the catheter out of the child's body by hand.

> *Kristin's Broviac removal wasn't too bad. They gave her Fentanyl ahead of time, so she was fairly relaxed. I wished that they had offered me a sedative as well. One of the nurses had her hand on Kristin's shoulder and quietly talked to her to try to keep her focused elsewhere. I held her legs, and my wife held her hand. The doctor put one hand on her chest, and pulled on the tubing with the other. It only took about two seconds to come out. There was little blood; they just put a Band-Aid on the site and sent us home.*

Implanted catheters such as the Port-a-cath are removed surgically in the operating room. Children are generally given general anesthesia, and the operation takes less than half an hour. Only one incision is made, usually just above the port at the same place as the scar from the implantation surgery. The sutures holding the port to the underlying muscle are cut, and the port with tubing is pulled out. The small incision is then stitched and bandaged. When the child begins to awaken, he is brought out to the parent(s). The family then waits until the surgeon has approved their departure. Often, the wait is short, for as soon as the child is awake enough to take a small drink or eat a popsicle, he is released. If your child becomes nauseated from the anesthesia, the wait can be several hours until he is feeling better.

Brent had a very easy time with his port-removal surgery. We sched-uled him to be the first patient early in the morning, so there was no delay getting in. Then the anesthesiologist asked him what flavor gas he wanted, which he liked. They brought him out to us while he was still groggy, and he woke up feeling goofy and happy. We went home soon there-after. It felt more like the ending then than on the last day of treatment.

Ceremonies

Some families enjoy having ceremonies to celebrate the end of cancer treat-ment. Especially for younger children who have spent much of their lives taking pills and having procedures, ceremonies can help them grasp that it is truly over. Here are ideas from many families on how to commemorate this important occasion:

- Take "good-bye" pictures of the hospital and staff.

- Take a picture of your child taking his last pill.

- Give trophies to your child and siblings.

   We had a big party during which my husband Scott stood up and called for everyone's attention. He gave a talk about how proud we were of Jeremy and handed him a big trophy. It had the victory angel on top and was engraved with "Jeremy, we are so proud of you and your victory. Love, Mom and Dad." We gave a plaque to his brother Jason for being the world's most supportive brother.

- Ask the clinic to present your child with a certificate.

- Let your child throw away or flush down the toilet all of the leftover pills.

   We waited for six months to celebrate, because we just didn't feel safe until then. But on his six-month anniversary we had a "toilet flushing party." Shawn threw every pill, and poured the liquid meds, saline, and mineral oil down the toilet, and just flushed and laughed. It was such a howl, I really wished we had videotaped it.

- Throw a big party for friends and family.

   Erica ended treatment in December, and we threw a big party at the church. We called it a "Celebration of Life." We invited all of the families that we had become so close to through the support group. We especially wanted the families who had lost their children to cancer, and they all came. My normally even-tempered husband gave a talk about Club Goodtimes (the support group) and how it was a club that no one ever wanted to join. When he talked about the many wonderful people we met there, his voice shook with emotion. Then the preacher prayed for the children who weren't with us. We ate a huge cake, and the children were entertained by a clown. It was both moving and fun.

- Throw a big party at school.

  When Joseph finished treatment he was in kindergarten, but the kids had gone through almost an entire year with him and they had known all about his treatments and frequent hospitalizations and had talked as a group about it when we made a presentation to the class, and at other times as well. It seemed appropriate to have an "all done with treatment" celebration. We even had his two best friends who go to different schools come over to join us, and big brother Nate came down from his class to share in the fun.

  It was a very joyous occasion, and we made it as much like a birth-day party as we could. I made cupcakes and juice and we played games. A friend who leads the story hour at our children's bookstore came and did some songs and stories with the kids, and I even sent each classmate home with a treat bag. At the end, right before time to go home, Joseph pulled out several cans of his favorite hospital discovery, and the kids took turns blasting a shower of silly string on everyone else! We all clapped and cheered, and Joseph's wonderful teacher and I had a chance to have a good celebratory cry while the kids put on their things to go home. Clean-up wasn't too darn bad, and it meant a lot to all of us.

  There's still a tiny remnant of green silly string on one of the fluores-cent light fixtures, and my big second-grader likes to go down and admire it when he visits his old kindergarten teacher.

- If your child has been seeing a counselor, schedule a visit to talk about the accomplishment.

- Have friends and family send congratulations cards.

- Ask the surgeon to give your child her port or Hickman line.

  I know that this may sound odd, but my six-year-old daughter hated her port and talked incessantly about getting it out. She even told me that *she was going to slice it out herself with a knife. I told her it would be better to wait until the doctors put her to sleep, but I promised her that she could have it after the operation to do with as she wished. That idea brought a smile to her face. She came out of the recovery room clutching a baggie with the port inside. Once we were home, she carried it around for weeks, jumped on it, hit it with a hammer, and finally cut it to pieces. That port really symbolized all of the painful things that had happened to her, and it made her feel better to hurt it back.*

- If consistent with your beliefs, have a religious ceremony of thanksgiving.

    I preached the sermon at church after Kristin ended treatment. It was the first Sunday of Lent, and I related our experience to that. Other than that, we didn't celebrate, because it's still not over. We still have to go every month for blood work and need to be vigilant. Ending treatment was a big milestone, but it paled in comparison to having the line pulled. We all have so much more freedom: no more lines to flush, changing bandages, or wrapping up for baths and swimming.

- Go on a trip or vacation to celebrate.

    All of the parents of children with leukemia in our community have become very close. When nine-year-old Brent finished his treatment, I called to congratulate him. He was so excited telling me about it, but then his voice started to shake and he cried when he told me, "My two aunts gave me a card with money inside to go to a motel with a pool for the weekend. They gave it to me because I had leukemia. Can you believe that?"

Some parents do not feel comfortable celebrating the end of treatment. One mother described her feelings this way:

> *We did nothing because we knew so many kids who relapsed. I didn't even throw away the pills for a year because I didn't trust that we were really done.*

As you have read so often in this book, every child, parent, and relative reacts differently to treatment. The differences do not matter. What is important is that you feel free to express your feelings, whatever they may be. You may be joyful, relieved, fearful or terrified, but end of treatment is emotionally charged for every member of the family.

What is normal?

After years of treatment, families grapple with the idea of returning to normal. Unfortunately, most parents don't really know what "normal" is any longer. Parents realize that returning to the carefree pre-cancer days is unrealistic, that life has changed. The constant interaction with medical personnel is ending, and a new phase is beginning in which routines do not revolve around caring for a sick child, giving medicines, and keeping clinic appointments. While it is true that the blissful ignorance of the days prior to cancer are gone forever, a different life—one often enriched by friends and experiences of the cancer years—begins.

I listened to several parents in our support group discuss "returning to normal" after treatment ended. I felt that, in a sense, they were wishing for a magic carpet ride back in time. However, I think that life is a series of evolutions. Even if we hadn't endured our oncology odyssey, our life would be different now than it was three years ago. I think that parents need to set goals, decide which direction they want to go after treatment ends, and make an effort to get there.

· · · · ·

It just seems like I can't leave it behind. If he gets diarrhea, I worry that it's a tumor. He has a bad skin rash now, and I keep thinking that it's cancer-related. My husband has terrible skin, so I know it's genetic, but there's a little part of my mind that keeps trying to connect it to leukemia. My son has been going to the playground; he's getting strong; he has rosy cheeks; he's just beautiful. When he has bruises on his legs, I automatically think his platelets are down. But when I look at the other kids, I realize that it's normal for active kids to have bruises on their knees. It's really hard to get used to. I still wake up at night, and the irrational side comes out. I'm just having a hard time letting go of it. I mean, I panicked when his feet were hurting, only to discover that his shoes were too small.

· · · · ·

We're a year off treatment, and I really don't think about relapse very often. I do occasionally find myself studying her to see if she looks pale, or I worry when she seems tired or her behavior is bad. Usually, I'm feeling safer. But honestly, I don't think any of us will ever go back to the days when we just assumed that our kids would grow up, that the parents would die first; that sense of security is probably gone forever.

· · · · ·

Shawn's six months off treatment, and he's just like a flower begin-ning to bloom. He's so happy and I try to be happy with him. I try very hard to put worries about the future out of my mind, because I feel that those thoughts will rob me of just being able to enjoy Shawn.

· · · · ·

For two months after ending treatment, Meagan was worried about everything that went in her mouth. She'd say, "Is this okay to eat? Will this hurt me? Am I safe? Am I going to get hurt doing this?" This para-noid phase just faded away.

· · · · ·

These first two months off treatment, I've noticed Kristin steadily gaining in self-confidence and composure.

Normal is a moving target—different for every person and family. No one can tell you what your normal will be. Normal is what keeps the family alive and planning and moving together to face their individual and collective futures. Normal is what feels right for the family now; what feels right for you now.

Many parents and children like to give back to the cancer community in some way. Helping others, for many people, is a satisfying way to reach out or bring closure to the active phase of cancer treatment. Helping others can create something enormously meaningful out of personal tragedy. Some examples of reaching out are:

- We started a Boy Scout project to keep the toy box full at the clinic.
- My children are counselors at the camp for kids with cancer.
- After my son died, I gave up my parish to begin work as a hospice chaplain.
- We organized a walk to raise funds for the Ronald McDonald House.
- We (a group of parents of children with leukemia) requested and were granted a conference with the oncology staff to share our thoughts on ways to improve pain management and communication between par-ents and staff. It was very well-received.

- We circulated a petition among parents to request increased hospital funding for psychosocial support staff. We presented it to the director of the Hematology/Oncology service.

- I started a Candlelighters group and organized meetings, conferences, and picnics, and write a quarterly newsletter.

- I requested that the clinic and local pediatricians refer newly diagnosed families to me if the parents wanted someone to talk to. I remembered how impossible it was to go to meetings in the first few months, and how desperately I needed to talk to someone who had already traveled the same road.

- We held a bone marrow donor drive.

- I give platelets and blood regularly.

- I took all of our leftover Hickman line supplies to camp and gave them to a family who needed them.

- The family of one child started a nonprofit company which produces beauty products. All proceeds, no strings attached, go to the local children's hospital for cancer research.

- Grace Ann Monaco, whose four-year-old daughter died in 1970 from ALL, was a founding member of a support group which grew into the Candlelighters Childhood Cancer Foundation. Her work with CCCF for 25 years and continued support is a gift from her daughter Kathleen Rea to parents and survivors. Grace Ann continues her involvement in childhood cancer through the Childhood Cancer Ombudsman Program, a service of the Childhood Brain Tumor Foundation, which provides free medical option review and help with insurance, employment, education access, and discrimination to families and survivors.

The possibilities are endless. Parents use whatever talents they have to help others, from designing head coverings to writing newsletters.

An equally healthy response to ending treatment for cancer is to put it behind you. Many families, after years of struggles, just want to enjoy a sense of normalcy. They don't want constant reminders of cancer, and feel that it's not good for children to be reminded of those hard times.

> I realized that it was time to put it behind us when I watched my two children playing house one day. There was only one adult and one child in the family. I asked what happened to the rest of the family and they both

said, "Cancer, they died." I didn't want them to have any more cancer in their lives. They had enough. I know people who worry all the time about the leukemia returning, and it is not healthy for them or their children. I decided to get out of the cancer mode, and back to being my usual upbeat self. I feel that we are finally back to normal, and it's a good place to be.

Parents and children need to talk to one another, examine their emotions, decide what course they want to chart, and work together toward a healthy life after cancer.

One year after treatment

After a year has passed since the end of treatment, parents have a different perspective. For some, the thoughts of cancer have receded, and life has resumed a predictable pattern. For others, fear is still a constant companion. The following are a sampling of comments from parents one year after the end of their child's treatment for leukemia:

> *He still eats like a bird.*

· · · · ·

> *She went back to eating a balanced diet a couple of months after treatment ended.*

· · · · ·

> *Her appetite has vastly improved, but she still has taste aversions, and only eats a few types of food.*

· · · · ·

> *It's been a year since treatment ended, and I don't think I'm obsessed with worry anymore, but in my quiet moments, I still get nauseated when she coughs (she had pneumonia at diagnosis).*

· · · · ·

> *I had to learn to stop referencing everything to the illness all of the time. For instance, I found myself saying things like, "Before you were sick" or "While you were sick." My six-year-old daughter finally pointed it out to me and asked me to stop. Now I use her age as a reference point.*

· · · · ·

I still worry and think in terms of the illness. For instance, he had to have some teeth pulled, and my first thought was to go get his counts checked to make sure that his platelets were high enough. Then I told myself that I was being ridiculous. I let him go in like a normal kid, and it was fine.

· · · · ·

I feel worse off therapy, as if I have something hanging over my head. I still get very worried and fretful whenever he gets a fever, but going to the clinic for checkups no longer bothers me. But I still do things like calling the doctor in an absolute panic when he has a red stool, only to find out that my husband fed him beets for lunch.

· · · · ·

I feel that the leukemia was almost a gift. We could have been like any other couple seeking the "American Dream" with both of us working and John in day care. But our priorities changed. I stay home, my husband began a home business, and we live every day to the fullest. Our time is spent loving and appreciating each other and every moment we have. I take nothing for granted—every smile, every hug, every "I love you" gets my undivided attention.

· · · · ·

Shawn is a year off treatment and I find myself letting go of the bad memories more and more. They are just fading away. What I am left with is awe, admiration, and amazement that my son handled all of the hardships of treatment and survived. He's very determined and strong-willed, and I'm so proud of him. When people say to me, "Oh, you were so strong to make it through that," I respond, "All I did was drive him to the appointments, he did the rest."

This experience has really changed me and my entire family. My marriage is much better, my other sons are stronger and closer to us, and Shawn has shown us all how tough a little kid can be. We take each precious day, one at a time, and try to get the most out of it. I so appreciate life and my family.

Possible long-term side effects

Dr. Giulio J. D'Angio, MD, wrote, "Vigilance is essential if the blossoms of success in pediatric oncology are not to bear bitter fruit. Cure is not enough." At diagnosis, parents do not know what price their child will ultimately pay for reprieve from leukemia. For the majority of children with low or intermediate ALL, the price is low. Short-term effects are discomfort, a bald head, and occasional school absences. Long-term effects—sometimes none. For children with high-risk ALL, AML, CML, or those who have relapsed and require more intensive treatment, the price for life may be higher: subtle or pronounced learning disabilities, impaired endocrine system, growth difficulties, and many other possible consequences.

Descriptions of a few of the possible long-term effects follow.

Female fertility

Younger girls are more resistant to damage to the ovaries from chemotherapy than are older teenagers. There have, however, been rare cases of ovarian failure in young girls who have been given high doses of cyclophosphamide as part of their treatment for leukemia. Additionally, one study discovered damaged ovaries in a percentage of girls who received spinal radiation. In the vast majority of cases, prepubertal girls who have been treated for leukemia exhibit normal growth, sexual development, and fertility.

Most teenagers who are treated after puberty for leukemia retain normal ovarian function. If teenagers do not resume having periods after treatment ends, or if they develop symptoms such as hot flashes or breast discharge, a pediatric endocrinologist should be consulted.

The chances of becoming pregnant and having a normal pregnancy and birth after treatment for leukemia are excellent. Data from the National Cancer Institute shows that offspring born to cancer survivors have the same risk of birth defects as the general population. However, all women treated with chemotherapy drugs which can cause cardiovascular damage (doxorubicin, daunomycin, cyclophosphamide) or who had radiation to the chest or spine should be monitored closely during pregnancy and delivery.

Fertility issues for children or adolescents who have undergone bone marrow transplants are covered in Chapter 20, *Bone Marrow and Stem Cell*

Transplantation. Precocious and delayed puberty are covered in Chapter 12, *Radiation*.

Male fertility

Use of methotrexate, vincristine, cytoxan (cyclophosphamide), and prednisone causes a rapid decrease in sperm count in teens or men who have passed puberty. Normal sperm production and motility generally return in the second year of maintenance.

After treatment for leukemia, males rarely have difficulty going through puberty. This does not mean that males are fertile. Males have cells that produce testosterone and cells that produce sperm. Therefore, a male could have normal testosterone-producing cells but abnormal sperm-producing cells. Patients who received cyclophosphamide or radiation to the testes should have testosterone levels and sperm count checked.

For all sexually mature males, sperm banking should be discussed with the oncologist prior to treatment. Sperm can be kept viable for ten to fifteen years, and this may allow some teens the opportunity to become fathers later in life.

Cardiovascular disorders

Heart problems may occur months or decades after treatment with anthracyclines (adriamycin, idarubicin, or daunomycin), high-dose cyclophosphamide, or chest irradiation. Symptoms include shortness of breath, fatigue, poor exercise tolerance, rapid heartbeat, and irregular heartbeat.

The heart damage is usually related to the cumulative dose of anthracyclines, and can range from mild electrocardiogram changes to sudden death from cardiac failure (very rare). For adults, the dose at which incidence of heart failure begins to increase is 550 mg/m^2, but there is growing evidence that for children who have received multiple chemotherapeutic agents including cyclophosphamide, the critical total anthracycline dose may be 350 to 400 mg/m^2 or lower.

Any child whose total dosage of doxorubicin and daunomycin exceeds 350 mg/m^2, who had chest radiation (not routine diagnostic x-rays), or who received high-dose cyclophosphamide prior to bone marrow transplantation is at risk for future cardiovascular problems. Because early diagnosis and prompt treatment are crucial, many authorities now recommend that any child who has received potentially cardiotoxic therapies should undergo an annual exam, including a physical examination, thorough history, chest x ray, 12-lead electrocardiogram, and echocardiogram.

In addition, for those children whose cardiac monitoring the first year off treatment is normal, the Children's Cancer Group recommends an EKG and echocardiogram every two to three years. Any pregnant woman with a history of anthracycline treatment should have her heart function followed closely throughout the pregnancy.

Whether survivors who were treated with high doses of anthracyclines should engage in isometric exercise (weight lifting, wrestling, football, rock climbing) is controversial. Consult with your oncologist if your child or teen wishes to engage in these activities.

> *My daughter's high-risk protocol required an echocardiogram before treatment began, and periodically during treatment. When I asked why she never had one after the baseline, I was told by the fellow that she needed the drugs so it didn't really matter if she had cardiac changes. When I asked at end of treatment about the echocardiogram, I was told that since she only received a total of 175 mg/m², an echocardiogram would only be given if symptoms developed. When I pulled out the Children's Cancer Group's recommendations on the subject and handed them over to my hometown pediatrician, he ordered an echocardiogram for her.*

Dental abnormalities

Dental abnormalities can be a side effect of treatment for leukemia, especially for children who are treated with cranial radiation. The most common problems are failure of the teeth to develop (agenesis), arrested root development, microdontia (unusually small teeth), and enamel abnormalities. Several parents report difficulties in insurance covering dental or orthodontic problems caused by radiation and/or chemotherapy. If you are a member of this group, collect articles on the studies which show that a relationship exists between treatment for leukemia and dentofacial development, and bring them to your child's oncologist. Ask the oncologist to write a letter to the insurance company using the research to support his position that the dental work is cancer-treatment related. The journal articles on this topic at *http://www.patientcenters.com/leukemia/* have dozens of such articles listed in their bibliographies.

> *Jeremy has had many dental problems. He lost his gums in front of his lower front teeth. To correct this, they took skin from the roof of his mouth and did a skin graft. He also had an eyetooth that just broke off at the root and fell out.*

· · · · ·

> *Gina needed oral surgery to expose one of her molars. She also needed extensive work on her bite and wore braces and appliances. Another molar has a hook on the root and the braces could not budge it, so that will require more surgery. This will be followed by another round of extensive orthodontic work. My other three children had minimal orthodontic work for cosmetic reasons only.*

Persistent weakness

Most children are remarkably resilient, and after treatment ends they resume normal activities at age-appropriate levels. But there are some children, particularly those who received cranial radiation, who have chronic problems with strength and coordination. As the population of leukemia survivors grows, it is hoped more attention will be focused on studying persistent weakness and investigating ways to prevent or overcome it.

> *When my daughter Christine ended treatment at age six, she was very weak, and had trouble with balance and coordination. For instance, she couldn't walk a balance beam holding an adult's hand, she couldn't skip or play hopscotch. She decided to take ballet and gymnastics, and we took her for many long walks and bike rides (with training wheels) to help her regain her strength. We made physical activities fun. I talked to her school gym teacher, her ballet instructor, and gymnastics teachers, and asked them to be supportive and encouraging. It's been a year since she ended treatment, and although she still has training wheels on her bike, she walks a balance beam with grace and assurance, can dribble a basketball, and is able to do almost all of the movements for ballet.*

· · · · ·

> *Judd finished his treatment at age six and had some muscular weakness. He tried organized sports, but preferred individual sports like skiing.*

Over several years, he gradually regained his strength and coordination so that his athletic ability was average.

• • • • •

We had Justin tested through the school district, and the district is giving him his physical therapy. He's weak in the hips and walks with his feet turned out. He's resistant to taking physical risks; for instance, he sits down and slides off things rather than jumping off. He just loves to go to physical therapy.

• • • • •

Rachel is two years off treatment and starting kindergarten. She has trouble skipping and galloping, and cannot hop on one foot. I worry about competitiveness during gym classes.

Learning disabilities, delayed growth, and premature or delayed puberty are most commonly associated with cranial radiation and are covered in Chapter 12. Coping strategies for dealing with learning disabilities are explored in Chapter 15, *School*. For detailed information on possible late-effects from childhood cancer read, *Childhood Cancer Survivors: A Practical Guide to the Future*, by Nancy Keene, Wendy Hobbie, and Kathy Ruccione.

The above information is about infrequent long-term effects from cancer treatment. Certain groups of children and teenagers are more, or less, at risk for side effects than others. The risk for your child depends on many factors, including the type of leukemia, total dosage of individual drugs, combinations of different types of chemotherapy, location and dose of radiation, and age at diagnosis. As with all the information contained in this book, please consult with your oncologist if you have any questions or concerns. The field of cancer treatment is constantly evolving and improving, and the experts in the field are years ahead of the published material. They can explain to you the reasons for their recommendations, and should show you the books or articles that support their position if you ask to see them.

An essential aspect of survivorship is making healthy choices. Good health habits and regular medical care help to protect survivors' health as well as lessen the likelihood of late effects from cancer treatment. A sizable number of adult cancers are linked to lifestyle choices. Eating a healthy diet, staying physically active, using sunscreen, avoiding excessive alcohol consumption, maintaining a healthy weight, and not smoking all help to keep survivors healthy and cancer-free. Wearing bike or motorcycle helmets, using seat belts, and calling a cab if the person driving has had too much to drink protect survivors from injury. Survivors have little or no control over genetic make-up or the environment in which they live. But making healthy choices on how to live the rest of their lives gives them control over some of their own destiny.

Follow-up care

In the past, survivors of cancer were on their own after treatment ended. With increasing numbers of long-term survivors, it became apparent that these young men and women often faced complex medical and psychosocial effects from their years of treatment. As a result, many institutions began late-effects clinics to provide a multidisciplinary team to monitor and support survivors. The nucleus of the team usually includes a nursing coordinator, pediatric oncologist, pediatric nurse practitioner, radiation oncologist, endocrinologist, school liaison, social worker, and psychologist.

The follow-up programs usually include a review of treatments received, counseling regarding potential health risks (or lack thereof), and case-specific diagnostic tests such as cardiac evaluations, hormonal studies, or testing for learning disabilities. These follow-up clinics not only provide comprehensive care for long-term survivors, but participate in research projects that track the effectiveness and side effects from various clinical trials. In addition, the follow-up clinic acts as an advocate for survivors with schools, insurance agencies, and employers.

If your institution does not provide comprehensive, long-term follow-up care, there are several issues that should be addressed at the end of treatment. A discussion of some of these follows.

Follow-up schedule

Protocols for clinical trials require specific follow-up schedules. For instance, after treatment for average-risk ALL, your child may need monthly physical exams and a monthly CBC for the first year off treatment, and a less frequent schedule for the following years. Find out from the oncologist what the required schedule is, and where the appointments will be. Make sure that your child understands that after treatment ends doctor appointments and blood draws will still be an occasional necessity.

Immunizations

If your child was diagnosed prior to receiving all of her immunizations, ask the oncologist when you should resume the regular schedule for immunizations.

> My doctor said to wait a year before beginning to catch up on shots. It was nice for her to get a long break before any more pokes.

Risks of smoking

Teens need continuing counseling on problems associated with smoking (cigarettes or marijuana) or engaging in other high-risk behaviors. Any child or teen who received anthracycline therapy (adriamycin, daunomycin, or idarubicin) is at risk for damage to the muscle of the heart. Smoking not only impacts the lungs, but it makes blood vessels hard, further decreasing the heart's ability to pump. The combination of heart damage from chemotherapy and smoking vastly increases the chance of heart disease, heart attack, congestive heart failure, stroke, cancer of the mouth, throat, and lungs, or death from sudden cardiac failure. An article on survivors and smoking contained in the Candlelighters Winter 1994 youth newsletter ends with these words:

> If you've had cancer and your friends haven't, they don't face the same risks from smoking that you do. You've fought hard for your life. Don't put it out in an ashtray.

Safe sex

Every teen and young adult who has survived cancer should be counseled about safe sexual practices. Despite the prevalence of sexual messages in our culture, most teens are woefully underinformed about the facts. Many survivors think, erroneously, that if they are infertile, they do not have to be concerned about the use of condoms or other birth control. However, all sorts of diseases, some potentially fatal (hepatitis C, HIV/ARC/AIDS) and some not (genital herpes, genital warts, gonorrhea), can be transmitted through sexual intercourse.

One nurse practitioner at a large follow-up clinic stated:

*I tell every teenager who comes through the door, regardless of their medical background, that I think that he or she is too young to have sex, and I explain why. But then I say, in the event that you do choose to become sexually active, you **always** need to use a condom, and not just any condom. I tell them to only use a latex condom with a spermicide, which is the most barrier-protective. I explain that no sex is the only guarantee to avoid the many diseases out there, but a latex condom with spermicide offers the next best protection. And I really stress that this should be done whoever the partner is, and for whatever type of sex. So many teenagers think that diseases only happen to other kinds of kids.*

Keeping the doctor informed

For a variety of reasons, many children and young adults are no longer cared for by pediatric oncologists who are familiar with their history. Additionally, when treatment ends, many patients and parents are not adequately informed on the risks of developing physical difficulties months, years, or decades after treatment ends. The risks of such delayed effects are real. Moreover, many primary care physicians—pediatricians, family practice doctors, internists, gynecologists—are not fully aware of all the different treatments used for the multitude of childhood cancers and their late effects.

It is imperative that survivors be informed advocates in their own healthcare. They need to be educated, in a supportive and responsible way, of the risk for future physical adversities, so that if a problem does arise, it will be recognized early and receive prompt attention. Young adults who have survived childhood cancer need to be fully cognizant of their unique medical history and able to share this information with all future doctors who will care for them.

Figures 18-1 and 18-2 chart the possible late effects of treatment for ALL and ANLL and the methods used to screen for them. Survivors of the chronic leukemias require frequent follow-up from their bone marrow transplant center. If your child is not being followed in a late-effects clinic, you may wish to photocopy this information to share with your child's current doctor or to send to your child if she is already living away from home. These charts are reprinted from *Survivors of Childhood Cancer: Assessment and Management.*

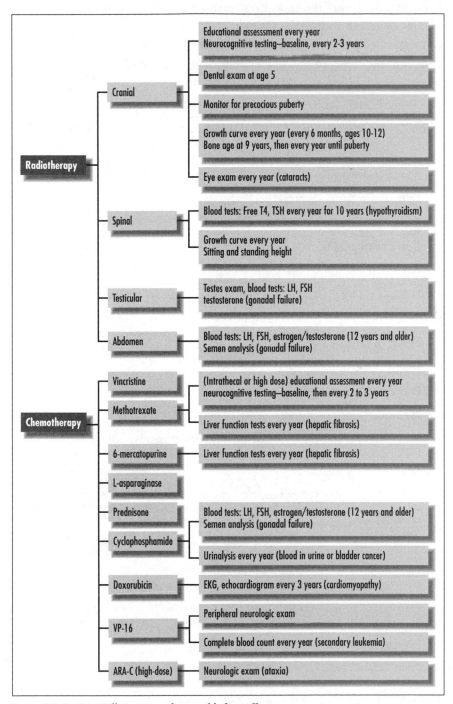

Figure 18-1. ALL: Follow-up test for possible late effects

A few months before the end of treatment, ask the oncologist to fill out the booklet bound in this book. This health history will become an indispensable part of your child's medical records for the rest of her life. It should be kept in a safe place and a copy should be given to each medical caregiver. When your child leaves home to begin her adult life, this booklet should go with her.

If you do not have a copy of the health history booklet, write down the following important information that should be in your child's health history:

- Name of disease

- Date of diagnosis and relapse, if any

- Place of treatment

- Dates of treatment

- Names of attending oncologist and primary nurse

- Names and total dosages of chemotherapeutic agents used

- Type, areas treated, and amount of radiation used

- Name of radiation center

- Date(s) radiation received

- Number of rads and to what location, e.g., whole body, cranial, etc.

- Dates and types of any surgeries

- Date and type of bone marrow or stem cell transplant, if any

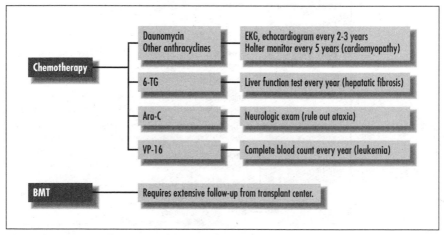

Figure 18-2. ANLL: Follow-up test for possible late effects

- Any major treatment complications

- Any persistent side effects of treatment

- Recommended medical follow-up

- Contact numbers for treating institutions

If your child will not be periodically examined at a long-term follow-up clinic, write down this information, and make sure that your child has a copy to give to any future doctor who will be treating her.

Employment

The population of adults who have survived childhood cancer is growing at a rapid rate. It is estimated that by the year 2000, 1 in every 900 young adults will be a cancer survivor. Thousands of survivors are staying well, growing up, graduating from college, and successfully entering the workforce. Survivors of childhood leukemia are educators, sports figures, radio announcers, doctors, social workers, dancers, lawyers, professionals of all types.

Diane Komp, MD, in *A Child Shall Lead Them*, writes:

> *I lecture about long-term survivors to each new group of medical students that comes through pediatrics at Yale. I can see from their faces that most of them prefer memorizing the odds that someone will make it than tasting the sweetness of individual victories. "That's very nice, but how representative is that case?"*

> *Not all of them feel that way, though. I watch their faces and can now pick out from their ranks a special type of young person who is being seen in increasing numbers in medical classrooms. Although their classmates cannot tell who they are, I can spot a long-term survivor of childhood cancer five minutes into that lecture.*

Despite their numbers, some survivors still face job discrimination due to fears about cancer and its treatment. Under federal law, and many state laws, an employer cannot treat a survivor differently from other employees because of a history of cancer except in certain circumstances involving health, life, and disability insurance. The Americans with Disabilities Act (ADA) prohibits many types of job discrimination by employers, employment agencies, state and local governments, and labor unions. In addition, most states have laws that prohibit discrimination based on disabilities, although what these laws cover varies widely.

The Americans with Disabilities Act of 1990 (ADA) prohibits discrimination based on actual disability, perceived disability, or history of a disability. Any employer with fifteen or more workers is covered by the ADA. The ADA requires that:

- Employer may not make medical inquiries of an applicant, unless:

    - Applicant has a visible disability, e.g., amputation, or

    - Applicant has voluntarily disclosed his cancer history.

    Such questions must be limited to asking the applicant to describe or demonstrate how she would perform essential job functions. Medical inquiries are allowed after a job offer has been made or during a pre-employment medical exam.

- Employer must provide reasonable accommodations unless it causes undue hardship.

- Employer may not discriminate because of family illness.

- Employer is not required to provide health insurance.

The Equal Employment Opportunity Commission (EEOC) enforces Title 1 (employment) of the ADA. Call (800) 669-4000 for enforcement information and (800) 669-3362 for enforcement publications. Other sections are enforced or have their enforcement coordinated by the US Department of Justice (Civil Rights Division, Public Access Section). The Justice Department's ADA website is at *http://www.usdoj.gov/crt/ada.html*.

In Canada, the Canadian Human Rights Act provides essentially the same rights as the ADA. The act is administered by the Canadian Human Rights Commission. You can get further information by calling the national office at (613) 995-1151.

If you feel that you have been discriminated against due to your disability or a relative's disability, contact the EEOC or the Canadian Human Rights Commission promptly. In the US, a charge of discrimination generally must be filed within 180 days of the notice of the discriminatory act.

Cancer survivors should not lie about a cancer history during a job interview. However, they should understand the consequences of voluntarily revealing a cancer history prior to receiving a job offer.

If a survivor of cancer or a member of the family feels that he has been denied a job, fired, forced from a job, denied reasonable accommodation, or discriminated against for promotions or medical leave because of cancer history, contact the Childhood Cancer Ombudsman Program for help (see Appendix C, *Resource Organizations*).

This program provides outside review by experts in medicine, disability rights, insurance, and employment. Areas in which access or discrimination are reviewed follow:

- Treatment plans
- Insurance
- Employment
- School access or IEP

The program also provides the following additional services related to above areas:

- Assistance in obtaining information needed
- Assistance with filing appeals
- Assistance with filing complaints
- Assistance on survivor response on job applications and at interviews

The military

Some survivors of childhood cancer wish to enlist in the military, or qualify for ROTC, the reserves, or the service academies. Grace Ann Monaco wrote in an article in *Pediatric Clinics of North America*:

> The laws and regulations relating to admission to the armed services are permissive, not mandatory. This means that each of the armed services can enforce these laws and regulations if the service wishes to do so. Usually, taken on a case-by-case basis, survivors of childhood cancer who meet the requirements of the particular service and who are "otherwise physically fit for service" are eligible for a medical waiver to serve in the armed forces, reserves, and ROTC, and to obtain admission to service academies if the survivor is free of cancer and, generally, has completed therapy five years previously.

Waivers are granted for survivors: a female neuroblastoma survivor was granted a waiver and entered the US Naval Academy. The Childhood Cancer Ombudsman Program can research federal regulations and research previous cases to aid the applicant to the military.

Insurance

Job discrimination can spell economic catastrophe for cancer survivors because most health insurance is obtained from employment. As survivors mature, seek employment, and move away from home, many encounter barriers to obtaining health insurance, such as rejection of application based on cancer history, policy reductions, policy cancellation, preexisting condition exclusions, increased premiums, or extended waiting periods. As current discussions about national healthcare reform are extremely contentious, it seems unlikely that major reforms of the American health insurance system will occur in the near future.

However, many states do offer high-risk individuals, like survivors, access to comprehensive health insurance plans (CHIPS). CHIPS, also called "high-risk pools," are a means for individuals to obtain insurance regardless of their physical condition or medical history. For more information on CHIPS, call your state Office of the Insurance Commissioner. The NCI publication *Facing Forward* lists contacts by state for insurance coverage for the hard to insure. See Appendix D, *Books and Online Sites*, for ordering information.

Although neither the states nor the federal government mandate a legal right to insurance, there are some legal remedies to insurance discrimination:

- COBRA. The Comprehensive Omnibus Budget Reconciliation Act (COBRA) is a federal law which requires public and private companies employing more than twenty workers to provide continuation of group coverage to employees if they quit, are fired, or work reduced hours. Coverage must extend to surviving, divorced, or separated spouses, and to dependent children. You must pay for your continued coverage, but it must not exceed by more than 2 percent the rate set for your former co-workers. By allowing you to purchase continued coverage, you have time to seek other long-term coverage.

- ERISA. The Employee Retirement and Income Security Act (ERISA) is a federal law which protects workers from being fired because of the cancer history of the employee or beneficiaries (spouse and children). ERISA also prohibits employers from encouraging a person with a cancer history to retire as a "disabled" employee. ERISA does not apply to job discrimination (denial of new job due to cancer history), discrimination which does not affect benefits, and employees whose compensation does not include benefits.

- **Health Insurance Portability and Accountability Act of 1996.** This law allows individuals to change to a new job without losing coverage if they have been insured for at least twelve months. It prevents group health plans from denying coverage based on medical history, genetic information, or claims history, although insurers can still exclude those with specific diseases or conditions. It also increases portability if you change from a group to an individual plan. The full text of the law is on the Internet at *http://epn.org/library/h3103.txt.*

ERISA, COBRA, and parts of the Health Insurance Portability and Accountability Act of 1996 are enforced by the Pension and Welfare Benefits Administration of the US Department of Labor in Washington, D.C. 20210, (202) 219-8776.

For detailed information on the ADA, COBRA, ERISA, and the Health Insurance Portability and Accountability Act of 1996, read *A Cancer Survivor's Almanac: Charting Your Journey,* edited by Barbara Hoffman, JD.

Appendix C lists organizations that can help if you or your child faces job discrimination or problems with insurance due to treatment for cancer.

Lisa N. Ellis, a survivor of ALL, included the following essay in her application to law schools. Lisa, who began law school in 1997, gives much of the credit for her success to her educational consultant, Joanne Holt.

> *Frustrated by my earlier performance on the LSAT, I began a search this year to uncover possible meaning in the gap between my actual test scores and my capabilities. My search led me to a rather unpredictable place: the sixth floor of Children's Hospital in Seattle, the same wing where I had received treatment for leukemia twenty-three years ago. Prompted by information received from a family friend who was also a former cancer patient, I started to explore the connection between my cancer treatment and my learning.*

From the colorful murals on the walls to the confusing floor plan of the building, much about the hospital looked the same to me. However, this time I was twenty-three years older and so was my oncologist. I approached her for information to help me further my career just as she was phasing out of hers. The information I hoped to receive would resolve some of the misgivings about my abilities on standardized tests and open new doors for me to retake the LSAT with enhanced opportunities.

The cancer-related information that wasn't revealed to me during my years of treatment was laid out on the table for me now. I was told that I was diagnosed at the same time the medical profession was starting to experience some significant breakthroughs in the treatment of childhood cancer. Stringent protocols involving chemotherapy, high doses of cranial and body radiation and painful procedures like spinal taps and bone marrow aspirations were beginning to produce positive results: more children were surviving what was previously viewed as a terminal disease. Caught in this watershed of medical breakthroughs, my cancer quickly responded and went into remission. Yet, I was informed that the same treatments that saved my life may also have affected my learning.

The statistics spelled out various side effects the treatment could have on former patients. Cited studies showed that some patients had difficulties with academic subjects like math, writing, and reading. Other research pointed to differences in processing speeds; including the inability to process information at a rapid pace or difficulty maintaining concentration for extended periods. Because I was only three years old when I was diagnosed, it was impossible to determine my cognitive makeup before treatment. Now, later in life, I had the opportunity to pinpoint the relevance these statistics had upon me.

I elected to go through an evaluation process which disclosed my educational strengths and weaknesses. Overall, the results indicated that I have strong intellectual ability. In particular, I demonstrated strong aptitude in vocabulary, comprehension, and verbal reasoning sections. Despite these encouraging results, scores for short-term sequential memory and processing speed sections were discrepant from my overall assessment. Yet, for me, the most significant impact these lower scores have posed is a greater challenge with timed standardized tests. At the advice of an educational consultant, I unofficially took the LSAT under untimed conditions. *The substantial improvements in my scores (169 instead of 150) confirmed my ability to deduce logical answers to test questions given adequate time.*

The results of this recent evaluation process validated my earlier conceptions about my academic profile. Sophomore year in college, I developed an understanding that I had to study harder than some of my classmates to learn the material and achieve good grades. Yet, instead of feeling defeated, I rose to the challenge. I look back on my college experience and believe that I benefited immensely from my extra efforts. I utilized the knowledge and guidance of my professors to discuss issues and write effectively. I also became highly organized, allowing me the ability to participate in sports, attain school leadership positions and maintain a solid grade point average. At Whitman College, I completed rigorous courses, consistently achieved a competitive grade point average, and received academic distinction with a minimum of accommodations.

Combined with my successful college performance is relevant and challenging work experience. I've held positions at several public law organizations which have utilized my abilities to communicate articulately, analyze complex issues, and develop rapport with diverse populations in multiple settings. Recently, I have been a Legal Extern for low-income persons at the Legal Action Center. I have direct experience analyzing evidence, interviewing clients, investigating case backgrounds, researching laws, and advocating for clients both orally and in writing.

With a history of academic and professional accomplishment, I have promising potential as a law student. In the past, I have adapted my learning style to overcome academic or work-related challenges. Now, I have gained insight and knowledge of my learning skills which will carry me with confidence through the demanding field of law.

CHAPTER 19

Relapse

Hold fast to dreams
For if dreams die
Life is a broken winged bird
That cannot fly.

—Langston Hughes

PARENTS FREQUENTLY DESCRIBE the return of their child's leukemia as more devastating than the original diagnosis. Parents feel betrayed. They think that they put their child through a hell for nothing. They are scared, for they know that any recurrence is serious. The anger is back—since they did everything the doctors said, why did the cancer return? They are afraid that if the first battery of treatments didn't work, what will? And the unspoken but most crushing feeling of all: If my child dies, how will I survive?

If your child has relapsed, one point that is well worth remembering: You are not the same person that you were at diagnosis. You've been through this before so you know how to get medical and emotional support. You have a relationship with the medical team, and you can speak the language now. You have developed friendships with other families of children with cancer. You know that something that seems insurmountable can be overcome, one day at a time.

This chapter explains how doctors determine if a relapse has occurred, emotional responses of the parents, and how to decide on a treatment plan.

Signs and symptoms

Although relapse can happen years after treatment ends, it most commonly occurs during treatment or in the first year off treatment. In fact, most treatment centers do not consider children to be long-term survivors of leukemia until they have been off treatment for at least two years.

The signs and symptoms of leukemia relapse include all of the same telltale warnings that occurred prior to diagnosis. These are:

- Fatigue
- Fevers
- Night sweats
- Bruises
- Pale skin
- Back, leg, or joint pain
- Loss of appetite
- Enlarged lymph nodes in the neck or groin
- Enlarged abdomen caused by a large spleen or liver
- Changes in behavior, such as excessive irritability — *not wanting to go to school.*
- Dizziness
- Headaches

Remember that many of these symptoms are also seen with normal childhood illnesses. However, persistent loss of appetite or fatigue or unusually severe symptoms require a call to your oncologist.

In some cases, parents have no warning. After they bring their child in for a routine bone marrow aspiration or spinal tap, they receive a totally unexpected telephone call from the doctor with the news.

> *I am a long-term survivor (30 years old), who first was diagnosed with ALL at age eight and subsequently relapsed three times, at ages thirteen, fifteen, and sixteen. The first relapse was by far the worst to deal with emotionally. It had been five years since my diagnosis, so I went in for my last spinal tap and bone marrow. I had been off treatment with good counts for two years. My mother and I didn't even wait for the test results; we went out to lunch and went shopping. Later that day, I called the clinic, and my doctor told me the bone marrow was fine, but she needed to talk to my mother. I heard my mother say, "No, no, oh no," and she started to cry. I just stood there feeling numb, knowing the news was bad. The cancer had returned to my central nervous system. We held each other and cried.*

The three most common sites for relapse are the bone marrow, the central nervous system, and the testes. Bone marrow relapse is the most common form of recurrence of leukemia. Achieving a prolonged second remission or cure after a bone marrow relapse is becoming more commonplace since the use of bone marrow transplantation has increased. Allogeneic transplants from an HLA-identical sibling (see Chapter 20, *Bone Marrow and Stem Cell Transplantation*) that is performed early in a second remission has resulted in longer leukemia-free survival when compared with chemotherapy. The value of autologous and matched unrelated bone marrow transplantation for relapsed ALL is uncertain.

Treatment for relapsed AML depends on prior treatment and other considerations. Options include clinical trials using new chemotherapy combinations and/or biologic agent studies, and bone marrow transplantation.

Since the use of central nervous system prophylaxis was initiated, the likelihood of CNS relapse has dramatically decreased. Currently, CNS relapse is seen in less than 10 percent of young patients. There are various of ways of treating CNS relapse, depending on the amount of prior radiation and intrathecal medication given. Usually, treatment plans include aggressive systemic and intrathecal therapy combined with craniospinal radiation.

Only 1 percent of boys with leukemia suffer a testicular relapse. Treatment for this type of relapse includes radiation to the testes (2400 cGy to both testes) and chemotherapy. Radiation to the testes at these doses usually causes sterility, and may cause hormonal abnormalities as well.

Occasionally leukemia recurs at other sites, such as the ovary or eye. These cases are usually treated with local radiation to the relapse site, and intensification of chemotherapy.

Refer to the PDQ for health professionals for the most up-to-date treatments and clinical trials for relapsed leukemia. These can be obtained by calling (800) 4-CANCER or on the Internet at *http://cancernet.nci.nih.gov/clinpdq/ soa.html.*

> *Right before Stephan went to camp, he went in for his maintenance spinal tap. I got a bill from a different specialist, and when I asked the oncologist about it, he said that Stephan had a few white cells in his fluid that he wanted to get another opinion on. He assured me that everything was okay, but I just had that feeling that something was about to go wrong. At his next spinal, his count was 88 in the cerebrospinal fluid. A central nervous system relapse.*

· · · · ·

Jody was complaining about pain and a feeling of pressure in his leg bones. I kept bringing him back to the oncologist, saying that something was wrong, that he was in great pain, but the doctor kept insisting that it was just growing pains. He didn't even examine his legs for a month. When he did, he could feel parts of the bone radiating heat. The bone scan showed the cancer in the exact spots that Jody had pointed out.

· · · · ·

Greg was in school, on maintenance, looking great. The night before a routine doctor's appointment, he started crying in the bathroom. But only half his face was crying. It was obvious that something was wrong. The next morning I was watching the doctor as he walked into the room, and when I saw his face I knew that we were in big, big trouble. Greg had Bell's palsy: the lumbar puncture showed that he had relapsed in his central nervous system.

· · · · ·

JaNette was diagnosed with AML with the Philadelphia chromosome. Four months into treatment, after a routine bone marrow aspiration, I got a phone call from the doctor saying that she had relapsed. I remember going to the hospital where they did another bone marrow. At exactly four o'clock in the afternoon, they gave me a relapse protocol to read. I was sitting on the floor in the hallway reading it, and it was so horrible because I knew what it meant! I understood what we were in for, and I started to bawl and couldn't stop.

Emotional responses

Parents who have children with leukemia in remission think or speak of relapse with an almost palpable dread. Just the thought can cause the emotions which surged in them at diagnosis to erupt. The depth of the emotions generated by relapse is very hard for parents and survivors to relive and describe. As one survivor of relapse said in a shaky voice when being interviewed, "It's been eleven years since I finished treatment, but talking about it shows that you scratch the surface and those overwhelming feelings are still right there."

Parents feel a wide array of emotions at relapse: numbness, guilt, dread, anger, fear, confusion, denial, and grief. Physical symptoms such as dizziness, nausea, fainting, and shortness of breath are common. Parents wonder how they can ask their child to endure it again. They wonder how they will survive it themselves. They oscillate between optimism and panic.

I found that relapse was far worse than the original diagnosis. At diagnosis, after a certain period of adjustment, you think that treatment has a beginning, a middle, and an end. But relapse creates a bigger burden to accept. You begin to feel that maybe the disease is more powerful than the medicine. I found that for awhile I just stopped functioning and thinking rationally. I felt that all the hell of treatment had been just a waste of time. I felt guilt and a tremendous sense of loss of control. I felt like I was on a runaway freight train, hurtling towards an end that didn't look so good anymore. This is the point at which people are willing to use any type of unconventional therapies because they are desperate. I know one mom in our support group who was even willing to try coffee enemas. She looks back on it now and says, "I just went crazy."

• • • • •

My first relapse was the worst emotionally. Neither my parents nor I ever thought that after five years it would be back. I also had been so young when I was first treated that I didn't really think of leukemia as cancer and didn't understand that I could die from it. But at thirteen, I remembered clearly what I had been through and all I could think was that it hadn't worked. I told my parents that I wouldn't do it again. My father sat me down and gave me a reality check. He explained that I would die if I didn't get treatment. He said, "If you don't do it for yourself, please do it for me and your mom." The next morning I went into the clinic and started all over again.

• • • • •

Jesse relapsed four times, and in some ways it got harder and in other ways it got easier. We knew each time that her chances for survival were fading, and that was hard. But each time we grieved and worked through the feelings, and our skills at handling relapse improved. I turned to God for comfort, and I think that helped me feel that I was standing on a rock out in the ocean, rather than thrashing around in the water. My faith gave me solace. Jesse handled the relapses better than anyone else in the family. She would calmly listen to the doctors' explanations, then she would say, "Okay, what do we have to do?" She was never angry. She was sometimes sad, but mostly accepting.

Deciding on a treatment plan

A rapid response is necessary when faced with a recurrence of childhood leukemia. Treatment plans for a first relapse may be specified in your child's protocol, or your physician may suggest a different approach. Suggestions for treatment may include radiation to the head and spine, radiation to the testes, more intensive chemotherapy, or bone marrow transplantation.

Physicians make recommendations based on knowledge, experience, and consultations with other experts in the field. Do not hesitate to ask your physician why she has suggested a certain approach to your child's relapse. Ask your doctor about treatment goals, methods, and possible side effects. Ask your doctor if she has consulted with others in the decision-making process, and if so, whom. Older children and teens need to be involved in decisions regarding their care and treatment choices.

Health Canada's publication, *This Battle Which I Must Fight: Cancer in Canada's Children and Teenagers*, states:

> This [relapse] is a time of crisis and ambivalence. The decision to be made is whether to continue to try to achieve a remission or to replace this hope with the hope for comfort for the child and a special time together. Each parent, and the child who is old enough to understand, requires differing amounts of time to reach a decision about how to proceed. Careful and frequent discussions with the medical team, as well as with trusted friends and relatives, may help clarify issues and bring some peace of mind.

Just like at diagnosis, time is a pressing concern. Parents know that treatment should begin as soon as possible. But beware rushing into a new treatment plan if you feel uncomfortable. Your child needs to know that you are 100 percent in favor of proceeding, and children have radar for parents' feelings. There is always time for answers to all of your questions and time to get a second opinion.

Refer to Chapter 6, *Forming a Partnership with the Medical Team,* for ways to obtain a second opinion. One excellent resource is the Childhood Cancer Ombudsman Program (see Appendix C, *Resource Organizations*). Panels of volunteer pediatric oncologists give second medical opinions or medical record reviews at the request of families or the treating oncologist. The program is particularly valuable in helping families make well-informed treatment choices, as well as becoming comfortable with the therapeutic approach chosen.

The information gleaned from second opinions and/or research may reinforce what your doctor recommended, or it might provide you with some additional treatment options. Either way, it may increase your comfort level during the treatment planning process. The following are questions that you might want to ask your doctor when discussing the treatment plan:

- What is the goal of this treatment? Is it likely to cure my child, or is it just for comfort?

- Why do you think that this treatment is the best option? What are the other choices, and why did you choose this one?

- Have you consulted with other physicians? If so, whom? Did you all agree on this treatment, or was there a range of choices suggested?

- Is there a standard treatment for this type of relapse? What is it?

- What clinical trials are ongoing for this type of relapse?

- Explain the potential benefits and possible side effects of the suggested treatment.

- What are the known or potential risks of the treatment?

- How often will my child need to be hospitalized?

- How long will my child need this treatment?

- If the treatment is investigational, is there scientific evidence that it works for leukemia?

- Will my child benefit, or is the study to advance medical knowledge?

- Does insurance cover this type of investigational treatment?

> After his CNS relapse while on maintenance, Stephan (eight years old) received cranial and spinal radiation and went through another induction, and they started to give him spinals with ARA-C, methotrexate, and hydrocortisone. Even with ondansetron it's bad. He's very sick to his stomach, and just feels queasy all of the time. After the reinduction, he went back on his maintenance schedule, and will finish at the expected time. But it's much harder for him now. His ankle bones ache, he's limping, and he can't run. Six days after vincristine, he gets severe back pain, like someone is pounding on his back hard. If he is bumped or jarred, he cries out in pain. He creeps along looking like an old man.

When Greg relapsed, they threw his protocol in the trash can, and our oncologist started making phone calls to other doctors in the Children's Cancer Group network to decide on a plan. Greg was put successively on three different relapse protocols in an attempt to keep him in remission. When his counts went down, the blasts would temporarily disappear, but when his counts rose, the blasts would creep back. His CNS relapse was followed by a bone marrow relapse, and the only option left was a bone marrow transplant, but we didn't know if he would be strong enough to survive it.

Christie was standard-risk ALL, so when she relapsed six months into treatment, they put her on a high-risk protocol, then when she relapsed again, she was put on even higher doses of chemotherapy. We finally went to them and said, "What are our options here?" They decided to give higher doses to try to get her in remission for a BMT, but by then she had serious heart damage from the ARA-C and was no longer an acceptable risk at most transplant centers. She ended up going to a center 3,000 miles from home which took high-risk cases.

After another relapse, they wanted to try a chemotherapy with limited possible results, and we really didn't want our eleven-year-old Caitlin to go through any more. But she talked it over with the doctor and concluded, "Of course I have to do it, I'm a fighting Irish."

When older children and parents disagree on the details of how to proceed, use the hospital social worker or psychologist to help you negotiate and make compromises. These discussions will help clarify each family member's thoughts and feelings, and will allow the child's emotional and physical well-being to be part of the equation.

In the Spring 1995 issue of the Candlelighters newsletter, Arthur Ablin, MD (Director Emeritus of Pediatric Clinical Oncology at the University of California, San Francisco) writes of the importance of goal-setting in the decision-making process after relapse:

Before determining which treatment is to be chosen, a decision must be made to determine the goal of treatment—in other words, what is it that we are trying to achieve. This crucial first step is the basis upon which any decision concerning treatment must be made. But it is too often omitted from consideration and/or discussion, even by the most experienced. The frustrations accompanying the previous failure of treatment, the fear of the loss of the hope for cure, the pressure of urgency to find solutions, the new awareness of the possibility or probability of death, lead us all to want to consider treatments first rather than these more difficult considerations involved in establishing goals. These also force us to deal with reality earlier, which could mean the almost intolerable confrontation with the death of a very-much-loved child, a tragedy to be avoided at all cost.

After you have set goals, received answers to all of your questions, obtained a second opinion if desired, and decided on a treatment plan, it is time to proceed. Your knowledge and experience may prove to be a double-edged sword. You have no illusions about the difficulties ahead because you've done it before, but you also will be strengthened by your ties with the cancer community, your comfort with your physicians and hospital routines, and your ability to "work the system" to get what your child needs. Many parents shared how their child took the lead about relapse treatment. While the parents agonized, their child said simply, "Let's just do it." And they did.

I encourage people to try to keep things in perspective. Attitude is a big part of survival. As difficult as it is, try to maintain a good attitude and keep focused on the future. I always thought, "I have cancer, this is a bad thing, but I am going to beat it." My analogy was a boxing match. When I relapsed, I was knocked down. But I always got up and kept fighting.

I had a total of three relapses, two of which were on treatment. Every time we relapse, statistics say our chances of survival are less likely. But I survived those three relapses, and now I live a life as normal as if cancer never touched it. After cancer, I finished high school and went to college. I gave birth to a beautiful, healthy baby girl. My daughter (still beautiful) is now seven years old, and with her I'll have a chance to relive some of the childhood I missed. For me, life does go on after cancer.

CHAPTER 20

Bone Marrow and Stem Cell Transplantation

*The courage of life is often a less dramatic
spectacle than the courage of the final
moment; but it is no less a magnificent
mixture of triumph and tragedy.*

—John Fitzgerald Kennedy
Profiles in Courage

BONE MARROW TRANSPLANTATION (BMT) AND STEM CELL TRANSPLANTATION (SCT) are complicated procedures used to treat leukemia, other cancers, and some blood diseases that were once considered incurable. In these procedures, the patient's bone marrow is totally destroyed by high-dose chemotherapy, with or without radiation. Normal marrow or stem cells are then infused into the patient's veins. The marrow or stem cells migrate to the cavities inside the bones where new, healthy blood cells are then produced.

Such transplants, although frequently life-saving, are expensive, technically complex, and potentially life-threatening. Understanding the procedures and their ramifications at a time of crisis can be tremendously difficult. This chapter will present the basics of bone marrow and stem cell transplantation in simple terms, as well as share the experiences of several families.

If a bone marrow or stem cell transplant has been recommended for your child, Appendix D, *Books and Online Sites*, lists several easy-to-read publications that provide more in-depth coverage of the subject. A bibliography of technical articles on the topic is available online at *http://www.patient-centers.com/leukemia*.

When are transplants necessary?

At present, some types of leukemia cannot be cured with conventional doses of chemotherapy and/or radiation. These cancers may be sensitive to extremely high doses of chemotherapy, but these doses permanently damage normal bone marrow. A bone marrow or stem cell transplant allows the delivery of such high-dose, potentially curable therapy after which bone marrow or stem cells are reinfused to rescue bone marrow function.

BMT or stem cell transplants are usually recommended for children with CML in the chronic phase, CMML after diagnosis, or AML in first or second remission. Transplant is recommended for some children with very high-risk types of ALL (e.g., Ph+ ALL) in first remission and usually in second remission in ALL if a matched sibling donor is available. Guidelines change over time as new information becomes available, and practices vary among institutions as well.

If a transplant has been recommended for your child or teenager, you may want to get a second opinion before proceeding. Chapter 19, *Relapse*, and Chapter 6, *Forming a Partnership with the Medical Team*, give several methods for obtaining an educated second opinion. In addition, to fully understand the issue, you may want to ask the oncologist some or all of the following questions:

- What are all the treatment options?
- For my child's type of cancer, history, and physical condition, what chance for survival does he have with a transplant? With other treatment?
- What are the risks from the transplant? Explain the statistical chance of each risk.
- What are the benefits of this type of transplant?
- What will be my child's short-term and long-term quality of life after the transplant?
- How long will she have to take medicines after the transplant?
- What are the side effects of these medicines?
- Is this transplant considered to be experimental, or is it accepted clinical practice?

> My daughter was six years old when she was diagnosed with AML. When she relapsed four months into treatment, an allogeneic bone marrow transplant was her only hope.

· · · · ·

After my son's second relapse from ALL, the doctors told us that a BMT was his last option for a cure.

· · · · ·

The day my daughter was diagnosed with CML, they told us her only chance for a cure was a BMT.

Types of transplants

Under certain circumstances, BMT or SCT is the treatment most likely to provide a cure for some children with leukemia. However, there are several different types of transplants available, and it is important to understand the types of transplant to better enable you to evaluate what has been proposed for your child.

What are HLA antigens?

Every individual has proteins, called human leukocyte-associated (HLA) antigens, on the surface of their cells. These protein markers allow the person's immune system to distinguish the body's own cells from those of another person. Scientists look at six different HLA antigens to determine a person's HLA type. Two people are considered to be a match if all six antigen sites are identical. If five or less sites match, it is called a mismatch or partial match.

HLA genes are inherited, so close relatives, especially siblings, are the most likely candidates for a six-antigen match. The odds of obtaining an unrelated (from a person not in the immediate family) matched bone marrow were once slim, but are now much improved due to the rapid expansion of persons typed and listed on various national and international marrow registries.

Allogeneic

Allogeneic BMTs are those in which donor bone marrow is transplanted into the patient. The marrow usually comes from a brother or sister with a matching tissue type or from a parent or sibling whose tissue type nearly matches the patient (a mismatched donor). Sometimes an matched unrelated donor (called MUD) can be located through the US National Marrow Donor Program or similar donor registries in the US or other countries. The risk of complications increases if the donor is mismatched or unrelated.

In an allogeneic BMT, the patient's bone marrow is destroyed through a combination of total body radiation and chemotherapy, or high-dose combination chemotherapy alone. The donor's marrow is dripped into the patient's vein in a manner similar to a blood transfusion. The donor marrow enters the cavities in the patient's bones, and if it engrafts properly, begins to produce new and healthy blood cells.

> Adele's transplant was almost two years ago, June 16, 1997. She was five and a half years old at the time. Donor marrow was harvested from Ben, two and a half at the time. Harvesting took approximately one hour, and after it was prepared for infusion, Adele received it (about 45 minutes later). The actual infusion was very simple—just hanging an IV bag. The doctor and nurses were, understandably, extremely careful with it, and it was very dramatic!

> One hour after completion, Adele could get up, and she and Ben immediately went running to the playroom! She had not crashed yet from the preparative chemotherapy, which had just been completed two days before. Just like her response to most of the treatment, however, this was not the norm. The nursing staff said they'd never seen a kid who felt well enough to do that following a BMT.

> Adele first showed something above a zero ANC on day T+15 (fifteen days after transplant). From then on, she improved quickly and steadily. She was released about six weeks after transplant, and met her goal of being at home and better (at least not sick!) for her sixth birthday. She did so well, that she was off all medication except for prophylactic Bactrim by the end of October. Because Adele showed basically no signs of graft-versus-host disease, she was taken off of almost all meds early. She returned to school in January.

The primary life-threatening complications of an allogeneic bone marrow transplant are graft-versus-host disease (GVHD) and infection. GVHD affects approximately 30 to 50 percent of patients who have undergone an allogeneic transplant, with a higher percentage of cases occurring after a transplant using mismatched marrow or marrow from an unrelated donor. While GVHD is a serious complication, it may decrease the likelihood that the child will relapse. This not-well-understood phenomenon is called the graft-versus-leukemia effect. GVHD is discussed in detail later in this chapter.

Transplant centers use different and various methods to reduce the risk of infection. The most effective methods are single-room isolation, thorough hand washing, and screened and irradiated blood products. Other infection control methods—air filters, requirements to cap and gown before visiting the patient, prohibiting live plants, fruits, and vegetables in the patient's room—remain unproven.

Autologous marrow transplant

During an autologous bone marrow transplant, the patient's own marrow is withdrawn (harvested) from the large bones of the hips. Some transplant centers use various methods to purge the marrow prior to freezing in order to kill any remaining leukemic cells. There are ongoing studies to evaluate the risks and benefits of purged versus unpurged autologous transplants and whether autologous transplant is better than conventional chemotherapy.

After the marrow is harvested and treated, it is cryopreserved (a type of freezing). The patient then undergoes radiation and chemotherapy or high-dose chemotherapy alone to kill all of his existing marrow. The frozen marrow is then thawed, and reinfused into the child or teen intravenously.

Children undergoing autologous transplants do not develop graft-versus-host disease and are therefore usually less susceptible to infection. This is because the GVHD suppresses the immune system, decreasing resistance to infection. But patients who undergo autologous transplants have higher relapse rates because of residual leukemic cells in the marrow or, perhaps, because there is no graft-versus-leukemia effect from GVHD. Patients who develop GVHD after an allogeneic transplant have lower relapse rates than those children who have an autologous or syngeneic transplant.

Syngeneic

Syngeneic bone marrow transplants are those in which the donor is the patient's identical twin. Because the marrow exactly matches the patient's, the major life-threatening complication of graft-versus-host disease (GVHD) is prevented. As with autologous transplants, any possible graft-versus-leukemia (GVL) benefit is absent in syngeneic transplants.

Jeremy had a syngeneic transplant from his identical twin brother as his donor to treat his secondary AML after treatment for Ewings. He received cytoxan and radiation in his conditioning regimen. One of the worst side effects he experienced was the nausea and vomiting. He was released from the hospital on day 9, readmitted on day 11 because of an infection, and discharged again on day 12. We stayed near the hospital and then we were allowed to go home on day 30. He has done very well.

Peripheral blood stem cell transplant (PBSCT)

When doctors aspirate liquid bone marrow from the cavities in bones, it is full of stem cells—cells from which all other cell types evolve. Stem cells can also be found in the circulating (also called peripheral) blood, although in a much less concentrated form.

In a peripheral blood stem cell transplant (PBSCT), the leukemia patient's own stem cells are harvested in a procedure called apheresis or leukapheresis. Patients are given GCSF prior to pheresis to stimulate stem cell production. Blood is removed through a central venous catheter or a catheter placed in a vein in the arm and circulated through a machine which extracts the stem cells. The blood is then returned to the patient. Each pheresis session lasts two to four hours, and generally from four to six sessions are required to harvest enough stem cells for a PBSCT. The stem cells are frozen until the transplant is performed. As with bone marrow, these stem cells are infused intravenously after high-dose chemotherapy.

Placental blood/umbilical cord blood stem cell transplant

Umbilical cord blood is a rich source of stem cells. Some institutions are conducting transplants using the umbilical cord blood obtained during the birth of a sibling or from preserved unrelated donor cord blood. The number of stem cells are usually sufficient for most children, but may not be adequate for adults, depending on their size. In some cases, engraftment, particularly of platelets, is delayed in this type of transplant.

> *Our fifteen-month-old son Garrett was diagnosed with AML M4 and had CNS involvement. He relapsed on treatment and the doctors recommended a cord blood transplant. There was one perfect match in Barcelona, Spain. It matched six out of six and was also a molecular match. I wanted to fly to Barcelona and hug everyone I could see.*

*He was so sick during treatment, including a trip to the ICU and
several periods of extended hospitalization for complications, that the
transplant was almost anticlimactic. He had cranial radiation, TBI, then
chemotherapy. He engrafted on day 12 and was out on day 21. He did
wonderfully—he only got one fever, no GVHD, no other problems. He has
not been inpatient since, and it's been fourteen months.*

Preliminary results suggest that graft-versus-host disease occurs less frequently in fully matched sibling placenta transplants although GVHD is still a problem in mismatched placental blood transplants. In addition, cord blood is rarely contaminated by viruses such as cytomegalovirus (CMV) or Epstein Barr virus (EBV) that can cause life-threatening complications after a BMT. Placental blood stem cell transplantation is one of many promising new directions in the research efforts of scientists studying ways to improve bone marrow transplantation.

Bone marrow transplant protocols vary among institutions, and are constantly evolving. Many aspects of bone marrow transplantation, for example, the graft-versus-leukemia effect, are not well understood, but are under intense scientific scrutiny. Research is also underway to identify those children most likely to benefit from a BMT, the best time to transplant, which new drugs best reduce the likelihood of infection, and the best methods to reduce post-transplant relapse.

For more information on types of transplants, write or phone the *Blood and Marrow Transplant Newsletter*, 2900 Skokie Valley Road, Highland Park, IL 60035, (888) 597-7674 or (847) 433-3313, fax (847) 433-4599, and ask for one of the following:

- "BMTs for AML," September 1994 issue
- "BMTs for ALL," November 1994 issue
- "BMTs for CML," March 1995 issue
- "Cord Blood Transplants," January 1996 issue

The *BMT Newsletter* is also published on the Internet at *http://www.bmt-news.org*.

Finding a donor

Finding a bone marrow donor can be a stressful and time-consuming task. The search may begin after relapse for children with ALL, in first remission for children with AML or some types of high-risk ALL, during the chronic phase for children with CML, and soon after diagnosis of children with CMML. In some lucky families, tests show that a sibling or parent is a partial or identical match. Other patients, especially those from minority groups not well-represented in the donor files, can spend months or years searching for a match.

> My advice to parents just beginning the process is do not rely on anyone else to make all the arrangements for a donor search and financial arrangements with the transplant center. We were focused on my son's relapse treatment and thought a donor search was ongoing. We then found out that over two precious months had been lost in a delay for financial approval. I foolishly relied on my doctor and his staff to make arrangements and follow through, and it just slipped through the cracks. I should have been on the phone several times a week making sure that the search had begun and that the transplant center was happy with the financial arrangements. I have a lot of guilt over whether those months made a difference in my son's outcome. I'll never know.

The first step in determining if a person is an HLA match is obtaining a sample of blood and sending it to a laboratory for analysis. Each member of the family is HLA typed, and if a match is not found, then the search widens to the donor marrow registries or placental blood banks. Appendix C, *Resources Organizations* lists registries, foundations, and programs that can assist you in finding a donor.

> Christie had a rare Mediterranean trait, and we could not find a match in all the registries worldwide. We decided that we had to do it on our own and began a donor drive in our town, which is predominantly Italian. The Red Cross discouraged us, saying that we probably wouldn't get a good response, that they could not process the blood without the money ($45 per person) in hand, and it would be better to spend quality time with Christie. But when the community of Rochester found out, it just snowballed. Dave and I went on TV and advocated for Christie, stressing the importance of Christie's bone marrow drive, and told people that this might help their own child one day. The first day of the drive, people lined up outside and stood for hours in the freezing rain and cold. The response was so overwhelming that late in the day they ran out of supplies. Large corporations became involved; GRC did a telethon that raised over $50,000. We typed over 4,000 people from Rochester and

received letters from all over the country. It was just a beautiful thing. Christie was such a powerful little person, and she came to represent so much to our community.

• • • • •

We felt that it was an omen that Jody's older sister and younger brother were perfect matches. They chose Marieke because she was older, but after all of the workup and tests, they discovered that she was CMV (cytomegalovirus) positive so they used two-year-old Christoph's marrow. Marieke was very disappointed.

• • • • •

While they were trying to find a match for JaNette, the church started a fundraiser and donor sign-up drive. They signed up over 600 people in two days, and United Blood Service had matching funds available to offset some of the costs. Meanwhile, we found an unrelated donor who lived in Milwaukee. She donated the marrow there, and a nurse from UCLA flew out to pick it up.

If a child needs a marrow transplant from an unrelated donor, the national and international registries are asked to conduct a computerized search of their databases. This will identify any donors with the same HLA type as the child. The registry contacts the potential donor to ask if he will donate more blood samples for additional tests.

If the testing shows compatibility, the donor is given an extensive explanation of the entire donation procedure and a complete medical exam. The donor must then make a final commitment to provide marrow for the child in need.

Choosing a transplant center

Choosing a transplant center is a very important decision. Institutions may just be starting a BMT program, or they may have vast experience. Some may be excellent for adults, but have limited pediatric experience. Some may allow you to room in with your child, while others may isolate the child or teen for weeks. Protocols vary among institutions, as well. The center closest to your home may not provide the best medical care available for your child or allow the necessary quality of life (rooming in, social workers, etc.) that you need.

To obtain a list of transplant centers, call for the current "Transplant Center Access Directory" from the National Marrow Donor Program (NMDP) Office of Patient Advocacy. The directory lists all BMT centers affiliated with the NMDP that perform unrelated BMTs. The directory includes the location of the center, diseases treated, and costs. To obtain a free copy, call 1-800-526-7809.

More than 450 transplant centers from 48 countries are listed on the web site of the Autologous Blood and Marrow Transplant Registry at *http://www.ibmtr.org* (click on transplant centers). The Oncology Nursing Society also has a list of transplant centers online at *http://www.ons.org*.

To help you learn about the policies of different transplant centers, here are some questions that you might ask:

- How many pediatric transplants did the institution do last year? How many of the type recommended for my child?

- How successful is your program? What are the one-, two-, and five-year survival rates? (Remember that some institutions accept very high-risk patients, and these statistics would not compare to a place that only performs less risky transplants.)

- What are the antigen match requirements? (Some institutions require a six-antigen match, others require five out of six, others permit a minor mismatch at the A or B antigen site, but not at other antigen sites.)

- What is the nurse-to-patient ratio? Do all the staff members have pediatric training and experience?

- What are the institution's rules on parents staying in the child's hospital room?

- What are the institution's anti-infection requirements? Isolation? Gown and gloves? Washing hands?

- Describe the BMT procedure in detail. Is radiation part of the pretransplant treatment?

- Explain the risks and benefits of this procedure.

- Assuming all goes well, how soon could my child leave the hospital? Leave the area to go home?

- What will his life be like, assuming all goes perfectly? If there are problems?

- What are the long-term side effects of this type of transplant?

- What long-term follow-up is available?

- Explain the waiting list requirements.

- What support staff is available (educator, social worker, child life therapist, chaplain, etc.)?

- How much will this procedure cost? How much will my insurance cover?

Many transplant centers have videos and booklets for patients and their families to explain services and describe what to expect before, during, and after transplant. Call any transplant center that you are considering, and ask them to send you all available materials.

To explore more fully what questions to ask various transplant centers, obtain the *Candlelighters Guide to Bone Marrow Transplants in Children* (listed in Appendix D). This excellent book has an entire chapter devoted to questions to ask to find the best transplant center for your child.

To obtain additional information on how to choose the appropriate transplant center, write or phone the *BMT Newsletter* to obtain the January 1994 issue "Choosing a BMT Center."

> *The head of oncology at UCLA comes to our city every two months to follow up on the kids who have been treated there. It was a big draw to us to have post-transplant follow-up at home, rather than having to travel a great distance to get back to the center. The other thing was that children are not put in laminar air flow, and families weren't required to cap and gown, only scrub their hands. Since I'm allergic to those hospital gloves, this allowed me to stay with my daughter throughout. We did, however, call around to several centers to compare facilities, costs, and insurance coverage.*

Making an informed consent is serious for a life-threatening procedure such as a bone marrow transplant. Do not hesitate to keep asking questions until you fully understand what is being proposed. Ask the doctor to use plain English if she has lapsed into medical jargon. Bring a tape recorder or friend to help remember the information. And include your child or teen in the discussion and decision-making process if she wishes. Do not sign the consent form until you feel comfortable that you understand the procedure and have had all of your questions answered.

Paying for the transplant

Bone marrow transplants are expensive, averaging from $150,000 to $200,000 for the transplant, hospitalization, and follow-up care. Fees for the donor search, donor blood tests, donor physical exam, and bone marrow harvest can total more than $30,000. Most bone marrow transplants for leukemia are no longer considered experimental, so many insurers cover the procedure without problems. However, not all insurers cover the donor-related costs.

Most insurance plans have a lifetime cap, and many only pay 80 percent of the costs of the transplant up to the cap. Often, transplant centers will not perform the procedure without all of the money guaranteed. With time of the essence, this can cause great anguish for families who struggle to raise funds or mortgage all of their belongings to pay.

> Our first quote from the transplant center was $350,000, but we were able to negotiate for a lower price.

· · · · ·

> My son died soon after the transplant. I hate to talk about the money, because I don't want people to think I begrudge spending it. I know that I would feel differently if the transplant had been successful, but I honestly think that we were misled about the real chance of success for his type of disease. We spent the equity on our house, plus took out a second mortgage. We will be paying it off the rest of our lives.

If you are having difficulty getting your insurance company to pay for the transplant, the Blood and Bone Marrow Newsletter provides a free referral service to attorneys and not-for-profit organizations who may be able to help you. Fill in the form at *http://www.bmtnews.org* or phone (847) 433-3313.

> When our son needed a transplant for AML, the insurance company kept refusing to pay because they said it was "experimental." So my wife became good friends with the catastrophic caseworker. The caseworker was extremely helpful. When it was disallowed again, she was upset and called my wife and said, "I'm going to tell you how to get this thing approved." She dictated two letters to my wife: one for unrelated transplant and one for cord blood. The doctor sent them in and they quickly approved the unrelated transplant but denied the cord blood again as experimental although our doctor thought cord blood was his best hope.

With some more coaching from the caseworker, a third attempt at a cord blood approval was successful. The caseworker even called my wife with the good news before she alerted the hospital. Her help most likely saved my son's life.

If you are not insured (or are underinsured) and must raise all or part of the necessary funds, refer to the organizations listed under "Financial and insurance help" in Appendix C. They may be able to offer some financial help, and can supply advice on how to quickly and effectively raise funds. Before working with any of these organizations, ask for all printed information available, and ask questions about any fees or costs associated with their services. Make sure that when the treatment is completed or if the child dies, any remaining funds may be applied to outstanding medical debts.

You might also call the *BMT Newsletter* and ask for the November 1993 issue, "Successful Fundraising" or read it online.

Our HMO refused to pay for our daughter's bone marrow transplant because it required an unrelated donor, which they considered to be "experimental." Her oncologist and several doctors from the transplant center gathered data and presented it to the insurance board. The HMO reversed its position and paid for the transplant, but not for the donor search, donor fees, donor harvest, or having the marrow transported from London. It cost us approximately $25,000.

Donating the marrow

Marrow is withdrawn (harvested) from the large bones of the hips. While the donor or patient (for autologous transplant) is under general anesthesia, the doctor inserts a large needle into the bones of the hips and withdraws bone marrow. This procedure is done up to fifty times to draw out a total of one to two pints. The entire process takes less than one hour. After marrow donation, some hospitals keep the donor overnight, while others discharge the same day if the donor is not in pain.

Because the amount of marrow that is removed contains less than five percent of the donor's developing blood cells, it only takes a few days for the body to replace the marrow. The donor or child is usually sore for a day or two, and may feel a bit tired for several days. The recovery time varies from donor to donor.

After no match was found for Christie in the 4,000 donors that we signed up and typed, I became her donor. We were just a partial match. Being her donor was just wonderful. It was Mother's Day weekend, and I was just full of faith and love. I thought this is it, God has given me a second chance to give life to this child. I had a very powerful feeling that it was so special that I could do this for my daughter. I really felt that this was it, it was going to work.

It was uncomfortable for a couple of days, and I was a little bruised. But the people there were wonderful, and they really followed me closely. I'm still on the registry; if someone called me tomorrow, I'd be on a plane. It's a very rewarding feeling, a gift from God.

• • • • •

Jody's two-year-old brother Christoph was a perfect match. I stayed with him when he donated marrow, and my husband stayed with Jody. Christoph seemed to handle the marrow donation easily. Although he had some nausea in the recovery room, he was up and running around late that afternoon saying, "I the donor." He felt very proud. I knew he was somewhat sore because he said, "My diaper hurts."

The transplant

Prior to the actual transplant, the patient's bone marrow is destroyed using high-dose chemotherapy with or without radiation. This portion of treatment is called conditioning. The purpose of the high-doses of chemotherapy and radiation is to kill all remaining cancer cells in the body and make room in the bones for the new bone marrow or stem cells.

Conditioning regimens vary according to institution and protocol, and also depend on the medical condition and history of the patient. Typically, the chemotherapy is given for two to six days, and radiation (if part of conditioning) is given in multiple small doses over several days.

They got JaNette into her second remission in December, then gave her maintenance drugs to keep her there until they were ready to start transplant conditioning in April. So, unlike some of the other kids, she went to transplant healthy and strong. JaNette had 1200 rads of total body radiation in five increments—two the first day, two the second day, and one the third day. Then she had two days of incredibly strong chemotherapy, one day of rest, then the transplant.

The transplant itself consists of simply infusing the marrow or stem cells through a central venous catheter or IV into the patient, just like a blood transfusion. The marrow or stem cells travel through the blood vessels, eventually filling the empty spaces in the long bones. Engraftment is when the new marrow begins to produce healthy white cells, red cells, and platelets. This typically occurs from two to six weeks after transplantation. Complete recovery of all components of immune function can take from one to two years.

I couldn't believe how beautiful the bone marrow was—a bag of shimmering red liquid. It just glistened. It meant life.

• • • • •

My dad donated marrow for my transplant. He said he was sore and doing the "bone marrow hop," but he made it to my room that day to see his marrow transfused into me. I really felt different as I was getting the bone marrow, like I was getting so much more energy.

• • • • •

I cannot say enough good things about the transplant center. They were very family-oriented, allowed us in the room 24 hours a day. I was allowed to sleep in bed with her (I just told the nurses to make sure to poke her and not me). The nurses were wonderful, and I still think of them as family. We didn't get very close to the other families; we tended to stay in our own child's room. One day a family would be there, then the next day they would be gone. I got to the point where I just didn't want to know.

• • • • •

The transplant went well except that he was 50 days in the laminar flow room so that we couldn't touch him. Five years old and we couldn't touch him. We had these gloves that we could use to reach in. But Jody was such an accepting kid, he adjusted. We played a lot of cards and at night we'd turn off the lights, and he'd imagine soaring out the tenth floor window. He'd just fly out of that room. He was on hyperal (IV nutrition) and lots of prednisone and other drugs, and he had a few tantrums. Once he pulled out all of his needles and threw them against the wall. I thought that it was a pretty healthy response, but the social worker showed up immediately.

• • • • •

We were prepared to stay five months in or near the transplant center, but we went home after only two and a half. She had the normal nausea, so she was on TPN (total parenteral nutrition) from transplant May 5 until the end of June. Until she could take her medications by mouth, I did some IVs at home. She had her last platelet transfusion in July. It took until the following June for her counts to normalize, and for her to start producing T cells. We feel lucky that things went so well.

Donor and patient confidentiality are closely guarded. The NMDP allows letter exchanges or meetings if both donor and recipient express a strong desire to do so, but only after a year has passed since the transplant.

Emotional responses

Bone marrow transplant takes a heavy emotional toll on the child, the parents, and the siblings. It can be a physically and mentally grueling procedure, with the possibility of months or years of aftereffects. Most transplant team members are extensively trained to meet the needs of the patient and family during the transplant and long convalescence. The team includes physicians and nurses, as well as psychiatrists, social workers, chaplains, educators, nutritionists, and child life therapists.

Christie had many painful complications after the unmatched allogeneic transplant. I remember lying next to her and saying, "Christie, if Mommy could take this away from you I would." She looked at me and said, "Mommy, I love you so much, I would never want you to go through this." But then she went on to say, "It's not so bad, I met a lot of people, we got to travel, Daddy didn't have to work, Danielle and Nicole got to spend time with Daddy." She just saw something positive in everything, even this terrible disease.

Christie was also very, very funny. She loved having me be the donor, and she started calling me her "blood sister." She kept saying, "Ma, when am I going to start being funny like you?" and I'd tell her that she was way beyond me. Her humor was contagious.

· · · · ·

Leah was feeling good and was very healthy when she went into the laminar air flow room. We lived near the transplant center, and she had at least twenty visitors a day. I think the visits and the nonstop telephone conversations really kept her spirits up.

I think the hardest part of the transplant was being in the laminar air flow room (LAF). They gave me a sterilization wash, put me in some boots, and told me I couldn't touch anything. I felt like a space person. Then I went into the room for two months. I really missed touching people. I cried when I got out and hugged my mom.

· · · · ·

What helped me the most was the decorations and having a positive attitude. My mom decorated the area outside the LAF room with balloons, cards, and posters. It was hard to take the medicine, so my mom made a huge poster to mark off how well I did. Every time I took my medicine, I got a sticker. When I got one hundred stickers, I got some roller blades.

· · · · ·

I felt great during the transplant and at the center, but when we came home it was very, very difficult. We had just moved before my daughter was transplanted, so we didn't have a good support system in place. She had been in the hospital, then transplant center for almost a year, and then we had to stay at home for another year. For a few months she would spike a fever every time someone who was not in the family came in the house. So my young son could never go to friends to play or have friends over. We just stayed home. It was very hard, and we all felt very isolated.

Often so much time and energy is focused on the child who needs the transplant that the needs of the sibling donor are overlooked. Siblings need careful preparation for what is about to occur, and all questions need to be answered and concerns addressed. Parents need to be careful that the sibling donor realizes that the results of the BMT are out of everyone's control, and that the sibling is not responsible for either her brother's life or death.

Organizations that can offer emotional support to families during the transplant are listed in Appendix C.

Complications

Some children have a smooth journey through the transplant process, while others bounce from one life-threatening complication to another. Some children live, and some children die. There is no way to predict which children or teens will develop problems, nor is there any way to anticipate whether the new development will be merely an inconvenience or a catastrophe. This section will present some of the major complications that can develop post-transplant, and the experiences of several families in facing these problems.

Failure to engraft

Engraftment is when the donated marrow takes up residence in the patient's bones and begins to produce healthy blood cells. In cases where a child has received HLA-matched marrow from a sibling, engraftment failure is less than 5 percent. In contrast, children receiving marrow from partially HLA matched family members or unrelated donors, graft rejection occurs in 5 to 25 percent of patients.

Infections

Most infections following transplant come from organisms within the body (e.g., CMV, gut bacteria). Good handwashing and adequately controlled ventilation can help minimize infections with staph and fungi.

The immune system of healthy children quickly destroys any foreign invaders; not so with children who have undergone a bone marrow transplant. The diseased immune system of these children has been destroyed by chemotherapy and radiation to allow the healthy marrow or stem cells to grow. Until the new marrow or stem cells engraft and begin to produce large numbers of white cells (two to six weeks), children post-transplant are in danger of developing serious infections.

To prevent and combat bacterial infections, children receive large doses of several kinds of antibiotics if their temperature goes above 101°F (38.5°C) any time in the first weeks after transplant. Ironically, the antibiotics used to treat bacteria allow fungi to flourish. Fungal infections often follow prolonged neutropenia and antibiotics and can't be prevented easily.

> Leah had so many problems with infections and getting her counts back up that she spent two years on steroids, cyclosporin, and monthly gammaglobulin.

· · · · ·

*During the related mismatched allogeneic transplant, I developed no
mouth sores, no infections, no GVHD. Just a headache the whole time. I
do miss being an athlete, I do miss the friends that I lost, and I do miss my
blond hair (it came back in brown, so I tried to dye it blond and it turned
bright, fluorescent red). But I can deal with those things. To survive I
think you need luck, a positive attitude, and a decorated room to help you
stay cheery.*

After the first month post-transplant, children are also susceptible to serious
viral infections, most commonly herpes simplex virus, cytomegalovirus, and
varicella zoster virus, particularly if they have GVHD. These can occur up to
two years after the transplant. Viral infections are notoriously hard to treat,
so many centers use prophylactic acyclovir or granciclovir or immunoglobu-
lin to prevent these infections.

CMV is usually preventable if the patient and donor are both CMV-negative
and all transfused blood products are CMV-negative or filtered to remove
white blood cells.

Interstitial pneumonitis, a sometimes fatal form of pneumonia, is most common the second or third month post-transplant. It is very uncommon after
autologous transplants and is most often associated with GVHD after allogeneic transplants.

Preventing infections is the best policy for those children who have had a
bone marrow or stem cell transplant. The following are suggestions to minimize exposure to bacteria, viruses, and fungi:

- Medical staff and all family members must wash their hands before
  touching the child.

- Keep your child away from crowds and people with infections.

- Do not let your child receive live virus inoculations until the immune
  system has fully recovered. Your child will need complete reimmuniza-
  tions. The timing of these will be directed by the doctor.

- Keep your child away from anyone who has recently been inoculated
  with a live virus (chicken pox, polio).

- Keep your child away from barnyard animals and all types of animal
  feces.

- Avoid home remodeling while your child is recovering.

- Call the doctor at the first sign of a fever or infection.

For more information on infections, obtain the September 1993 *BMT News-letter,* "Infections," or read Chapter 8 of *Bone Marrow Transplants: A Book of Basics for Patients,* by Susan Stewart (see Appendix D).

Graft-versus-host disease (GVHD)

Graft-versus-host disease is a frequent complication of allogeneic bone mar-row transplants. It does not occur with autologous or syngeneic transplants. In GVHD, the bone marrow or stem cells provided by the donor (graft) attack the tissues and organs of the BMT child (host). Approximately 30 to 50 percent of persons who have a related HLA-matched transplant develop some degree of GVHD. The incidence and severity of GVHD are increased for those children who receive unrelated or mismatched marrow, but are decreased if cells that cause GVHD are reduced prior to infusion. The major-ity of GVHD cases are mild, although some can be life-threatening.

There are two types of GVHD: acute GVHD and chronic GVHD. Patients can develop one type, both types, or neither. Acute GVHD usually occurs at the time of engraftment or shortly thereafter. Donor cells identify the patient's cells as foreign, and may attack the patient's skin, liver, stomach, or intes-tines. Allogeneic BMT patients are given drugs before and after transplant in an attempt to prevent GVHD. Symptoms of acute GVHD can range from mild skin rash to severe, sometimes fatal infections, or liver, stomach, and intestinal problems. Acute GVHD is treated with cyclosporin and steroids (prednisone, dexamethasone). Methotrexate may be given to prevent GVHD.

> JaNette's transplant was on May 5 and her ANC was up to 1000 on May 30. That's when her graft-versus-host started. It doesn't look like a regular rash, more like pinpoint red dots under the skin. It's very itchy, and then it starts to peel. She looked like she had leprosy! She had very little internal graft-versus-host disease. She's a year and a half post-transplant, and she still broke out in a rash the last time they tried to taper her off the cyclosporin.

· · · · ·

> Ryan died from acute graft-versus-host disease. It destroyed his liver. It was a hard death, and we felt that it robbed us of whatever time he would have had left if he didn't have the BMT.

Chronic GVHD usually develops after the third month post-transplant. It primarily affects the skin (itchy rash, discoloration of the skin, tightening of the skin, hair loss), eyes (dry, light-sensitive), mouth and esophagus (dry, tooth decay, difficulty swallowing), intestines (diarrhea, cramping, weight loss), liver (jaundice), lungs (shortness of breath, wheezing, coughing), and joints (decreased mobility). This list may seem overwhelming, but remember that only some patients develop chronic GVHD, and those who do may experience all, a few, or only one of these symptoms.

> A year and a half after the transplant, they tried to taper my daughter off the cyclosporin. Her liver function counts went way up, and she broke out in a rash all over her body. The bottoms of her feet were so blistered that she couldn't walk. She has permanent dark splotches all over her torso, but the ones on her face and neck gradually faded away.

· · · · ·

> I wasn't supposed to go out in the sun after my transplant, but I did anyway. The sun aggravated the mild GVHD that I had and I turned blotchy. I had itchy light and dark patches on my stomach and face. I had to go back on steroids.

Veno-occlusive disease

Veno-occlusive disease (VOD) is a complication that can occur after bone marrow or stem cell transplantation in which the flow of blood through the liver becomes obstructed. Children who have had more than one transplant or previous liver problems are more at risk to develop VOD. It can occur gradually or very quickly. Symptoms of VOD include jaundice (yellowing of the skin), an enlarged liver, pain in the upper right abdomen, fluid in the abdomen, and unexplained weight gain. Treatment includes fluid restriction, diuretics (such as furosemide), anti-clotting medications, and removal of all but the most essential amino acids from IV nutrition (hyperalimentation).

Long-term side effects

Increasing numbers of children are being cured of their disease and surviving years after a bone marrow or stem cell transplant. The intensity of the treatment prior to, during, and after transplant can cause major effects not apparent for months or years. This section will describe a few of the major long-term side effects that sometimes develop after a bone marrow transplant.

Relapse

Despite the intensive chemotherapy and/or radiation given prior to the bone marrow or stem cell transplant, some children suffer a recurrence of the original disease. This is most likely to occur in the first several years post-transplant.

> *Jody had his transplant in October, and we thought he was doing wonderfully. In June he just started getting tired and slowing down. We brought him in and found out that he had relapsed. They said there was no hope for a cure, but they thought that they could get him into remission again. He lived for another fifteen months.*

Problems with the eyes

Most children treated with total body radiation develop cataracts. How the radiation is administered affects the child's chance of developing this complication. If the total body radiation (TBI) is given in one dose, approximately 80 percent of children develop cataracts. If the TBI is given in smaller doses over several days (fractionated), the chance of developing cataracts is much lower. Almost all protocols now use fractionated TBI.

> *My eight-year-old daughter is six years out from the full body radiation used to prepare her for bone marrow transplant. She had the first of two cataract surgeries Tuesday. It was an outpatient procedure and she was a real trooper. The doctor was able to insert a permanent replacement lens, which is a good thing since it means we don't have to do the contact lens thing. I can't wait for the day when radiation is no longer a treatment for cancer. Until then I have to acknowledge begrudging thanks because it saved my baby's life.*

Decreased tear production is common in those children with chronic GVHD, but is also seen in patients with no GVHD.

Growth and dental development

Irradiation can affect growth. If your child had prior cranial radiation, or total body radiation (TBI) as part of preparation for the BMT, she should be closely monitored for learning disabilities, dental problems (facial bone and jaw growth, delayed development of permanent teeth, incomplete root development), and growth hormone deficiency resulting in delayed or decreased growth.

Aseptic necrosis

Long-term use of high-dose steroids can cause, in some people, a problem called aseptic necrosis. This condition is caused by the death of the small blood vessels that nourish the bones. Pain and loss of mobility result.

> Leslee was an athlete who played three sports prior to her AML diagnosis and bone marrow transplant. The steroids saved her life, but destroyed her bones. She has had surgery on her shoulders, hips, and knee joints. Her shoulders and hips are much better, but her knees are still painful, and she has trouble getting around. The surgeon is hoping that soon he will be able to use live bone in experimental surgery to help her.

Thyroid function

Children who receive chemotherapy only do not develop thyroid deficiency as a result of treatment. Those children who receive TBI do, however, have a 25 to 50 percent chance of having low thyroid function due to a decreased production of thyroid hormone. Tablets containing thyroid hormone usually are effective in treating the problem.

Puberty and sterility

Children who had only chemotherapy during the conditioning regimen usually have normal sexual development, though not always. Those who had total body irradiation, however, are particularly at risk for delayed puberty (the incidence is lower if the radiation was given in several smaller doses). All children treated by transplantation should be followed closely by a pediatric endocrinologist, who can prescribe hormones (testosterone for boys, estrogen and progesterone for girls) to assist in normal pubertal development. Girls are more likely to need hormonal replacement; boys usually produce testosterone but not sperm.

Children who receive total body radiation usually (but not always) become sterile, that is, after growing up, girls will not be able to become pregnant, nor will boys be able to father children. Ability to have a normal sex life is not affected. Some children treated only with chemotherapy have remained fertile, and to date all offspring have been healthy.

Secondary malignancy

Children who receive a BMT or stem cell transplant have a small risk of developing a second malignancy (cancer), particularly if total body irradiation was used in the preparative regimen. Since transplants are relatively new treatments for children and teens with cancer, the overall impact and long-term effects are not yet clear. Your doctor can explain your known risks given your disease and treatment.

The transplant center was very clear about all of the potential problems. That was good, for it prepared me. My attitude is watch for them, hope they don't happen, if they do, then live with them. JaNette has lost about 50 percent of her lung capacity, probably from the radiation. She has to do daily treatments to keep her lungs from tightening up. She still is on cyclosporin one-and-a-half years later and flares up with the GVHD rash periodically. She can no longer tolerate gamma globulin, so her counts go down sometimes and she gets pneumonia. I know that she may get cataracts, develop heart problems, and many other things. But she had an easy time with the transplant, she's a happy third-grader, she's alive, and we feel so, so very lucky.

CHAPTER 21

Death and Bereavement

*The loss of my son has illuminated for me the
true definition of love: the giving of oneself,
body and spirit, to another. His death, like
that of any child, is a story of withered hopes
and unfulfilled dreams. In this book I have
tried to capture a few remembered strains of
the brief, glad music of his life. These are all I
have of him now, and they comfort me
even as they break my heart.*

—Gordon Livingstone, MD
Only Spring

THE DEATH OF A CHILD CAUSES almost unendurable pain and anguish for loved
ones left behind. Death from cancer comes after months or years of debilitating treatment, emotional swings, and financial crises. The family begins the
years of grief already exhausted from the years of fighting cancer. It is truly
every parent's worst nightmare.

In this chapter, many parents share their innermost thoughts and feelings
about deciding to end treatment, dying at home or in the hospital, and grief.
It didn't matter whether the parents had recently lost their child, or whether
it had happened decades ago—tears flowed when talking about it. Because
family members and friends can be strong sources of support or casualties of
the grieving process, parents describe things that really helped them, and
they make suggestions on what to avoid. Grief has as many facets as there
are grieving parents, so what follows are the experiences of a few.

Making the decision to end treatment

For children who have had a series of relapses, medical caregivers and parents need to decide when to end active treatment and begin to work toward
making the child comfortable for his remaining days. This is an intensely

personal decision. Some families want to try every available treatment and exhaust all possible remedies. Others reach a point where they feel they have done all they can and they simply do not want their child to suffer any more. They hope for time to share memories, express love, and prepare for death.

> *After Christie came home from the transplant center, she started to perk up and feel a bit better. But she had pretty massive problems with graft-versus-host disease, infections, fragile bones, and a very weak heart. She had a stomach abscess that they thought was causing her vomiting and eating problems, so they decided to biopsy it. They came out and said they found a cluster of tumors on her ovary, which turned out to be malignant leukemic cells. In my rational mind, I knew it was time to stop. I could imagine stopping the treatment, but I just couldn't picture life without her.*

Dr. Arthur Ablin, Director Emeritus of Pediatric Clinical Oncology at the University of California, San Francisco, wrote in the Spring 1995 Candlelighters newsletter about the difficulties of deciding to end active treatment:

> *All too often, the decision to abandon the goal for cure and, reluctantly, accept the reality of inevitable death of a child is too painful and, therefore, never made. This paralyzing pain occurs with equal frequency, perhaps, for the family and the doctor. We of the medical profession have no equal in our ability to prolong dying. We have a powerful array of mechanical, electronic, pharmaceutical, and biotechnical interventions at our command. We can keep people dying for months and even years. Applying or withholding this armamentarium is an awesome responsibility and it requires infinite wisdom to know how to manage wisely and correctly. We can do great good by applying these tools correctly but can also do incalculable harm through over-utilization. Physicians and families alike must work together to avoid the possible pitfalls....When cure is beyond all of us, then the challenge is to make the rest of life as worthwhile and rich as possible. There is much to do for the terminally and critically ill child and his or her family. They have that right, we have the privilege, to be of service.*

Many children know when it is time to stop. In the Spring 1995 issue of the Candlelighters newsletter, Grace Monaco describes how her four-year-old daughter told her, "I don't think I can come home, Mommy! All my machinery is worn out, and I don't think they have any more parts."

When my six-year-old son Greg was in the hospital in intensive relapse treatment, he would repeat over and over again, "I want to go home." When he was finally well enough to come home for awhile, he kept saying, "I want to go home." In frustration, I said, "Greg, you are home, why do you keep saying that?" He looked up and quietly said, "I want to go to my heavenly home. I want to go to God." I said, "Honey, please don't say that," and, knowing how much we loved him, he replied, "Okay, Mom, I'll fight, I won't go." And he did fight hard for several more months. But he was way ahead of us in acceptance, he was at peace, and he knew it was time to let go.

· · · · ·

The history of Jody's battle with leukemia is long, and to me, marked with his resilience, strength, and incredibly strong spirit. He was diagnosed with ALL shortly after his second birthday. He relapsed just before he turned three, then not again until he was five and a half, seven months after he went off chemotherapy treatment. He underwent a bone marrow transplant approached with the good omen of having a perfect match with both his older sister and younger brother, and thrived until another relapse at age six and a half. Realistic hope for Jody's long-term survival was dashed at that time. Jody achieved another remission which lasted for several months, then experienced a bone marrow relapse. We realized that the disease was systemic, and all conventional means of treating the leukemia were, finally, hopeless.

While the doctor was ready to present us with medical options that Thursday afternoon, we already knew our decision. It was rational: Jody should go off all chemotherapy treatment. Jody's leukemia was clearly very resistant to chemotherapy drugs. It was ethical: With no chance of further good health and high-quality living, allowing death to come naturally was surely the best choice. It was humane: Jody would be treated for pain, and we would bring him home to die in familiar surroundings with his family. And it was sad: Jody's laughter wasn't to be heard again, he wasn't to feel good again, he was to become sicker and sicker and die. The unfathomable reality of life without Jody's presence was marching to meet us without reprieve.

When it is clear that death is inevitable, parents struggle with the thought of how to "tell" the ill child and siblings. All too often in our culture, children are perceived as having to be protected from death, as if this somehow makes their last days better. On the contrary, any pediatric nurse or social worker can tell you that children, often as young as four, know that they are dying. If the parents are trying to spare the child, an unhealthy situation develops. The child pretends everything is okay to please the parents, and the parents try to mask their deep grief with a false smile. Everyone loses.

This scenario is replayed on a daily basis at hospitals all over the country: scared, lonely children dying without being able to tell the people they love the most how they are feeling. This type of denial keeps children and parents alike from finishing up business—distributing belongings, telling each other how much they love one another, saying good-bye. It also strips parents of their ability to prepare their child for the journey from life to death. Children need to know what to expect. They need to know that they will be surrounded by those they love, and that their parents will be holding them, and they need to know what the family's beliefs are about what happens after death.

> *Jennifer contracted a respiratory fungal infection that resulted in her being hospitalized on a ventilator. She was given lots of morphine so that she wouldn't feel air hungry. She was alert off and on for a few days. We read to her and played tapes. After one week on the respirator she took a turn for the worse. She didn't respond to me after that. Her kidneys were ceasing to function, and she started to get puffy. Her liver was deteriorating, and her painful pancreatitis had come back. After ten days on the respirator, I couldn't bear it any longer. I lay down in her bed, took her in my arms, and kissed her at least 200 times. I talked to her for a long time, and told her that we would take care of her cats, and that I was sorry that she had to suffer so much, and how beautiful Heaven is. I told her to go be with Jesus, her Grandpa, and her dog. I also told her how much we all loved her and how proud we were of her. I got off the bed to change positions, and the nurse rushed in. Her heart had suddenly stopped the second I got up. I believe she heard me and just needed to know it was okay to go. She didn't want to leave until she knew her Mommy was ready.*

> *Because of her Christian upbringing, Jennifer knew all about Heaven. She had told me that she wasn't afraid to die, and this has been a great source of comfort to us. I believe that she was preparing for her death, even as we hoped for her remission. Before she went to the hospital, she spent all her money, gave away some of her possessions to her sisters, and said a final goodbye to her home, cats, teachers, and friends.*

· · · · ·

After Caitlin decided she wanted no more treatments, we brought her home. She asked me to give her clothes to the poor, and her special things to her brothers. She gave them the last of her money, saying she no longer had any use for it. She had already bought them Christmas presents for the coming Christmas and given them ahead of time. Her affairs were oh so in order. She asked my friend to make me laugh after she died. She told me that it wasn't dying she minded, because her friend who had already died had come in a dream and told her that heaven was a good place, but she did not want to leave her father and me. They were agonizing conversations, yet I am so glad that we were able to have them.

Supportive care

In the US, there is a very active and effective hospice system. Hospices ease the transition from hospital to home and provide support for the entire family. Hospice personnel ensure adequate pain control, allow the patient to control the last days or weeks of his life, and provide active bereavement support after death.

Usually, if the family wishes the child to die at home, a smooth transition occurs from the oncology ward to hospice care. Unfortunately, sometimes pediatric patients are not referred to hospice, and the parents are left to deal with their child's last days at home with no experienced help and no clear idea of what is to come. Before you leave the hospital, it is wise to find out the name of a contact person at the agency that will be taking over the home care of your child.

When Jody came home, he was assigned both a pediatric visiting nurse and a hospice nurse. On their first visits, I was handed a great deal of literature to read, including a whole notebook from hospice. I lacked both the desire and energy to read the literature and learn a whole new medical system—let alone two. I just wanted one phone number to call for help, with two or three consistent people to answer.

In actuality, the care we received was wonderful. The primary nurse would call, offer to visit if we wanted it, assess Jody's condition over the phone, handle any questions we had, and would ask if we wanted a call the next day. She would tell us who would be calling if she was not working at the appointed time. Interestingly, the service that I found most beneficial at that time was the nurse running interference for us with the doctor. The pain medications needed to be adjusted and changed at times; advice was needed about his intake, his mouth sores, and his hand and foot inflammation. As I, along with Jody, became quieter and more removed from outside activities, even the thought of calling the clinic and being made directly aware of the bustle and demands of that world was very unappealing.

If you have questions about hospice or what support is available, you can contact Children's Hospice International at (800) 24-CHILD.

Dying in the hospital

Some children die in the hospital suddenly, while others slowly decline for weeks or months. If your child is slowly dying, you may have choices about where your child will spend her last days. There are no right or wrong choices. Much depends on the number of people available to provide care at home, and how comfortable they are doing so. Many parents ask their child where they prefer to be. Some like to be with the nurses in a hospital environment, while others want to stay at home with brothers, sisters, friends, and pets. Parents, children, and staff need to talk honestly to decide on the appropriate place for the child, and then obtain the support (hospice, private nurses in the hospital, family members) needed to make the choice a comfortable reality. Remain flexible so that as the situation changes, options remain open.

Although we had been advised that it didn't look good for Greg, we were trying one last time to get him to transplant. He was sleeping quietly in his hospital bed. He had been complaining of severe head pain, and was on a low morphine drip. The afternoon nurse woke him to take vitals, and he chatted with her. He told me, "Mom, I'm going to go back to sleep, I love you." Two hours later the night nurse tried to wake him up to give him some medicine, and she couldn't wake him. They called the doctor in from his home, and he ordered a CAT scan. When the film came up to the floor, the doctor took me out in the hall and said, "He's not going to live through the night." He held up the film showing a massive cerebral infarction; Greg was bleeding into the brain. He quietly died less than an hour later. Family and staff were in total shock. Nobody expected it. But, looking back, Greg had decided that he had had enough, he was ready to go. I am grateful that he didn't die on a transplant floor in a strange city. We were able to call in friends and family, and we were surrounded and supported by the wonderful nurses whom we knew so intimately. I couldn't leave him until three nurses promised to stay with him and escort him to the morgue. They are still dear friends.

. . . . .

I felt bad for my daughter, because like any good child, she wanted permission, even to die. My husband had promised her that he would never give up. He kept on saying, "Fight. Fight. Don't give up, don't leave me. We'll do another transplant, we'll try different medicine. It's too early to give up." I looked at him and said, "She's not going anywhere until you tell her that it's okay." Then he told her, and she took her last breath. He still feels guilty to this day because of his promises. He just doesn't understand that it was time; that she needed to know that it was okay with us.

Parents of children who died in the hospital stressed the importance of clear communication. Parents need to be strong advocates for adequate pain control, and they need to clearly tell the staff how they would like things to be. For instance, in most hospitals, patients are routinely resuscitated using CPR and electric shocks to the heart (this is called a "code"). Parents need to discuss their wishes with the oncologist and ensure that an order of "no code" is put in the chart and on the child's door. Parents also should discuss whether they want nurses or doctors present when their child dies. Many families feel very close to the hospital staff and feel supported by their presence, while others prefer to have only family and close friends at the bedside. Advance planning helps to ensure that as death approaches, the family's wishes are understood and respected.

Dying at home

A child's death at home can be a peaceful or a frightening experience, depending on the preparation and support provided to the family.

It was scary to be taking Caitlin home to die, but she was so happy to be there. Her brother was fourteen years old, six-foot-three, and he carried her everywhere she wanted to go. We let her be in charge, whoever she wanted to see would be allowed in. My parents bought her a television and a VCR, each with remotes. She'd sit in bed with a remote in each hand, glad not to have to compete with her brothers, and say, "I got the power."

The night of her death her vomiting was too bad for us to stay at home. We brought her to the hospital in our car; we fixed a bed for her in the back with me and her aunt on the floor and her dad driving. She was taken directly to the pediatric floor, where they started an IV and gave her something to stop the vomiting. My husband and I were in such denial that we had packed enough for at least a two-week stay. No one on the staff had told us that her death was very near.

Ten days after her death we had to return to the pediatric floor with our son, and one of the doctors asked me if I had known Caitlin was dying when we came in with her. I said, "No, did you?" He replied, "Yes, because her breathing had changed." This new information hurt me deeply. It would have been good to have been told that her death was near and been given some choices about how we would like to handle it. I truly believe this could have been done quickly and as gently as all of her care had been given. I would like to have had the chance to hold Caitlin in my arms as she left our world, cradling her as closely as possible for the last time. Instead, I was hanging over the railing, holding her hand.

· · · · ·

We decided to bring Jody home to die for several reasons. First of all, the medical profession was offering no more realistic hope. Secondly, Jody was young enough and small enough to be easily held, carried, cared for by us. Thirdly, nothing violent or terrifying happened [at home], which made us seriously debate whether to go back in the hospital with him.

I saw many life values in a new way from the experience of Jody dying at home. What comes to my mind is a sunny, breezy afternoon, September 13. Only Jody and I were home. I held him outside under the plum tree for perhaps an hour and a half or longer. I couldn't support him well and read to him at the same time, so we didn't do anything. I spoke to him some, but mostly just held him quietly. I was aware as I looked up into the sky that my normal reaction on such a day would be to want to be hiking, biking, "doing" something. A surprise recognition burst and spread gently through my consciousness: I was exactly where I wanted to be and no doing of anything could mean as much as being there with Jody.

Jody's last day, September 16, was peaceful. A spiritual healer, whom Jody had known for two years, came and spent time with him. A massage therapist/healer/friend, who had visited him several times during the five

weeks he was home, gave him a long, gentle massage. My husband Tom
stayed home from teaching that day (by chance?). Jody lay in his arms or
on my lap most of the day. The visiting home nurse came by briefly,
offered to stay, but we preferred to be alone. I was holding Jody; Tom was
next to me holding his feet. Jody's breathing became labored and irregu-
lar. His eyes were unblinking long before he took his last breath, then a
heartbeat, then another, then silence.

Siblings

Whether your child is dying at home or in the hospital, if there are siblings they should be included in the family response. Being part of things, having jobs to do, helps brothers and sisters remain involved, contributing members of the family. Young children can answer the doorbell, go on errands, or make tapes to play for the sibling. Older children can help with meals, stay with the ill child to give parents a break, answer the phones, or help make funeral arrangements. These jobs should not be "make-work"—children should truly be helping. This allows them not only to clarify their role in the family, but helps them to prepare for the death as well as have an opportunity to say goodbye. These jobs help siblings feel themselves to be a useful part of the family rather than a forgotten and perhaps less loved brother or sister.

The Compassionate Friends (see Appendix C, *Resource Organizations*), has dozens of resources to help all members of the family.

The funeral

Funerals and related rituals (memorial services, wakes, burial, shiva) are important not only as a time to say good-bye and to begin to accept the reality of death, but they also provide an opportunity to recognize the relationships and impact that the child or teen has had on others. Funerals allow a gathering together to share memories and to show support for the remaining family members. A funeral is a tangible demonstration of love.

We had Greg's minister, godparents, and kindergarten teacher come
to our house to help plan the service. We did not want it to be scary,
because we wanted all of his young friends to come. They needed to say
good-bye, too, and above all, we wanted them to be comfortable. During

the service several songs were sung, and the minister didn't stand up at a pulpit. He stood on our level with his hand on Greg's casket, and talked about Greg's life. It was simple and good. On the way to the cemetery it rained lightly, and the sky was filled with three rainbows. Sadness and hope.

Children of all ages should be allowed to attend the funeral if they wish, but only after they have been prepared first about what to expect. They need an explanation of where they will be going (funeral, shiva, wake, memorial service, burial) and what these words mean. They need to know what type of room they are going to, if the casket will be there, if it will be open, if there will be flowers, who will be there, how the mourners will be acting, who will stay with the them, what they will be expected to say, and how long they will be there. All questions should be answered honestly and children's feelings respected.

Many siblings also benefit from giving one last gift to the departed, such as writing a private note and dropping it in the casket, or bringing some of their sister's favorite flowers to put in her hands. If you have any questions or concerns about what to tell the remaining children or whether they should attend the services or burial, read *How Do We Tell the Children? A Parent's Guide to Helping Children Understand and Cope when Someone Dies* by Dan Schaefer and Christine Lyons.

One of our pastors was a very close personal friend who stayed with us for the last three days in the hospital at Jesse's bedside. When she died, we were physically and emotionally weary; we just couldn't think. He and the other pastors planned the whole service and walked us through it.

There were hundreds of people there—Jesse had touched so many lives. The pastors had known Jesse her whole life and they loved her, truly loved her. They told personal stories; reminisced about the last hugs they had shared with her. They told the story of her faith and of her death, which comforted many of those who attended. Each family member walked up during the service and brought some of her favorite flowers.

We had given our children free rein to pick out the clothes that Jesse would be buried in. They made very thoughtful choices: her favorite, very comfortable pajamas with little tea cups on them, and her teddy bear. The service was very special: a celebration, a testament to her faith and ours.

Ministers, priests, and rabbis have a unique opportunity to provide support, love, and comfort to the grieving family and friends. They usually know the family well, and can evoke poignant memories of the deceased child or teen during the service. Members of the clergy often have excellent counseling skills, and can visit the family after the funeral to provide ongoing help during mourning.

The role of family and friends

Family members and friends can be a wellspring of deep comfort and solace during grieving. Some people seem to know just when a hug is necessary or when silence is most welcome. Unfortunately, in our society there are few guidelines for handling the social aspects of grief. Many well-meaning persons voice opinions concerning the time it is taking to "get over it" or question the parents' decision to not give away their child's clothing. Others do not know what to say, so they are silent, pretending that life's greatest catastrophe has not occurred. Many friends never again mention the deceased child's name, not knowing that this silence, as if the cherished child never existed, only adds to parents' pain. Holidays can become uncomfortable, as they bring sadness as well as joy.

In an attempt to alleviate these difficulties, bereaved parents helped compile the following lists of what helps, and what does not, in the hope that it may guide those family members and friends who deeply care, but just don't know how to help. These suggestions are offered with the understanding that what works for one person may not work for another. Try to use your knowledge of the bereaved family to choose options that you think will make them comfortable. If in doubt, ask them.

Things that help

The long lists of things that help from Chapter 5, *Family and Friends*, (e.g., keeping the household running, feeding the family, and helping with bills) are still appropriate here. The following lists are specific suggestions for grief.

Helpful things to say:

- I am so sorry.

- I cannot even imagine the pain that you are feeling, but I am thinking about you.

- I really care about you.

- You and your family are in my thoughts and prayers.

- We would like to hold a memorial service at the school for your son if you think that it would be appropriate.

- I will never forget John's sunny smile.

- I will never forget Jane's gentle way with children and animals.

Parents also offer a list of helpful things to do:

- Go to the funeral or memorial service.

  We were overwhelmed and touched by all of the people who came to the funeral. Even people that I had not seen in years—like some of my college professors—attended. Her oncologist and nurse drove 100 miles to be there.

- Show genuine concern and caring by listening.

  What has helped me the most is for people to just listen. Finding time to remember and reminisce is sometimes very difficult and painful, yet other times I feel much pride and happiness. Friends whose children also have cancer have been the greatest help to me during my daughter's illness and after her death.

- Help the siblings.

  When Jody was dying, his two well siblings, ages nine and four, presented concerns. I witnessed extremely tender moments, also flares of anger and hurt feelings. I assumed they felt neglected as I spent more and more time with Jody, just being his companion and caretaker. Christoph, four, wanted to be near, to talk, to play. His energetic pace and my feelings of guilt became nearly intolerable to me the last ten days or so. I decided to get the help of close friends and relatives to play with and lovingly attend to Christoph as many hours as possible when Tom was not home. Often they were in the same room with Jody and me.

  · · · · ·

  We had friends just call and say, "We will pick up Nick on Saturday and take him to Water World, then to our house for dinner. We were hoping he could spend the night. Will that be all right?" They did this many times, and it not only was fun for him, but it gave us a chance to be alone with each other and our grief.

The day my daughter died, a close friend—herself a bereaved parent—did something wonderful. She took over my three kids, and prepared them for the funeral. She sat down with them and they read a book entitled, "Today My Sister Died," and talked about it. She described in great detail what would happen at the funeral, and more importantly, she prepared them for some of the not-so-helpful comments that they would hear. So, when the first person said, "You're the big sister now," they had a response. She listened to them and prepared them and it truly helped them cope.

- Write the parents a note instead of sending just a preprinted sympathy card with your signature. Include special things you remember about their child or your feelings about their child. Letters, poems, or drawings from classmates and friends allow children to share their feelings with the family of the deceased, as well as provide poignant testimonials that the family will cherish.

- Talk about the child who has died. Parents forever carry in their heart cherished memories of their child and enjoy hearing others' favorite recollections.

Months after the funeral, we gathered family members and some close friends to share memories on tape. We did a lot of laughing as well as shed a few tears. But I will always cherish those tapes.

· · · · ·

I think most of all parents want their child to be remembered. It really comforts me to go to Greg's grave and find flowers, notes, or toys left by others.

- When parents express guilt over what they did or did not do, reassure them that they did everything they could. Remind them that they provided their child with the best medicine had to offer.

- Remember anniversaries. Call or send a card or flowers on the anniversary of the child's death.

- Respect the family's method of grieving.

- Give donations in the child's name to a favorite charity of the child or parents, for instance, the child's school library, Candlelighters, the local children's camp, the Leukemia Society, American Cancer Society, or hospice.

Every year we still get a card saying that Caitlin's occupational therapist donated money to Camp Goodtimes. It makes me feel good that she is remembered so fondly and that the money will help other kids with cancer and their brothers and sisters.

- Commemorate the child's life in some tangible way. Examples are planting trees, shrubs, or flowers, erecting a memorial or plaque, displaying a picture of the child.

One of our Candlelighters fathers was on the city council. He encouraged the city to dedicate a new park to the children who had never grown up. They agreed, and named it "Children's Memorial Park." A local nursery offered to sell trees at a special discount for families or groups to buy and dedicate to a deceased child. A kiosk was built at the front of the park with the location of each tree and the name of the child to whom it is dedicated. Our Candlelighters board bought a grove of trees and a plaque with the names of the more than seventy children from our organization who have died since 1978 when we were founded. Last summer, we reserved the park for a "memorial picnic" and remembered and celebrated our departed children.

- Be patient. Acute grief from the loss of a child lasts a long, long time. Expectations of a rapid recovery are unrealistic and hurtful to parents.

- Encourage follow-up from medical personnel.

Caitlin had a very kind, very gentle radiation oncologist. I went back to see her after Caitlin died; she said, "We were so happy when we saw the progress that Caitlin made, from a stretcher to sitting to talking and walking again; and then our hearts broke when she relapsed. I wept." It was so human and so wonderful for her to let me know that she cared.

· · · · ·

We have had several phone calls from Jesse's oncologist, surgeon, and primary nurse. They were so wonderful to our entire family for years, and we miss them. We also had one call from the grief counselor at Children's, but we never heard from her again. We named our cat after one of the doctors, and it had been a running joke at the hospital. He wrote my children a funny letter about that. But, after the death of my child, I realized that they were busy and we really didn't have a relationship left. It is hard, after such intimacy. But my job now is grieving, and their job is trying to save other kids.

Things that do not help

Please do not say to the parents:

- I know exactly how you feel.
- It's a blessing her suffering has ended.
- Thank goodness you are young enough to have another child.
- At least you have your other children.
- Be brave.
- Time will heal.
- God doesn't give anyone more than they can bear.
- It was God's will.
- He's in a better place now.
- God must have needed another angel.
- It's lucky this happened to someone as strong as you.
- Don't worry, in time you'll get over it.
- Why did you decide to cremate him?
- How is your marriage holding up?
- You need to be strong for your other children.

Please do not say to the siblings:

- You need to be strong for your mom and dad.
- Don't cry, it upsets your parents.
- You're the man of the house now.
- How does it feel to be the big sister?

Even if a bereaved parent has deep religious faith, it is often tested by their child's death. Parents are not comforted by well-meaning friends who assume faith is making the grief bearable; indeed, many parents find it to be infuriating. It's better to just say "I'm sorry."

In the months and years following the child's death, any of the following might not be appreciated:

- Don't you think it's time to get over it?
- It's been six months; it's time to put the past behind you.

- Life goes on.

- You need to get on with your life.

- You shouldn't be feeling that way.

- Don't you think you should give away all of his clothes?

- Don't cry.

- Don't be sad.

- Don't worry.

- Doesn't it bother you to have her pictures around?

- Please don't talk about Johnnie, it just stirs up all those memories.

- It's not good to just sit around, you need to get out and have some fun.

Don't let your own sense of helplessness keep you from reaching out. Pretending that nothing is wrong or being afraid to talk about the child who has died hurts grieving parents.

The following are suggestions from parents on what not to do:

- Don't remove anything that belonged to the child who died, unless specifically asked to by the parents.

    One family member took my son's toothbrush out of the bathroom and threw it away. I missed it immediately. She probably felt that she was doing me a favor, but it made me so angry. I needed to keep things. I have his hair from the second time it fell out, because he wanted to save it, and I've kept his teeth which had to be pulled during treatment. I just need to have those things, and I resent people who insist you must clear out a child's things. Parents should be able to keep things or get rid of them—whichever is comfortable—regardless of others' opinions.

- Don't offer advice.

    Christie's room is still her room. We still refer to it as Christie's room. People just don't have the right to say you shouldn't leave that room empty: it's not empty, it's full of her life. I know that they are not trying to hurt us. It just bothers them to see that room. Sometimes it is just a reminder of death; yet, there are times when being in there and surrounded by all her things brings us closer to her and her time with us.

- Don't say anything which in any way suggests that the child's medical care was inadequate. Parents already feel intense guilt over what should have been or could have been.

  I can't tell you how many people said things like "If only you had gone to a different treatment facility," or, "if only you had used this or that treatment." What people need most is support for what they are doing or did do.

- Don't look on the bright side or find silver linings.

  I became unexpectedly pregnant the month after my daughter died. I can't tell you how many people said things like "The circle of life is complete," or, "God is taking one and giving you another," or, "God is replacing her." She can never be replaced. It was horrible to hear those things, and I felt it was unfair to both the unborn baby and to my daughter who died.

- Don't come and pray over the child who is dying unless you have been asked.

  The mother of one of my son's friends called and asked to pray. I said okay, but was surprised when she showed up in person with a friend, and in a very loud voice, began exhorting the devil to leave. My son was only seven and very sick, and it was scary for him.

  ⋅ ⋅ ⋅ ⋅ ⋅

  The sister of my son's bus driver, whom I had never met, came by the hospital with a bit of holy cloth to put under my son's pillow. It required us to say a special prayer over and over again. We declined, but it was awkward. People need to respect the parents' beliefs, not push their own.

- Don't drop bereaved parents from the support group. Talk about your options; grief-stricken parents have enough silence in their lives.

  When my daughter was terminal, in really bad shape, I went to the support group. We had all bonded and were very close. I felt guilty because I really wanted to cry and was trying to hold it back because I didn't want to upset everybody else. All of a sudden, I felt like I was the alien, like you feel when your child is diagnosed. Here I was in a room full of people I loved, where I had felt safe. Now I was alone again, this time with no hopes of Christie's recovery. It was truly the end. I never felt more scared or alone.

. . . . .

Our support group was run by two social workers from the two local hospitals. The rule was that bereaved parents could come for one visit after the funeral to say good-bye and that was it. They were out. Two parents in our group lost their children, and we had a struggle with the social workers about changing the rules. They were adamant that the two groups of parents should not mingle, that it would be too upsetting for the parents of kids on treatment. My son was on treatment, and I felt strongly that we shouldn't abandon our friends in their time of greatest need and that we would all benefit from sharing their experiences and grief. In the end, we compromised by having the bereaved parent/s stay in the group for a year, then they would become a member of the new bereaved group. Both groups meet at the same time and place, so we socialize together after the meetings.

. . . . .

We don't have a support group or a bereaved group per se, we just have frequent gatherings. So we all see each other almost monthly, and there is no issue of losing your friends if your child dies.

- Don't make comments about the parents' strength.

  People would say things to me like "You're so strong," or, "I just couldn't live through what you have." It makes me want to scream. Do they mean I loved my child less than they love theirs because I have phys-ically survived?

Sibling grief

Siblings are sometimes called the "forgotten grievers" because attention is typically focused on the parents. Children and teens hesitate to express their own strong feelings in an attempt to prevent causing their parents additional distress. Indeed, adult family members and friends may advise the brothers and sisters to "be strong" for their parents or to "help your parents by being good." These requests place a terribly unfair burden on children who have already endured months or years of stress and family disruption. Siblings need continual reinforcement that each of them is an irreplaceable member of the family and that the entire family has suffered a loss. They have a right to mourn openly and in their own way.

The family requires such reorganization after a child's death, and there is nowhere to look for an example. Each person in the family constellation has different feelings and different ways of grieving; there is just no way to reconcile all of this when the supposed leaders of the group are totally out of it. Not to mention the fact that both my husband and I wanted more understanding and compassion from each other than we were possibly able to give.

Children express grief in many ways, including physically (changes in eating habits, toileting, sleeping, stomach aches); emotionally (regression to earlier behaviors, risk taking); through fear (of the dark, being away from parents); through guilt (said "I wish you would die" to sibling, and sibling died); and with emotional changes (tantrums, crying, sadness, anxiety, withdrawal, depression).

Many families pull apart because it is too painful to share their deep, but different feelings of grief. Some parents worry that if they start talking, they will "break down" in front of the children. But children who are excluded from the family's mourning may begin to feel alienated from the family. Here are suggestions from families to help pull together while mourning:

- Let the siblings go to the funeral. They have suffered a loss; they need to say good-bye; they need support for their grief just as much as adults.

    I grew up going to my relatives' funerals. Having those positive experiences really helped me deal with the loss of my son. There is nothing more natural than to take a child to the funeral, where they are part of families loving each other, crying together, and laughing at some of the memories. Too many people try to protect kids from death and it does them a great disservice.

- Children and teens experience the same feelings as adults. By sharing your own feelings, it can encourage them to identify their own. (For example, "I'm really feeling sad today. How do you feel?")

- Some families establish a regular meeting time to talk about their feelings. Both tears and laughter erupt when family members talk about funny or touching memories of the departed child. One family even had theme nights, such as trying to remember every practical joke he ever pulled, or things that he did that were not so nice (it's not necessary to remember the child as a saint).

- Jointly discuss how holidays and anniversaries should be observed. Some families hang a Christmas stocking every year for the departed child, while others merely mention her name during the blessing. Each family devises different ways to handle the child's birthday and the anniversary of her death.

- Encourage all family members to join a group such as a Candlelighters bereavement group or Compassionate Friends (see Appendix C).

Parental grief

There are as many ways to grieve as there are bereaved parents. There is no timetable, no appropriate progression from one stage to the next, no time when parents should "be over it." Losing a child is one of life's most horrific and painful events.

The death of a child shatters the very order of the universe—children are not supposed to die before their parents. It seems unnatural, incomprehensible. Losing a child entails mourning not only the child herself, but all of the hopes, dreams, wishes, fantasies, and needs relating to her. When you lose a child, you lose part of yourself, part of your future.

This book will not go through the numerous psychological descriptions of the grieving process. There are excellent reference books available, several of which are listed in Appendix D, *Books and Online Sites*. Here, the parents themselves will tell you about grief.

I truly think that it is the worst thing in the entire world. Nothing worse can happen than losing your child. There is no reprieve. None.

· · · · ·

I was having a very hard time grieving when a wonderful therapist that I was seeing said to me, "You are beating yourself up about grieving. Think about it: When you enter marriage, what are you called? A wife. When your spouse dies, what are you called? A widow. When you don't have a home and you are living on the street, what is the name for that? A homeless person. When you lose a child, what's it called, what's the name?" I said, "I don't know." She said, "Exactly. There is not even a word in our vocabulary. That's how terrible it is. It doesn't even have a name."

. . . . .

The biggest thing that I had to learn was just to cope with whatever I was feeling on that particular day. When I feel angry, I just need to let myself be angry. If I need to cry all day, I do. I still have plenty of those days. If someone calls me and wants to take me out to lunch to cheer me up, I have learned to say no when I'm not feeling like going out. I know that it hurts other people to see me cry, but I need to do that sometimes. I just miss her so much.

. . . . .

Every day when I walk out of my house I tell myself to grab the mask. I feel like I walk different than everybody and talk different than everybody and look different than everybody. It's the worst part of bereavement, the isolation caused by people who just don't know how to talk to you, when really all they need to do is listen and remember with you.

. . . . .

I found myself getting busier and busier, thinking that I could outrun the pain. I realized that I couldn't avoid the hurt; I just had to grit my teeth, cry, and live through it.

. . . . .

My daughter was our firefly; she lit the whole scene up. When she died, that spirit was gone, and there was just a hole left. We just didn't feel like a family anymore.

. . . . .

I feel jealous when I hear about people who have lost their fear when their child dies. I became more fearful, of everything. I am a very strong person, but I really picked up a lot of fear, and, four years later, I still have it.

. . . . .

I felt like our sick daughter was the center of our universe for so long, that now I need to start feeling some responsibility for my other kids whom I've been away from for so long, both physically and emotionally. I told my husband the other night that I didn't even know if I loved the three kids anymore. I cannot feel a thing. Pinch me, I don't feel it. Hug me, I don't feel it. I'm numb.

· · · · ·

It's hard to admit, but there was an element of relief when my daughter died. Not relief for myself, but for her. I was almost glad that she wouldn't face a life full of disabilities. That she wouldn't face the numerous orthopedic surgeries that would have been required to repair the damage from treatment. That she wouldn't face the pain of not having children of her own. I just felt relief that she would no longer feel any pain.

· · · · ·

At first we didn't feel like a family anymore. Now it's better, but it's still not the family that I was used to, that I want. I still feel like the mother of four children, not three. I find it very hard to answer when someone asks me how many children I have. I also can't sign cards like I used to, with all of our names, so now I just write "from the gang." I guess that's not fair to the boys, but I just can't bear to leave her name off.

· · · · ·

I had a visual image of our family of five. When Jody died, it became this physical square thing with only mom, dad, boy, girl, and it bothered me so much.

· · · · ·

I thought this morning of how I used to listen to Jesse breathe. Now I can't hear her breathe or laugh. I can't feel her arms around me. I remember missed kisses and late-night times. I ache. Heaven seems so far away.

· · · · ·

It seems that sometimes she is still so near that during conversations I can hear her comments or answers, and yet I fear the memories might fade and I so cherish the nearness. We each wear articles of her clothes or jewelry every day. One daughter is sleeping on the floor in our room, and the other two are sleeping in her bed.

· · · · ·

The worst times were the first two Christmases. We had to grit our teeth, put our heads down, and just get through it. We had to keep moving, never stop moving. I would have ignored it altogether if I didn't have another child.

· · · · ·

Birthdays are hard for us. Greg's birthday was June 10, and his brother's is June 9. So it's pretty hard to ignore. On Greg's birthday and the anniversary of his death, we blow up balloons, one for every year he would have been alive, write messages on them with markers, and release them at his grave.

· · · · ·

It seems like just about every holiday has some difficult memory attached to it now. He was diagnosed on Easter, and then relapsed the next year on Valentine's Day. I hate them both now. Christmas is always hard. And Halloween is tough because he so loved to dress up. I see all those little ones in their costumes and I'm just flooded with pain.

· · · · ·

I keep wondering if I should have put a stop to the bone marrow transplant because I had no peace about it. I felt such fear and dread about her platelets and liver. And what I feared happened. I still pray to have peace over making that choice. To have peace over giving a teenager the weight of deciding all that herself. I still feel so guilty and know I'd still be kissing her goodnight if we hadn't gone forward—and how I miss those kisses.

· · · · ·

I feel like Job 3:25-26:

What I feared has come upon me; What I dreaded has happened to me; I have no peace, no quietness; I have no rest but only turmoil.

· · · · ·

This evening my heart was so saddened. I paced up and down in front of the mantel, pausing to look at each picture of my daughter. Something that I cannot describe catches in my chest, and I can't breathe right. I look at her face and try to will it to life for a kiss and a touch, for softly spoken endearments at night. How we love all of our children, yet one missing leaves such a stabbing pain.

· · · · ·

I worry that missing one child so desperately pervades my very ability to be a good mom to my other three. I so wish to find joy again, to find things in life to smile about. I so wish my children could see me smile again. I pray that God will give me this thing, because it is beyond my finding in this world.

. . . . .

I had always heard that time heals all things. I was afraid of healing, because I didn't want to feel any farther away than I felt when he died. It's been seven years, and he still feels really close, a presence. But I still ache to touch his body so, that little back and fat tummy.

. . . . .

It's been two years, and I still feel a lot of rage. I walk down the street and see kids hanging out, smoking, doing drugs, being rude, wasting themselves, and I am filled with rage that my son—such a straight arrow, so decent, so strong—is gone.

. . . . .

I feel strongly that parents should seek out other parents who have lost children. Nobody else understands as well. Nobody else is as comfortable with it. We have our own sense of humor, and we often laugh hard about things that make other people uncomfortable.

. . . . .

It's hard when people I have just met ask, "How many children do you have?" In the beginning I always felt that I had to explain that I had two but one died. Now I just say one. I don't want their sympathy, I don't want their pity, but most of all I just don't want to have to explain. After two years or so, I started to feel uncomfortable giving out my life history and then having to deal with other people's discomfort. So now I just say one, and yet it still feels like I'm betraying him every time I do it.

. . . . .

That one-year rule, when you are supposed to start feeling better, I've found to be true. Not that any of the pain is lessened, but I realized that I had managed to live through a year of holidays and anniversaries. I knew it was possible to do it a second, then a third time. One year isn't magic, but it does prove to you that you can survive.

. . . . .

On the anniversary of Ryan's death we all went to the cemetery, and his girlfriend's parents planted a cherry tree at the foot of his grave. That was on a Sunday. I woke up on Monday feeling just as bad as I did the day before. All I could think was, "Oh hell, I have to go through that whole cycle again." The first year did not bring me any peace.

This morning was the four-year anniversary of my daughter's death. While I was at church I wanted to write in the intentions book, "I want my daughter back," but then I didn't because nobody would understand. I guess I'm pretty unreal in my thoughts a lot of the time.

From the minute I turn the calendar over to August, I'm on a knife edge. The twentieth of August just pulses on the calendar. I become depressed, spacey, I'm just in a very bad mood. I get sick a lot those first three weeks of August. But when it's over, I begin to relax and look forward to fall.

At church, we always sit with the same group of close friends who helped us through Jesse's illness and are helping us grieve her death. If they begin to sing a hymn that reminds one of us of Jesse, we all start to cry, and someone produces a box of tissues which gets passed down the aisles. People must wonder at the group that sobs through services. But it has helped me so much to have a community of grievers, it's been a very cleansing thing. It has spread out the tears.

I think parents need to know that it hurts like hell and they will feel crazy. But it is a normal craziness. If they talk to other bereaved parents, they will know that pain, guilt, rage, and craziness are how normal human beings feel when their child dies.

Bereaved parents are frequently reassured that "time will ease the pain." Most find that this is not the case. Time helps them understand the pain; the passage of time reassures them that they can adjust and they will survive. The acute pain becomes more quiescent, but still erupts when parents go to what would have been their child's graduation, hear their child's favorite song, or just go to the grocery store. Grief is a long, difficult journey, with many ups and downs. But, with time, parents report that laughter and joy do return. They acknowledge that life will never be the same, but it can be good again.

Looking back after many years

Four parents whose children died many years ago share their thoughts on grief and how they changed:

> My fifteen-year-old son was diagnosed with leukemia in 1962, and he lived until February 1963. He was tall, sturdy, wonderful. He inspired us all. Although it was very painful when he died, I truly felt that I had done all that I possibly could. I had four younger children, and I'd parceled myself out as best I could. Jennifer was born in October 1965, and my mother always said David had asked Our Lord to send her "to help me mend my heart."
>
> I felt that I had done my best for David, he was at peace, and I also needed peace. Our deep faith greatly helped. David was strong enough to tell me, "I don't want you to worry, Mom, God knows what he is doing." I also had a flock of kids who were hurting and needed me. So I threw myself back into life and carried on.
>
> There are many imponderables that I think of. What would David be like if he had survived? Would the lives of his brothers and sisters have been different if they had not lived through his illness and death? How would my marriage have been different? What would I be like if he was still alive? These thoughts serve no purpose; you just have to give yourself credit for doing your best and leave it at that. But at times when I feel desperate, I simply look up at the night sky, and I know that one of those stars is mine.

· · · · ·

> My daughter died in March 1971. That feeling that I had a hole in my solar plexus and was walking around with a heart literally broken in two lasted for over a year. I didn't go to a movie for four years, and it was very difficult for me to find pleasure in anything. But I have healed and am again a fully functional person. I have fun, tell jokes, play guitar, make speeches, and love my children.
>
> There are many things that I did to heal. I linked up with another bereaved parent. Our relationship worked wonderfully; we clung to each other and we helped each other survive the holidays. During my daughter's illness and a catastrophic diagnosis of mental illness in my other

daughter, I began to take too many tranquilizers. So I entered a 12-step program, and think that it literally saved my life. I gave up pills, quit smoking, rediscovered faith, and learned a new way to live.

At that time I also became very involved in a church, which was perhaps the most comforting, healing thing of all. I decided never to visit my daughter's grave. I know it comforts some people, but not me. I never thought for a second that she was there, just her bones. She, I will meet again. And finally, I had more children. I caution newly bereaved parents to think long and hard about the timing of the next child. But I look at my children, and I thank God for them.

Grieving was such hard work. For years her birthday was a black time for me, but that has faded away with the years. For a long time I felt like I was only going through the motions of life. But I just decided to act cheerful, force myself to go out, count my blessings, and reach out to people who were less fortunate than me. It worked.

· · · · ·

Life does go on after the death of someone you love... even if it's your child. It isn't always easy or fun or purposeful, but it's like anything else... life is what you make of it.

My son Cory died on Mother's Day 1985 after five and a half years of battling leukemia. When he left this existence a big part of my heart died with him. At first, the sky wasn't as blue as it once was... the mountains weren't as majestic... the ocean wasn't as magnificent, and yeah, it was hard to get out of bed and put one foot in front of the other. But I had to do it. I had to go on, not only for my daughter, but for myself, too.

One day the fog lifted, and I knew in what remained of my heart that my little boy wanted me to continue on loving life and all it has to offer. Before he died, Cory told me, "Don't weep for me, Mama. Just remember me and all the love I brought with me. I chose this life to be with you, but I was never meant to grow up."

I wrote a poem based on the things he said to bolster my courage and to help me cope with his leaving. I hope anyone who reads it can derive some comfort from it as well.

The Freedom of Flight

Don't weep for me when I have gone away...
Death is not like the end of the play.
It's like the freedom of the butterfly's first flight.
I won't really be gone—only from sight.
All the love that I brought with me from birth,
Will always be with you, while you are on earth.
I will be back in God's loving embrace...
So please wipe those tears of sadness off of your face.

Be happy I'm free from pain and despair,
Free like the birds that soar through the air.
I will always be with you, in everything you see...
Wherever you look it will remind you of me...
A flower in bloom, a new bud on a tree...
Or even a dandelion growing in the lawn,
But please don't think of me as gone.
A kid's game of soccer, a familiar song you will hear...
Comic books, cartoons, and "Danger," my favorite bear.
Don't think of death as the end of me.
It's just the beginning of my flight to be free.
Don't mourn my passing, because I will be
As one with God, all knowingness and light.
I will dance on the stars that shine in the night,
Or glide like a leaf caught in a gentle breeze...
Or soar on the wind with a bird's grace and ease...
Maybe hitch a ride on the tail of a kite,
All with the magic and freedom of a butterfly's first flight.

I will never stop missing him. Thankfully he gave me the strength to move forward. Cory loved life so much and fought so courageously during the short time he was here, it would be an insult to his memory if I didn't cling to and enjoy life as tenaciously as he taught me to. The memories of the fun we had, the love we shared, and the vision of him dancing on the stars sustain me.

· · · · ·

The old adage that "time heals" is a myth. You need to choose to heal and then find out how to help yourself. As I look back on our journey, our first instinct was to huddle as a family; to bask in what was left. We were hurting together; we loved him; we missed him; we needed to celebrate who he was. We intuitively knew that we were going to make it, we just didn't know how.

When Donnie died thirteen years ago, we didn't know much about grief. There wasn't as much written about it then as there is now. But we were committed to healing individually and as a family. One of the important things that we did for one another was to give each other lots of space. My husband and I knew the distancing was necessary but temporary. We were on a teeter-totter. We each had a different schedule, a different way of handling pain. He allowed me my "craziness," and I respected his silence. I found that it helped me to wallow in it, to feel it all, to cry. I've grieved clean.

If you have children, learn about how kids grieve. They revisit their grief at each developmental stage. Keep the door open so that they can talk about it. After Donny's death, I found that I just had to be with kids. I volunteered at the school, and followed all of his friends until they graduated from high school. A friend carried his cap and gown, and they made a speech about how a very important person was missing from the ceremony. I cried, but it was good.

I think it is very important for people to choose to feel. If you attend a grief support group or Compassionate Friends, or read about the grief process, you will quickly realize that your feelings are normal and that each person goes through grief differently. Another good reason to go to a group is that other people can give voice to your feelings when you just don't have any words. In the beginning you are just a ball of pain. You learn that every person feels that way; that it is normal, human. Many people come to group and never speak, but they are comforted. I found it was far better for me to be in the same room with real people who had walked down the same road, rather than just to read about it in books. Feel the pain and you will heal.

I just wish that I had armfuls of time.

—Four-year-old with cancer
Armfuls of Time

Photographs of Our Children

Children during and after treatment

YOUR CHILD WILL PROBABLY be changed in appearance or attitude by the drugs that he takes for treatment. However, when treatment ends, your child's appearance, energy, and personality will recover. It's hard to tell yourself "this too will pass" when you are looking at a child who has lost his hair, is swollen from prednisone, and has frequent rages. The parents of the children below make these photos public so that you can more fully believe that you will "get your child back" after chemotherapy is over.

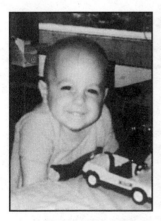 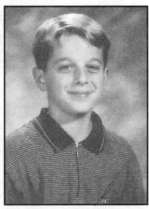

JEREMY

Kim

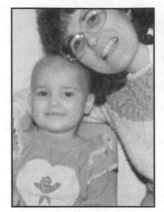 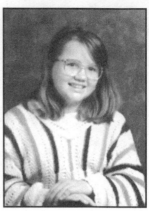

Judd

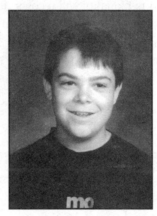

Kristin

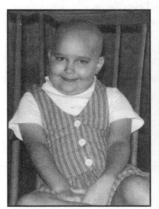 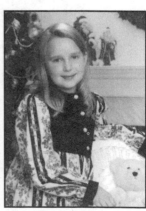

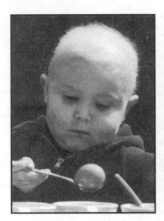 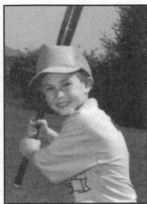 BRENT

JUSTIN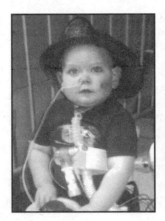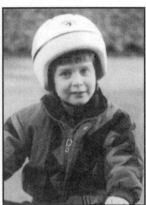

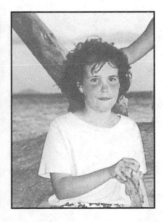 KATY

JOHN

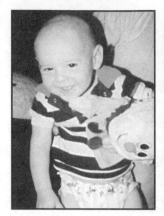 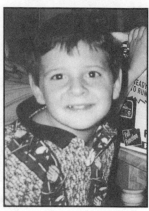

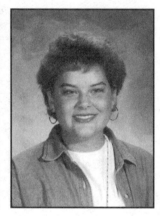 LESLEE

MEAGAN

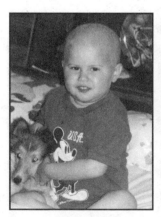 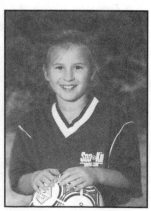

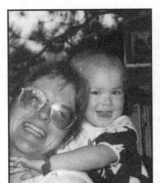
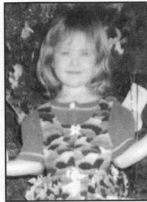

CARRIE BETH

GINA

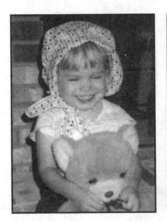
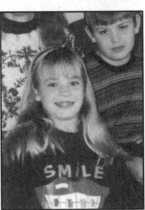

NAOMI

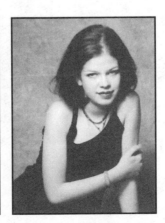

In Memoriam

Despite major advances in treatment, some children still die from childhood leukemia. Some of the grieving parents who helped create this book wished to share a photograph of their beloved child. In loving memory, we dedicate this page to them—departed but not forgotten.

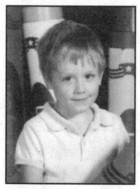

GREGORY SMITH

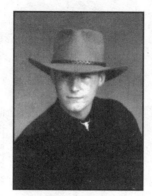

RYAN REDDELL

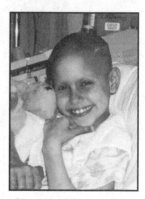

CHRISTIE SIMONETTI

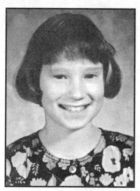

CAITLIN
McCARTHY-KING

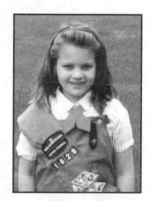

JENNIFER
HAWKINSON

Blood Counts and What They Mean

KEEPING TRACK OF THEIR CHILD'S BLOOD counts becomes a way of life for parents of children with leukemia. Unfortunately, misunderstandings about the implications of certain changes in blood values can cause unnecessary worry and fear. To help prevent these concerns, and to better enable parents to help spot trends in the blood values of their child, this appendix explains the blood counts of healthy children, the blood counts of children being treated for leukemia, and what each blood value means.

Values for healthy children

Each laboratory and lab handbook has slightly different reference values for each blood cell, so your lab sheets may differ slightly from those that appear later in this appendix (see figure B-1). There is also variation in values for children of different ages. For instance, in children from newborn to four years old, granulocytes are lower and lymphocytes higher than the numbers listed below. Geographic location affects reference ranges as well. The following table lists blood count values for healthy children:

Blood Count Type	Values for Healthy Children
Hemoglobin (Hgb.)	11.5–13.5 g/100ml.
Hematocrit	34–40%
Red blood count	3.9–5.3 m/cm or 3.9-5.3 x 10^{12}/L
Platelets	160,000–500,000 mm^3
White blood count	5,000–10,000 mm^3 or 5–10 K/ul
WBC differential:	
Segmented neutrophils	50–70%
Band neutrophils	1–3%
Basophils	0.5–1%
Eosinophils	1–4%
Lymphocytes	12–46%
Monocytes	2–10%
Bilirubin (total)	0.3–1.3 mg./dl
Direct (conjugated)	0.1–0.4 mg./dl

Blood Count Type	Values for Healthy Children
Indirect (unconjugated)	0.2–0.18 mg./dl
AST (SGOT)	0–36 IU./l.
ALT (SGPT)	0–48 IU./l.

Values for children on chemotherapy

Blood counts of children being treated for leukemia fluctuate wildly. White blood cell counts can go down to zero or be above normal. Red cell counts go down periodically during treatment, necessitating transfusions of packed red cells. Platelet levels also decrease, requiring platelet transfusions. Absolute neutrophil counts (ANC) are closely watched as they give the physician an idea of the child's ability to fight infection. ANCs vary from zero to in the thousands.

Oncologists consider all of the blood values to get the total picture of the child's reaction to illness, chemotherapy, radiation, or infection. Trends are more important than any single value. For instance, if the values were 5.0, 4.7, 4.9, then the second result was insignificant. If, on the other hand, the values were 5.0, 4.7, 4.6, then there is a decrease in the cell line.

The explanations below will describe each blood value. If you have any questions about your child's blood counts, ask your child's doctor for a clear explanation. Especially in the beginning, many parents agonize over whether the rapid changes in blood counts (often requiring transfusions, changes in chemo dosages, or whether the child can have visitors) are normal or expected. The only way to address your worries and prevent them from escalating is to ask what the changes mean.

What do these blood values mean?

The following sections explain each line of the above list of blood values. See Figure B-1 to get an idea of the different ways these values might be displayed on the actual lab reports prepared for your child.

Hemoglobin (Hgb)

Red cells contain hemoglobin, the molecules that carry oxygen and carbon dioxide in the blood. Measuring hemoglobin gives an exact picture of the ability of the blood to carry oxygen. Children may have low hemoglobin levels at diagnosis and during the intensive parts of treatment. This is because both cancer and chemotherapy decrease the bone marrow's ability to produce new red cells. During maintenance, your child's hemoglobin level will be higher than during induction and consolidation, but still lower than that of a healthy child. Signs and symptoms of anemia—pallor, shortness of breath, fatigue—may start to show if the hemoglobin gets very low.

Hematocrit (HCT); also called PCV (packed cell volume)

The purpose of this test is to determine the ratio of plasma (clear liquid part of blood) to red cells in the blood. Blood is drawn from a vein, finger prick, or from a Hickman or Port-a-cath and is spun in a centrifuge to separate the red cells from the

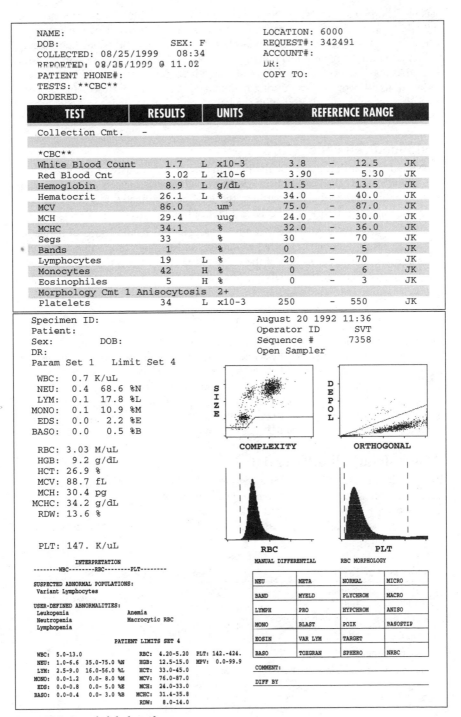

NAME:
DOB: SEX: F
COLLECTED: 08/25/1999   08:34
REPORTED: 08/25/1999 @ 11.02
PATIENT PHONE#:
TESTS: **CBC**
ORDERED:

LOCATION: 6000
REQUEST#: 342491
ACCOUNT#:
DR:
COPY TO:

TEST	RESULTS		UNITS	REFERENCE RANGE			
Collection Cmt.	–						
*CBC**							
White Blood Count	1.7	L	x10-3	3.8	–	12.5	JK
Red Blood Cnt	3.02	L	x10-6	3.90	–	5.30	JK
Hemoglobin	8.9	L	g/dL	11.5	–	13.5	JK
Hematocrit	26.1	L	%	34.0	–	40.0	JK
MCV	86.0		um³	75.0	–	87.0	JK
MCH	29.4		uug	24.0	–	30.0	JK
MCHC	34.1		%	32.0	–	36.0	JK
Segs	33		%	30	–	70	JK
Bands	1		%	0	–	5	JK
Lymphocytes	19	L	%	20	–	70	JK
Monocytes	42	H	%	0	–	6	JK
Eosinophiles	5	H	%	0	–	3	JK
Morphology Cmt 1 Anisocytosis	2+						
Platelets	34	L	x10-3	250	–	550	JK

Specimen ID:
Patient:
Sex: DOB:
DR:
Param Set 1   Limit Set 4

WBC: 0.7 K/uL
NEU: 0.4   68.6 %N
LYM: 0.1   17.8 %L
MONO: 0.1   10.9 %M
EDS: 0.0   2.2 %E
BASO: 0.0   0.5 %B

RBC: 3.03 M/uL
HGB: 9.2 g/dL
HCT: 26.9 %
MCV: 88.7 fL
MCH: 30.4 pg
MCHC: 34.2 g/dL
RDW: 13.6 %

PLT: 147. K/uL

August 20 1992 11:36
Operator ID   SVT
Sequence #   7358
Open Sampler

COMPLEXITY   ORTHOGONAL

RBC   PLT

INTERPRETATION
--------WBC--------RBC--------PLT--------

SUSPECTED ABNORMAL POPULATIONS:
Variant Lymphocytes

USER-DEFINED ABNORMALITIES:
Leukopenia   Anemia
Neutropenia   Macrocytic RBC
Lymphopenia

PATIENT LIMITS SET 4

WBC: 5.0-13.0   RBC: 4.20-5.20   PLT: 142.-424.
NEU: 1.0-6.6 35.0-75.0 %N   HGB: 12.5-15.0   MPV: 0.0-99.9
LYM: 2.5-9.0 16.0-56.0 %L   HCT: 33.0-45.0
MONO: 0.0-1.2   0.0- 8.0 %M   MCV: 76.0-87.0
EDS: 0.0-0.8   0.0- 5.0 %E   MCH: 24.0-33.0
BASO: 0.0-0.4   0.0- 3.0 %B   MCHC: 31.4-35.8
                              RDW: 8.0-14.0

MANUAL DIFFERENTIAL   RBC MORPHOLOGY

NEU	META	NORMAL	MICRO
BAND	MYELD	PLYCHROM	MACRO
LYMPH	PRO	HYPCHROM	ANISO
MONO	BLAST	POIK	BASOSTIP
EOSIN	VAR LYM	TARGET	
BASO	TOXGRAN	SPHERO	NRBC

COMMENT:

DIFF BY

Figure B-1. Sample lab data sheets

plasma. The hematocrit is the percentage of cells in the blood; for instance, if the child has a hematocrit of 30 percent, it means that 30 percent of the amount of blood drawn was cells and the rest was plasma. When the child is on chemotherapy, the bone marrow does not make many red cells, and the hematocrit will go down. The child may be given a transfusion of packed red cells when the hematocrit goes below 18 to 19 percent. Even during maintenance the bone marrow is partially suppressed, so the hematocrit is often in the low to mid-thirties. This results in less oxygen being carried in the blood, and your child may have less energy.

Red blood cell count (RBC)

Red blood cells are produced by the bone marrow continuously in healthy children and adults. These cells contain hemoglobin, which carries oxygen and carbon dioxide throughout the body. To determine the RBC, an automated electronic device is used to count the number of red cells in a liter of blood.

Red cell indices (MCV, MCH, MCHC) are mathematical relationships of hematocrit to red cell count, hemoglobin to red cell count, and hemoglobin to hematocrit. This gives a mathematical expression of the degree of change in shape found in red cells. The higher the number (low teens are fine), the more distorted the red cell population is.

White blood cell count (WBC)

The total white blood cell count determines the body's ability to fight infection. Treatment for cancer kills healthy white cells as well as diseased ones. Parents need to expect prolonged periods of low white counts during treatment. To determine the WBC, an automated electronic device counts the number of white cells in a liter of blood. If your lab sheet uses K/uL instead of mm^3, multiply by 1000 to get the value in mm^3. For example, on the lab sheet in Figure B-1, the total WBC is 0.7 K/uL. Therefore, $0.7 \times 1000 = 700$ mm^3.

White blood cell differential

When a child has blood drawn for a complete blood count (CBC), one section of the lab report will state the total white blood cell count and a "differential." This means that each type of white blood cell will be listed as a percentage of the total. For example, if the total WBC count is 1500 mm^3, the differential might appear as in the following table:

White Blood Cell Type	Percentage of Total WBC
Segmented neutrophils (also called polys or segs)	49%
Band neutrophils (also called bands)	1%
Basophils (also called basos)	1%
Eosinophils (also called eos)	1%
Lymphocytes (also called lymphs)	38%
Monocytes (also called monos)	10%

You might also see cells called metamyelocytes, myelocytes, promyelocytes, and myeloblasts listed. These are immature white cells usually only found in the bone marrow. They may be seen in the blood during recovery from low counts.

The differential is obtained by microscopic analysis of a blood sample on a slide.

Absolute neutrophil count (ANC)

The absolute neutrophil count (also called the absolute granulocyte count or AGC) is a measure of the body's ability to withstand infection. Generally, an ANC above 1,000 means that the child's infection-fighting ability is near normal.

To calculate the ANC, add the percentages of neutrophils (both segmented and band) and multiply by the total WBC. Using the example above, the ANC is 49 percent + 1 percent = 50 percent. 50 percent of 1,500 (.50 × 1,500) = 750. The ANC is 750.

Platelet count

Platelets are necessary to repair the body and to stop bleeding through the formation of clots. Because platelets are produced by the bone marrow, platelet counts decrease when a child is on chemotherapy. Signs of lowering platelet counts are small vessel bleeding such as bruises, gum bleeding, or nosebleeding. Platelet transfusions may be given when the count is very low (between 10,000–20,000 mm^3) or when there is bleeding. Platelets are counted by passing a blood sample through an electronic device.

Approximately one-third of all platelets spend a great deal of time in the spleen. Any splenic dysfunction such as enlargement may cause the counts to drop precipitously. If the spleen is removed, platelet counts may skyrocket. This transient thrombocytosis (elevated platelet count) will abate within a month.

Alanine aminotransferase (ALT)

ALT is also called SGPT (serum glutamic pyruvic transaminase). When doctors talk about "liver functions," they are usually referring to tests on blood samples that measure liver damage. If the chemotherapy is proving to be toxic to your child's liver, the damaged liver cells release an enzyme called ALT into the blood serum. ALT levels can go up in the hundreds or even thousands in some children on chemotherapy. Each institution and protocol has different points at which they decrease dosages or stop chemotherapy to allow the child's liver to recover. If you notice a change in your child's ALT, ask for an explanation and plan of action (for example, "John's ALT is now 450, what is your plan to reduce or stop the chemotherapy to allow his liver to recover?")

> I was very interested in my daughter's blood counts throughout her treatment. I also tried to get information without making people mad. If I asked a question and received an unsatisfactory answer, I would reply in a nice way, "I am worrying about this and would really appreciate a few minutes of your time to explain it to me." I found the attendings and clinic director to be the most willing to provide explanations. If you get a ridiculous reply (once a fellow patted me on the head and said, "It's our job to think about these things, not yours"), go find someone else to ask.

Aspartate aminotransferase (AST); also called serum glutamic oxaloacetic transaminase (SGOT)

SGOT is an enzyme present in high concentrations in tissues with high metabolic activity, including the liver. Severely damaged or killed cells release SGOT into the blood. The amount of SGOT in the blood is directly related to the amount of tissue damage. Therefore, if your child's liver is being damaged by the chemotherapy, the SGOT can rise into the thousands. In addition, there are other causes for an elevated SGOT, such as viral infections, reaction to an anesthetic, and many others. If your child's level jumps unexpectedly, ask the physician for an explanation and a plan of action.

Bilirubin

The body converts hemoglobin released from damaged red cells into bilirubin. The liver removes the bilirubin from the blood, and excretes it into the bile, which is released into the small intestine to aid digestion.

Normally there is only a small amount of bilirubin in the bloodstream. Bilirubin rises if there is excessive red blood cell destruction or if the liver is unable to excrete the normal amount of bilirubin produced.

There are two types of bilirubin: indirect (also called unconjugated), and direct (also called conjugated). An increase in indirect (unconjugated) is seen when destruction of red cells has occurred, while an increase of direct (conjugated) is seen when there is a dysfunction or blockage of the liver.

If excessive amounts of bilirubin are present in the body, the bilirubin seeps into the tissues, producing a yellow color called jaundice.

If your child's total bilirubin rises above normal levels, ask the physician for an explanation and plan of action.

Your child's pattern

Each child develops a unique pattern of blood counts during treatment, and observant parents can help track these changes. This appendix contains a record-keeping sheet that you can use to record your child's blood values (see Figure B-2). If there is a change in the pattern, show it to your child's doctor and ask for an explanation. Doctors consider all of the laboratory results to decide how to proceed, but they should be willing to explain their plan of action to you so that you better understand what is happening and worry less.

If your child is participating in a clinical trial and you have obtained the entire clinical trial protocol (discussed in Chapter 4, *Clinical Trials*), it will contain a section that clearly outlines the actions that should be taken by the oncologist if certain changes in blood counts occur. For example, my daughter's protocol has an extensive section which lists each drug and when the dosage should be modified. For vincristine it states:

Vincristine
　　1.5 mg/m^2 (2 mg maximum) IV push weekly × 4 doses days 0,7,14,21.
Seizures
　　Hold one dose, then reinstitute.

Blood Counts								
Date:								
WBC ref. range ———								
Neutrophils (polys or segs)								
Neutrophils (bands)								
ANC (polys + bands, multiplied by WBC)								
Hematocrit ref. range ———								
Platelets ref. range ———								
Chemistries								
Chemotherapy								
Side Effects								

Figure B-2. Example of a record-keeping sheet

Severe foot drop, paresis, or ilius

> Hold dose(s): when symptoms abate, resume at 1.0 mg/m^2; escalate to full dose as tolerated.

Jaw pain

> Treat with analgesics; do not modify vincristine dose.

Withhold if total bilirubin >1.9 mg/dL. Administer 1/2 dose if total bilirubin 1.5–1.9 mg/dL.

Resources

If you would like more information on laboratory diagnostic tests, two good books that can often be found in the reference section of your local library are:

Everything You Need to Know About Medical Tests, written by 70 doctors and medical experts. Springhouse, PA: Springhouse Corporation, 1996.

Sobel, David, MD, and Tom Ferguson, MD. *The People's Book of Medical Tests.* New York: Summit Books, 1985.

Resource Organizations

Service organizations

Candlelighters Childhood Cancer Foundation
7910 Woodmont Avenue, Suite 460
Bethesda, MD 20814
(800) 366-CCCF
Fax: (301) 718-2686
http://www.candlelighters.org
Email: *info@candlelighters.org*

Founded in 1970, Candlelighters has more than 40,000 members worldwide. Some of the free services provided by Candlelighters are a yearly bibliography and resource guide, quarterly newsletter, youth newsletter, and various handbooks to help families of children with cancer.

Candlelighters Childhood Cancer Foundation Canada
National Office
55 Eglinton Avenue E, Suite 401
Toronto, ON Canada M4P 1G8
(800) 363-1062 (Canada only)
(416) 489-6440
Fax: (416) 489-9812
http://www.candlelighters.ca/
Email: *staff@candlelighters.ca*

Provides the same services as US Candlelighters.

American Cancer Society
1599 Clifton Road NE
Atlanta, GA 30329-4251
(800) ACS-2345
http://www.cancer.org

Has a national network of employees and volunteers who implement research, education, and patient service programs. Although programs differ according to state and province, some widely available programs are patient-to-patient visitation, transportation to appointments, housing near treatment centers, equipment and supplies, support groups, literature on a large variety of topics, summer camps for children with cancer, research and educational programs.

Canadian Cancer Society
565 W. 10th Avenue
Vancouver, BC Canada V5Z 4J4
(604) 872-4400
http://www.bc.cancer.ca/

Provides same services as the US Cancer Society.

Childhood Cancer Ombudsman Program
P.O. Box 595
Burgess, VA 22432
Fax: (804) 580-2502
Email: *gpmonaco@rivnet.net*

This free service helps children with cancer and their families who are experiencing difficulties in gaining access to appropriate education, medical care, healthcare cost coverage, and meaningful employment. Services include medical library searches, a second opinion program, and help resolving problems with insurance or discrimination.

Leukemia Society of America
600 Third Avenue, 4th Floor
New York, NY 10016
(212) 573-8484 or 1-800-955-4LSA
Fax: (212) 856-9686
http://www.leukemia.org

This organization provides financial assistance to families (up to $750/year for outpatients), funds research, sponsors a national program in education for the public and the medical community, and publishes a large number of booklets on cancer-related topics.

Organizations that provide information

The Academy for Guided Imagery
P.O. Box 2070
Mill Valley, CA 94942
(800) 726-2070

This organization can assist in locating a professional in your area to help your child learn visualization.

The American Society of Clinical Hypnosis
33 West Grand Avenue, Suite 402
Chicago, IL 60610
(847) 297-3317

A membership organization for doctors, psychologists, and dentists who use hypnosis in their practices. For referral to a local member, send request with S.A.S.E.

The Disability Rights Education and Defense Fund
2212 Sixth Street
Berkeley, CA 94710
(800) 466-4232

Answers questions about the Americans with Disabilities Act, explains how to file a complaint, and provides dispute resolution.

Job Accommodation Network (JAN)
West Virginia University
918 Chestnut Ridge Road, Suite 1
P.O. Box 6080
Morgantown, WV 26516
(800) 526-7234 or (800) ADA-WORK

An international consulting service that provides free information about how employers can accommodate people with disabilities. The service also provides information on the Americans with Disabilities Act (ADA). In Canada, JANCANA is a service of Human Resources Development Canada and the Canadian Council on Rehabilitation and Work.

National Cancer Institute (NCI)
Cancer Information Service
Building 31, Room 10A16
9000 Rockville Pike
Bethesda, MD 20892
(800) 4-CANCER
Fax: (301) 231-6941
CANCERFAX: (301) 402-5874
http://www.nci.nih.gov

Provides a nationwide telephone service for people with cancer, their families and friends, and the professionals who treat them. The NCI answers questions and send out informational booklets on a variety of cancer-related topics. CANCERFAX provides treatment guidelines, with current data on prognosis, staging, and histologic classifications. To use CANCERFAX you need a fax machine with a telephone set to touch-tone dialing. A recording will give you instructions.

National Childhood Cancer Foundation
440 E. Huntington Drive
P.O. Box 60012
Arcadia, CA 91066-6012
(626) 447-1674
Fax: (626) 447-6359
http://www.nccf.org

Supports pediatric cancer treatment and research in more than 115 hospitals in North America and Australia. Their newsletter, *Childhood Cancerline*, provides information on new treatments and psychosocial support.

National Coalition for Cancer Survivorship
1010 Wayne Avenue
Silver Spring, MD 20910
(301) 650-8868
Fax: (301) 565-9670

An organization that addresses the needs of long-term cancer survivors and advocates for change in healthcare to maximize survivor's access to optimal treatment and support. Extensive publications list.

National Information Center for Children and Youth with Disabilities (NICHY)
P.O. Box 1492
Washington, DC 20013
(800) 695-0285

A clearinghouse that provides free pamphlets and information on disabilities and the rights of disabled children and their parents.

PDQ (Physician Data Query)
(800) 4-CANCER
http://cancernet.nci.nih.gov

PDQ is the National Cancer Institute's computerized listing of accurate and up-to-date information for patients and health professionals about cancer treatments, research studies and clinical trials.

Starbright Foundation
1990 S. Bundy Drive, Suite 100
Los Angeles, CA 90025
(310) 442-1560
Fax: (310) 442-1568
http://www.starbright.org

Co-chaired by Steven Spielberg and Gen. Norman Schwarzkopf, Starbright Foundation is best known for its online network of interactive, virtual-reality playgrounds where seriously ill, hospitalized children across the country meet, talk, and play to help cope with the pain, stress, and anxiety of treatment. For teens who are ill, "Videos with Attitude" offer guidance from peers who have "been there." The videos are free to families and come with a parent guide.

Organizations that provide emotional support

Association for the Care of Children's Health (ACCH)
7910 Woodmont Avenue, Suite 300
Bethesda, MD 20814
(609) 224-1742

A nonprofit, multidisciplinary organization of health professionals and parents that promotes psychosocial health of children and their parents. It sponsors conferences, provides advocacy resources, and publishes journals, newsletters, and booklets.

Cancer Care, Inc.
1180 Avenue of the Americas
New York, NY 10036
(800) 813-4673
(212) 302-2400
Fax: (212) 719-0263
http://www.cancercare.org

A national, nonprofit organization that provides referrals, one-on-one counseling, specialized support groups, and educational programs.

Cancer Cured Kids
P.O. Box 189
Old Westbury, NY 11568
(800) CCK-7525
(516) 484-8160
Fax: (516) 484-8160 (call first)

An organization dedicated to the quality of life of kids who have survived cancer. They supply information about educational and psychosocial needs.

Center for Attitudinal Healing
33 Buchanan Drive
Sausalito, CA 94965
(415) 331-6161

A nonprofit, nonsectarian group that sponsors local and national workshops for children with catastrophic or life-threatening diseases and their siblings. The center uses music and art in a supportive program to help children ages six to sixteen share their feelings about their situation. They have also published several excellent books.

Chai Lifeline/Camp Simcha
National Office
48 West 25th Street, 6th Floor
New York, NY 10010
(212) 255-1160 or (800) 343-2527
Fax: (212) 255-1495

A national, nonprofit Jewish organization that provides support service programs to children and their families in crisis, including medical referrals, support groups, visits to hospitalized and housebound children, financial aid, transportation, a kosher camp for kids with cancer, and more.

ChemoCare
231 North Avenue West
Westfield, NJ 07090
(800) 55-CHEMO (outside New Jersey)
(908) 233-1103 (within New Jersey)
Fax: (908) 233-0228

Provides one-to-one emotional support to cancer patients and their families undergoing chemotherapy, radiation, and/or surgery, from trained and certified volunteers who have undergone the treatments themselves.

Child Life Council
11820 Parklawn Drive, Suite 202
Rockville, MD 20852
(301) 881-7090
Fax: (301) 881-7092

Promotes the well-being of children and families in healthcare settings by supporting the development and practice of the child life profession with training conferences, publications, and information.

Children's Hopes and Dreams Foundation
280 Route 46
Dover, NJ 07801
(973) 361-7348

This organization operates a free, worldwide pen-pal program for children ages five to seventeen with disabilities, chronic illnesses, or life-threatening illnesses.

Coping Magazine
P.O. Box 682268
Franklin, TN 37068
(615) 790-2400
Fax: (615) 794-0179

A bimonthly publication for people whose lives have been touched by cancer.

Famous Phone Friends
9109 Sawyer Street
Los Angeles, CA 90035
(310) 204-5683

Links children who are confined to the hospital or home due to injury or illness by telephone with entertainers and athletes. Referral by physician, nurse, hospital volunteer, or treatment center social worker.

Friends Network
P.O. Box 4545
Santa Barbara, CA 93140
Attention: Kenon Neal

A national, nonprofit organization that distributes *The Funletter,* a full-color activities newsletter, to children with cancer.

Love Letters, Inc.
P.O. Box 416875
Chicago, IL 60641
(630) 620-1970

This free service, started by a mother whose son died of cancer, is run by a group of volunteers who send letters, cards, and gifts to catastrophically ill children. This is not a pen-pal organization. Confidentiality is guaranteed.

National Children's Cancer Society

(800) 532-6459

http://www.children-cancer.com

Helps children affected by childhood cancer and their families by providing financial assistance, advocacy, education, and emotional support.

Parents Caring and Sharing

c/o Chumie Bodek
109 Rutledge Street
Brooklyn, NY 11211
(718) 596-1542 or 596-9002 (call during business hours, Eastern time)

Provides outreach, a support network, and newsletter for Jewish Orthodox families with children with cancer. Holds monthly meetings and links families of children with similar diseases.

Songs of Love Foundation

P.O. Box 750809 Dept P
Forest Hills, NY 11375
(800) 960-SONG
http://www.songsoflove.org
Email: *SongsLove@aol.com*

A nonprofit organization with a volunteer group of more than 200 artists who produce personalized musical portraits for children with chronic or life-threatening diseases.

Bone marrow and stem cell transplantation

Additional resources for bone marrow or stem cell transplant families are listed at *http://www.bmtnews.org*.

The Barbara DeBoer Foundation

2069 S. Busse Road
Mount Prospect, IL 60056
(800) 895-8478 or (847) 981-0130

Helps identify and utilize resources in your community to raise funds for transplants.

Children's Organ Transplant Association

2501 Cota Drive
Bloomington, IN 47403
(800) 366-2682
http://www.cota.org

Provides fundraising help.

National Bone Marrow Transplant Link

29209 Northwestern Highway #624
Southfield, MI 48034
(800) LINK-BMT or (810) 932-8483

Provides a hot line, peer support, a library, a clearinghouse, and suggestions for financial assistance.

National Marrow Donor Program (NMDP)
3433 Broadway Street, NE, Suite 500
Minneapolis, MN 55413
Donor information: (800) MARROW-2
Patient search information: (800) 526-7809
Corporate recruitment programs: (800) 526-7809
Fax: (612) 627-8195
http://www.marrow.org

The NMDP has the world's largest computerized listing of potential bone marrow donors—3,500,000 in 1999. The NMDP has cooperative search arrangements with many other registries worldwide. They also provide information on transplant centers in the US.

Financial and insurance help

Cancer Fund of America
2901 Breezewood Lane
Knoxville, TN 37921
(800) 578-5284
Fax: (615) 938-2968

Helps defray cancer-related expenses not covered by insurance.

The National Transplant Assistance Fund
6 Bryn Mawr Avenue
P.O. Box 258
Bryn Mawr, PA 19010
(800) 642-8399 or (610) 527-5056
http://www.transplantfund.org

Provides fundraising assistance and donor awareness material to transplant patients nationwide.

Patient Advocacy Coalition
850 E. Harvard Avenue, Suite 465
Denver, CO 80210
(303) 744-7667
Fax: (303) 744-7876

Helps resolve insurance reimbursement problems.

Patient Advocate Foundation
780 Pilot House Drive, Suite #100-C
Newport News, VA 23606
(800) 532-5274 or (757) 873-6668
Fax: (757) 873-8999
http://www.patientadvocate.org
Email: *patient@pinn.net*

Publications, help with insurance problems, referrals to attorneys.

The Sparrow Foundation
1155 N. 130th, Suite 310
Seattle, WA 98104
(206) 745-5403

Provides help with fundraising for any medical needs.

Free air services

Air Care Alliance
(800) 296-1217
http://www.aircareall.org

ACA is a nationwide association of humanitarian flying organizations.

Corporate Angel Network, Inc. (CAN)
Westchester County Airport, Building 1
White Plains, NY 10604
(914) 328-1313
Fax: (800) 328-4226

A nationwide, nonprofit program designed to give patients with cancer the use of available seats on corporate aircraft to get to and from recognized cancer treatment centers. Patients must be able to walk and travel without life-support systems or medical attention. A child may be accompanied by up to two adults. This service will also fly donors. There is no cost or financial need requirements.

DreamLine, Inc.
Contact: Bob Iverson
1701 N. Clybourn
Chicago, IL 60614
(312) 202-9000
Fax: (312) 202-0188
http://www.bobiverson.com/dreamline.htm

Provides free airline travel for children with serious illnesses needing emergency medical treatment or to travel for vacation.

Mission Air Transportation Network
Proctor & Gamble Building
4711 Young Street
North York, ON Canada M2N 6K8
(416) 222-6335
Fax: (416) 222-6930

An organization that provides free air transport to Canadians in financial need who must travel from their own communities to recognized facilities for medical care.

National Patient Air Transport Hot Line
24-hour hot line: (800) 296-1217

Specialists refer callers to the most appropriate, cost-effective charitable or commercial services, including volunteer pilot organizations and special airline transport programs.

Wish fulfillment organizations

In addition to the large organizations listed below, there are many smaller and local organizations that grant wishes to seriously ill children. A more comprehensive list of wish fulfillment organizations can be found on the Web at *http://www.patient-centers.com/leukemia/*.

Children's Wish Foundation International
7840 Roswell Road, Suite 301
Atlanta, GA 30350
(770) 393-WISH
(800) 323-WISH
Fax: (404) 393-0683

US or Europe. Fulfills wishes of terminally ill children.

The Children's Wish Foundation of Canada
95 Bayly Street, Suite 404
Ajax, Ontario
Canada L1S 7K8
(905) 426-5656
Fax: (905) 426-4111

Their goal is to provide a once-in-a-lifetime experience for children ages three to eighteen with high-risk, life-threatening diseases. There are chapters throughout Canada. Parents can call for the location of the chapter nearest to them.

The Dream Factory, Inc.
P.O. Box 3942
Louisville, KY 40202
(800) 456-7556
Fax: (502) 584-0023

Chapters in 30 states. Grants wishes of children ages three to thirteen who are seriously or chronically ill.

Make-a-Wish Foundation of America
100 W. Clarendon, Suite 2200
Phoenix, AZ 85013
(602) 279-WISH or (800) 722-WISH
Fax: (602) 279-0855
http://www.wish.org
Email: *mawfa@wish.org*

US and international chapters and affiliates. Grants wishes to children under the age of eighteen with life-threatening illnesses.

The Starlight Foundation
International Headquarters
12424 Wilshire Boulevard, Suite 1050
Los Angeles, CA 90025
(310) 207-3558

Has chapters in the United States, Canada, Australia, and United Kingdom. Fulfills wishes for seriously ill children ages four to eighteen.

Sunshine Foundation
P.O. Box 255
5400 County Road 547 N
Loughman, FL 33858
(813) 424-4188 or (800) 457-1976

No geographic boundaries. Grants wishes to chronically or terminally ill children ages three to twenty-one.

Bereavement

The Centering Corporation
1531 N. Saddle Creek Road
Omaha, NE 68104
(402) 553-1200

Publishes a free catalog which contains an extensive listing of books, cards, and audio- and videotapes on death and grieving.

Children's Hospice International
2202 Mt. Vernon Avenue, Suite 3C
Alexandria, VA 22301
(703) 684-0330
(800) 24-CHILD

The Compassionate Friends National Office
P.O. Box 3696
Oak Brook, IL 60522-3696
(630) 990-0010
Fax: (630) 990-0246
http://www.compassionatefriends.org

A self-help organization that offers understanding and friendship to bereaved families through support meetings at local chapters and telephone support (they match persons with similar losses). It publishes a newsletter for parents and one for siblings, and offers a resource catalog with a comprehensive list of books, audio, and video materials on adult and sibling grief.

Books and Online Sites

A wealth of information is available through libraries and computers. This appendix briefly describes how to get the most from these resources and lists specific books and online sites that you might find helpful when researching your child's medical condition or treatment.

You might find there are some books you wish to own. If they are not in stock at your local or online bookstore, ask if they can be special-ordered for you. Most bookstores are happy to do this.

How to get information from your library or computer

Most libraries now have a computerized database of all materials available in their various branches. Some libraries may still use a manual card catalog system. Ask a librarian if you need help learning to use these systems. A librarian can also tell you how to request a book from another branch and how to put a book on hold if it is currently checked out.

If a book is not in your library's collection, ask the librarian if she can obtain it from another library by requesting an inter-library loan. This is a common practice, and you might be able to get medical texts from university or medical school libraries.

In addition to books, you can find relevant magazine and medical journal articles at the library. The librarian can show you how to use the database to search for relevant articles and where to find the periodicals. Public libraries usually subscribe to only the most popular medical journals such as the *New England Journal of Medicine*. If you are able to visit a university or medical school library, you will find many more medical journals available. To find the nearest medical library open to the public, call the National Network of Libraries of Medicine at (800) 338-7657. If you do not live close to one of these libraries, ask your local librarian if she can help you obtain copies of the articles you want.

There is an astonishing amount of information available through the Internet. Libraries from all over the world can be accessed, and you can download information in minutes from huge databases like MedLine or Cancerlit. Obtaining information from large medical databases, established journals, or large libraries is exceedingly helpful for parents at home with sick children. However, the huge numbers of people using the Internet has spawned chat rooms, bulletin boards, and thousands of FAQs (frequently asked questions), which may or may not contain accurate information. You may want to adopt the motto "Let the buyer beware."

If you do not have a home computer, many libraries provide Internet access. Ask the librarian to help you connect to MedLine, Physician's Data Query (PDQ), or other databases you wish to search. Don't hesitate to ask for assistance in finding web sites or whatever else you need on the Internet.

General

Information provided in this appendix has been organized by topic. If you cannot find a book in your bookstore or library, the following organizations may have copies available as well as additional resources for all age groups.

Candlelighters Childhood Cancer Foundation. *Bibliography and Resource Guide.* 1994 with an update in 1998. (800) 366-CCCF. Extensive listing of books and articles on childhood cancer, coping skills, death and bereavement, effects on family, long-term side effects, medical support, and terminal home care. Excellent resource.

Candlelighters Childhood Cancer Foundation Canada. *Resource Catalog.* 1999. (800) 363-1062 (Canada only) or (416) 489-6440. Extensive listing of books, articles, and videotapes on all aspects of childhood cancer. Excellent resource.

Centering Corporation. *Creative Care Package.* Lists more than 300 books and videos on coping with serious illness, loss, and grief. (402) 553-1200.

Compassionate Friends. *Resource Guide.* Contains hundreds of books, pamphlets, videos, and audiotapes on all aspects of grief. (630) 990-0010.

Reading

Bearison, David J. *'They Never Want to Tell You': Children Talk About Cancer.* Cambridge, Massachusetts: Harvard University Press, 1991. Several children and teenagers living with cancer candidly discuss their feelings. Written by a developmental psychologist.

Bombeck, Erma. *I Want to Grow Hair, I Want to Grow Up, I Want to Go to Boise.* New York: Harper & Row Publishers, 1989. Funny, touching book about children surviving cancer. This book is out of print, but may be in your local library.

Connolly, Harry. *Fighting Chance: Journeys Through Childhood Cancer.* Woodholm House, 1998. Contains more than 200 pictures of patients, families, and caregivers battling childhood cancer.

Cousins, Norman. *Head First: The Biology of Hope and the Healing Power of the Human Spirit.* New York: E.P. Dutton, 1989. After 25 years as editor of *Saturday Review,* Cousins spent a decade on the medical staff of UCLA researching the biological basis for hope. He presents the mounting volume of evidence that positive attitudes help combat disease. Also contains excellent information on enhancing the doctor/patient relationship.

Dorfman, Elena. *The C-Word: Teenagers and Their Families Living with Cancer.* Portland, Oregon: New Sage Press, rev. ed. 1998. A cancer survivor (treated from age sixteen to eighteen) spent four years interviewing and photographing the daily lives of five teenagers with cancer and their families. This book portrays in words and powerful pictures some of the deepest emotions experienced by teens with cancer and those close to them. Four of the five teens featured have leukemia.

Johnson, Joy, and S. M. Johnson. *Why Mine?: A Book for Parents Whose Child Is Seriously Ill.* Omaha, Nebraska: Centering Corporation, 1981. To order, call (402) 553-1200. Quotes from parents across the country make this a valuable book for families of seriously ill children. Addresses fears, feelings, marriages, siblings, and the ill child.

Krumme, Cynthia. *Having Leukemia Isn't So Bad. Of Course It Wouldn't Be My First Choice*. Winchester, Massachusetts: Sargasso Enterprises, 1993. To order, call (718) 729-9037; 14 Wildwood Street, Winchester, MA 01890. Personal story of Catherine Krumme, diagnosed with leukemia at age four, relapsed at age seven, finished treatment at age ten. Catherine is now working on a master's degree in special education.

Kushner, Harold. *When Bad Things Happen to Good People*. Boston: G.K. Hall, rev. ed. 1997. A rabbi wrote this comforting book on how people of faith deal with catastrophic events.

Lazlo, John, MD. *The Cure of Childhood Leukemia: Into the Age of Miracles*. Rutgers University Press, 1996. Fascinating book that describes researchers and scientific developments that resulted in the high rate of cures for childhood leukemia.

Lerner, Michael. *Choices in Healing: Integrating the Best of Conventional and Complementary Approaches to Medicine*. Cambridge, Massachusetts: The MIT Press, 1996. A comprehensive overview of both conventional and complementary approaches to cancer treatment, including nutritional therapies, physical therapies, psychological and spiritual approaches, traditional medicines from around the world, and methods for living with cancer. Compassionate and objective. It is also available online at *http://www.commonweal.org/choicescontents.html*.

National Institute of Health. *Young People with Cancer: A Handbook for Parents*. 67-page booklet. To obtain a free copy, call (800) 4-CANCER. This booklet describes the different types of childhood cancer, medical procedures, dealing with the diagnosis, family issues, and sources of information.

Online

CANSearch

http://www.cansearch.org/canserch/canserch.htm

A guide to cancer resources on the Internet, produced by the National Coalition for Cancer Survivorship.

GrannyBarb and Art's Leukemia Links

http://www.acor.org/diseases/hematology/Leukemia/leukmain.html

The best adult/child leukemia information on the Internet. It includes leukemia-specific information, leukemia organizations, and links to useful resources such as CancerNet, PDQ, abstracts, cancer literature, Internet support groups, bone marrow transplant sites, and cord blood transplant sites.

Pediatric Oncology Resource Center

http://acor.org/diseases/ped-onc

Edited by Patty Feist-Mack, this site is the best single source of information about pediatric cancers on the Internet. It contains detailed and accurate material on diseases, treatment, family issues, activism, and bereavement. It also provides links to helpful cancer sites.

Steve Dunn's CancerGuide
http://www.cancerguide.org

A great place to start when looking for information. Steve Dunn, a cancer survivor, clearly explains cancer types and staging, chemotherapy, pathology reports, and the pros and cons of researching your own cancer. He also recommends books and includes inspirational patient stories. He has links to many of the best cancer sites on the Web.

Reading for children/teens/siblings

Children

Crary, Elizabeth. *Dealing with Feelings. I'm Frustrated; I'm Mad; I'm Sad Series.* Seattle: Parenting Press, 1992. Fun, game-like books to teach preschool and early elementary children how to handle feelings and solve problems.

Foss, Karen. *The Problem with Hair: A Story for Children Learning about Cancer.* Centering Corporation, 1996. A poem/story about a group of friends and what happens when one of them loses her hair from chemotherapy.

Hairballs on my Pillow. CARTI. P.O. Box 55050, Little Rock, AR 72215. (800) 482-8561 or (501) 664-8573. Videotape interviews children with cancer and their friends about friendship and returning to school. $35 for video and newsletters for students, exercises and activities for students, and a teacher's notebook of information about cancer and its treatment, dealing with returning students, and additional resources.

Hautzig, Deborah. *A Visit to the Sesame Street Hospital.* New York: Random House, 1985. Grover, his mother, Ernie, and Bert visit the Sesame Street Hospital in preparation for Grover's upcoming operation.

Krisher, Trudy. *Kathy's Hats: A Story of Hope.* Concept Books, 1992. (800) 255-7675. A charming book for ages five to ten about a girl whose love of hats comes in handy when chemotherapy makes her hair fall out.

Leukemia Society of America. *I'm Having a Bone Marrow Transplant.* To obtain a free copy, call (800) 955-4LSA. Coloring book for young children helps to explain what to expect during the BMT for any type of cancer.

Leukemia Society of America. *Sam Fights Back.* To obtain a free copy, call (800) 955-4LSA. A coloring and activity book to help three- to six-year-old leukemia patients learn about leukemia and discuss their feelings.

Nessim, Susan, and Barbara Wyman. *Draw Me a Picture.* A coloring book for children with cancer (ages three to six). Marty Bunny talks about how it was when he was in the hospital for cancer and invites readers to draw about their experiences. Send $7.45 check to Cancervive, 6500 Wilshire Blvd., #500, Los Angeles, CA 90048.

Rogers, Fred. *Going to the Hospital.* New York: G.P. Putnam's Sons, 1997. With pictures and words, TV's beloved Mr. Rogers helps children ages three to eight learn about hospitals.

Rogers, Fred. *Some Things Change and Some Things Stay the Same.* American Cancer Society. Order by calling (800) ACS-2345. Very comforting book for preschool-age children with cancer and their siblings.

Mr. Rogers Talks About Childhood Cancer. 1990. Videotapes (2), guidebook, story-book. Forty-five minutes. VHS. Available from American Cancer Society. (800) ACS-2345. Mr. Rogers talks to children and uses characters from the Land of Make Believe to stress the importance of talking about feelings.

Richmond, Christina. *Chemo Girl: Saving the World One Treatment at a Time.* Jones and Bartlett Publishers, 1996. Written by a twelve-year-old with rhabdomyosarcoma, this book describes a superhero who shares hope and encouragement.

Schultz, Charles. *Why, Charlie Brown, Why?* New York: Topper Books, 1990. Tender story of a classmate who develops leukemia. Available as a book or videotape. For video availability, call the Leukemia Society of America, (800) 955-4LSA.

Teens

Childife Council. *For Teenagers: Visiting the Hospital.* 1996. Helps acquaint adolescents with hospital routines and policies, staff, and common medical terms. $2.00. Can order at *http://www.childife.org.*

Gravelle, Karen, and Bertram A. John. *Teenagers Face to Face with Cancer.* New York: Julian Messner, 1986. Seventeen teenagers talk openly about their cancer, including diagnosis, dealing with doctors, chemotherapy, relationships with others, planning for the future, and relapse. A heartfelt, honest, yet comforting book.

Lazar, Linda, and Bonnie Crawford. *My Journal: Reflections on Life.* Centering Corporation. (402) 553-1200. Journal for teens coping with life-threatening or terminal illness. Includes chapters called "Things Accomplished in My Life," "I've Been Thinking," and "Questions I'd Like Answered."

Richter, Elizabeth. *The Teenage Hospital Experience: You Can Handle It.* New York: Coward, McCann, and Geohegan, 1982.

Siblings

American Cancer Society. *When Your Brother or Sister Has Cancer.* To obtain a free copy, call (800) ACS-2345. This sixteen-page booklet describes the emotions felt by siblings of a child with cancer.

O'Toole, Donna. *Aarvy Aardvark Finds Hope: A Read Aloud Story for People of All Ages About Loving and Losing, Friendship and Hope.* Compassion Books, 1988. Aarvy Aardvark and his friend Ralphie Rabbit show how a family member or friend can help another in distress.

Peterkin, Allan. *What About Me? When Brothers and Sisters Get Sick.* Magination Press, 1992. Describes the feelings of siblings whose brother or sister is hospitalized.

Medical Treatment

Leukemia

Baker, Lynn, MD. *You and Leukemia: A Day at a Time.* Philadelphia: W.B. Saunders Company, 1988. Chapter 4 contains clear descriptions of procedures written for both children and adults.

Leukemia Society of America. *Acute Lymphocytic Leukemia. Acute Myelogenous Leukemia. Chronic Mylogenous Leukemia.* (800) 955-4LSA. Booklets that explain the diseases, symptoms, diagnosis, prognosis, and treatments.

Pizzo, Philip A., MD, and David G. Poplack, MD, eds. *Principles and Practice of Pediatric Oncology.* Philadelphia: Lippencott-Raven, 1997. Extremely technical.

Coping with procedures

Benson, Herbert, MD. *The Relaxation Response*. New York: Avon Books, 1990. This is an excellent resource for the relaxation method of pain relief.

Kuttner, Leora, PhD. *A Child in Pain: How to Help, What to Do*. Point Roberts, Washington: Hartley & Marks, 1996. With warmth and understanding, Dr. Kuttner explains the role and meaning of pain, how to assess pain, and many methods to alleviate it. Excellent, thorough resource.

Kuttner, Leora, PhD. *No Fears, No Tears*. Videotape. Available through the Canadian Cancer Society: 265 West Tenth Avenue, Vancouver, BC V5Z 4J4, Canada. Phone: (604) 872-4400; *http://www.bc.cancer.ca/* Documentary of eight young children and their parents as they learn how to manage the pain of cancer treatment. Runs 27 minutes.

Kuttner, Leora, PhD. *No Fears, No Tears—13 Years Later*. Videotape. To order, fax your request to (604) 294-9986 or send email to *leora_kuttner@sfu.ca*. Thirteen years after learning how to manage their painful cancer treatments, seven survivors of childhood cancer make sense of their early traumatic experiences and demonstrate the power of mind-body pain relief. Runs 46 minutes, 42 seconds.

Lewis, Sheldon, and Sheila Lewis. *Stress-Proofing Your Child: Mind-Body Exercises to Enhance Your Child's Health*. New York: Bantam Books, 1996. This book is highly recommended for all parents. It clearly explains easy ways to teach children techniques such as guided imagery, deep breathing, and meditation to decrease stress, increase a child's sense of control, and boost children's confidence. A wonderful, practical book.

Partnership with medical team

Center for Attitudinal Healing. *Advice to Doctors and Other Big People from Kids*. Berkeley, California: Celestial Arts, 1991. Book written by children with catastrophic illnesses offers suggestions and expresses feelings about health care workers. Wise and poignant, it reminds us how perceptive and aware children of all ages are, and how absolutely necessary it is to involve them in medical decisions.

Keene, Nancy. *Working with Your Doctor: Getting the Healthcare You Deserve*. Sebastopol, California: O'Reilly & Associates, Inc., 1998. Book provides practical guidance to help patients take an active role in maintaining health and steps to improve the doctor/patient relationship.

Komp, Diane M., MD. *Children Are Images of Grace: A Pediatrician's Trilogy of Faith, Hope, and Love*. Grand Rapids, Michigan: Zondervan Publishing House, 1996. Written by a Christian pediatric oncologist, this book combines three previous books that describe her feelings for her patients and her warm and loving approach to caring for children with cancer.

Leff, Patricia Taner, and Elanie H. Walizer. *Building the Healing Partnership: Parents, Professionals & Children with Chronic Illnesses and Disabilities*. Brookline, Massachusetts: Brookline Books, 1992. This book uses parents' and caretakers' personal stories to explore the feelings of both families and members of the medical team. Empathetic and practical guide for caring to children with chronic illnesses or disabilities.

Hospitalization

Keene, Nancy. *Your Child in the Hospital: A Practical Guide for Parents*. Sebastopol, California: O'Reilly & Associates, rev. ed. 1999. A pocket guide full of parent stories to help parents prepare their child physically and emotionally for hospitalizations.

Kellerman, Johnathan. *Helping the Fearful Child*. New York: W.W. Norton, 1981. Although this book was written as a guide for everyday and problem anxieties, it is full of excellent advice for parents of children undergoing traumatic procedures. Chapters 7, "Going to the Doctor," and 8, "Coping with Hospitalization," are full of real-life examples and methods to effectively help the child. This book is out of print, but may be available in your local library.

Clinical trials

Finn, Robert. *Cancer Clinical Trials: Experimental Treatments and How They Can Help You*. Sebastopol, California: O'Reilly & Associates, 1999. Excellent guide that explains the structure, ethics, and types of clinical trials. Also covers how to evaluate a trial and deal with financial issues.

McAllister, Robert M., MD, and Sylvia Horowitz, PhD. *Cancer*. New York: Basic Books, 1993. This book is divided into three parts: description of cancer, the cancer patient, and the ten most common cancers. Includes an excellent and detailed chapter on all aspects of clinical trials and a good basic description of how cancer cells operate.

National Cancer Institute. *What Are Clinical Trials All About?* To obtain a free copy, call (800) 4-CANCER. Twenty-two page booklet covers basic information about clinical trials.

The Centerwatch Clinical Trials Listing Service at *http://www.centerwatch.com* contains a searchable database of 7,500 current clinical trials in all areas of medicine, including cancer.

Chemotherapy

Dodd, Marylin J., RN, PhD. *Managing the Side Effects of Chemotherapy & Radiation Therapy: A Guide for Patients and Their Families*. UCSF Nursing, 1996. This book contains thorough explanations of possible side effects of chemotherapy and radiation and suggestions for managing them.

Leukemia Society of America. *Directory of Prescription Drug Patient Assistance Programs*. To obtain a free copy, call (800) 955-4LSA. Directory lists companies that provide prescription drugs to eligible patients either free or at minimal cost.

Leukemia Society of America. *Understanding Chemotherapy*. To obtain a free copy, call (800) 955-4LSA. Thirty-six-page guide includes general information on side effects of chemotherapy and detailed information on drugs used to treat leukemia, lymphoma, and multiple myeloma.

National Institutes of Health. *Chemotherapy & You: A Guide to Self-Help During Treatment*. To obtain a free copy, call (800) 4-CANCER. Fifty-six-page booklet includes answers to commonly asked questions about chemotherapy, its side effects, emotions while on chemotherapy, and nutrition.

Physicians' Desk Reference. Oradell, New Jersey: Medical Economics Data, 1996. Reference, issued yearly, lists authoritative information on all FDA-approved drugs. Technical language. Available at the reference desk in most libraries.

Pizzo, Philip A., MD, and David G. Poplack, MD, eds. *Principles and Practice of Pediatric Oncology.* Philadelphia: Lippencott-Raven, 1997. Chapter 9, "General Principles of Chemotherapy." Chapter 44, "Management of Nausea and Vomiting." Extremely technical.

USP DI, Volume II, *Advice for the Patient: Drug Information in Lay Language.* United States Pharmacopeial Convention, Inc., 1995. Contains detailed drug information in nonmedical language. Available in most libraries.

Radiation

McKay, Judith and Nancee Hirano. *The Chemotherapy and Radiation Survival Guide.* Oakland, California: New Harbinger, 1998. Basic, understandable guide to chemotherapy and radiation and their side effects.

National Cancer Institute. *Radiation Therapy and You: A Guide to Self-help During Treatment.* To order a free copy, call (800) 4-CANCER. Fifty-two-page booklet clearly defines radiation, explains what to expect, describes possible side effects, and discusses follow-up care.

O'Connell, Avice, MD, and Norma Leone. *Your Child and X-Rays: A Parents' Guide to Radiation, X-Rays, and Other Imaging Procedures.* Rochester, New York: Lion Press, 1988. Eighty-nine-page book explains x-ray treatments in easy-to-understand language.

Pizzo, Philip A., MD, and David G. Poplack, MD, eds. *Principles and Practice of Pediatric Oncology.* Philadelphia: Lippencott-Raven, 1997. Chapter 11, "General Principles of Radiation Therapy." Extremely technical.

Relapse

Adams, David, and Eleanor Deveau. *Coping with Childhood Cancer: Where Do We Go From Here?* Toronto: Kinbridge Publications, rev. ed. 1993. Contains an excellent chapter on relapse, which covers such topics as the impact of relapse, how relapse strikes, feelings, pain, siblings, adjustment to living, the adolescent patient, and some thoughts for single parents. This book is out of print, but may be available in your local library. It can still be ordered from Canadian Candlelighters.

National Cancer Institute. *When Cancer Recurs: Meeting the Challenge Again.* To obtain a free copy, call (800) 4-CANCER. Booklet describes different types of recurrence, types of treatment, and coping with the return of the cancer.

National Cancer Institute. *Advanced Cancer: Living Each Day.* To obtain a free copy, call (800) 4-CANCER. Thirty-two page booklet provides practical information to make living with advanced cancer easier.

Bone marrow and stem cell transplantation

Blood and Marrow Transplant Newsletter, (888) 597-7674. This extremely informative and up-to-date newsletter is written and published by a former BMT patient. It is published six times a year, and is available by writing or calling the above number.

It is also electronically published on the Internet at *http://www.bmtnews.org*. It is free, but donations are accepted (and appreciated). Includes articles on medical aspects of BMTs, personal stories, and reviews of books and videos on the topic.

Johnson, F. Leonard, MD, and 31 others. *The Candlelighters Guide to Bone Marrow Transplants in Children*. Bethesda, Maryland: Candlelighters, 1994. (800) 366-CCCF. Free to families. Straightforward, informative guide designed to educate parents about what a BMT is, types of BMTs, long-term medical effects, financial issues, psychosocial effects, impact on schooling and family life, what happens if the transplant fails, and seven family stories on their experiences.

National Cancer Institute. *Bone Marrow Transplantation and Peripheral Blood Stem Cell Transplantation*. 1994. To obtain a free copy, call (800) 4-CANCER and ask for NIH Pub. No. 95-1178. Excellent 50-page booklet covers the purpose of BMTs, the types of BMTs, complications, long-term effects, financial considerations, psychosocial considerations, the future of BMTs, clinical trials and PDQ, and resources.

Pizzo, Philip A., MD, and David G. Poplack, MD, eds. *Principles and Practice of Pediatric Oncology*. Philadelphia: Lippencott-Raven, 1997. Chapter 14, "Bone Marrow Transplantation in Pediatric Oncology." Extremely technical.

Stewart, Susan. *Bone Marrow Transplants: A Book of Basics for Patients*. Published by BMT Newsletter, 2900 Skokie Valley Road, Highland Park, IL 60035, (888) 597-7674 or (847) 433-3313. 170-page book clearly explains all medical aspects of bone marrow transplantation, the different types of transplants, emotional and psychological considerations, pediatric transplants, complications, and insurance issues. Technically accurate, yet easy to read. (An updated version is expected in 1999.)

Online medical resources

Alternative Medicine Homepage
http://www.pitt.edu/~cbw/altm.html

American Cancer Society
http://www.cancer.org
Provides useful information about cancer treatments, news, and research.

Canadian Cancer Society
http://www.cancer.ca/
Provides useful information about cancer and includes a link to its research partner, the National Cancer Institute of Canada.

CancerNet
(800) 4-CANCER
http://pdqsearch@icicc.nci.nih.gov/
Email: *CancerNet@icicc.nci.nih.gov*. Subject: none or use a dash if required. Message: help (if you use a signature, suppress it). You will receive a list of available publications and instructions on how to get the information you want. By far the most comprehensive and up-to-date source of information about cancer. It is maintained by the US National Cancer Institute. Many of the resources listed in this book are available from the database.

If you would like to be notified by email when CancerNet is updated each month, send email with the word *subscribe* or *subs* as the body of the message. CancerNet will then send you a message each month telling you what has been updated. To cancel this service, send email with the word *unsubscribe* or *unsubs* as the body of the message.

CancerWEB Online Medical Dictionary
http://www.graylab.ac.uk/omd/index.html
One of the most complete medical dictionaries available on the World Wide Web.

EMF-Link
http://infoventures.com/emf/

Hypermedia Clinical Practice Guidelines for Cancer Pain
http://www.statsci.com/talaria/talaria.html/

Med Help International
http://medhlp.netusa.net/
A nonprofit organization that provides medical information written in nontechnical language in order to support patients and their families. The all-volunteer staff is comprised of physicians and other healthcare professionals who are electronically connected.

Medicine Online
http://www.meds.com/
Provides patients and professionals with in-depth educational information on specific diseases. Also includes information on reimbursement and a treatment guide.

MedWeb: Oncology
http://www.medweb.emory.edu/MedWeb/

The Multimedia Medical Reference Library
http://www.med-library.com/medlibrary/

Oncolink
http://cancer.med.upenn.edu
A text and multimedia service available through the Internet. This service was started by E. Loren Buhle, Jr., PhD, the parent of a child with leukemia. Oncolink offers a wide variety of cancer-related information, including articles, handbooks, case studies, writings by patients and their families, and visual images, including a children's art gallery.

Oncolink, Pediatric Leukemia Page
http://cancer.med.upenn.edu/disease/leukemia
Contains a large amount of information on childhood leukemia, including bone marrow transplantation.

Patient Support.com
http://www.patientsupport.com

PharmInfoNet tm
http://pharminfo.com

Devoted to delivering useful, up-to-date, and accurate pharmaceutical information to healthcare providers, pharmacists, and patients.

Preventing Central Venous Catheter Infections
http://www.med.umkc.edu/cvcsite/

Designed to provide useful information to help reduce the risk of central venous catheter infections.

PubMed
http://www.ncbi.nlm.nih.gov/PubMed/

The National Library of Medicine's free search service provides access to nine million citations in MEDLINE and PREMEDLINE (with links to participating online journals), and other related databases. Also includes FAQs, news, and clinical alerts.

Rx List—The Internet Drug Index
http://www.rxlist.com

TeleSCAN-Telmatics Services in Cancer
http://telescan.nki.nl/

The first European Internet service for cancer research, treatment, and education, providing a hypermedia interface to primarily European information resources and services related to cancer.

Bone marrow transplantation
The Anthony Nolen Bone Marrow Trust
http://www.anthonynolan.org.uk/index.html

A leading research center and the United Kingdom register for potential donors. This site references other international BMT sites.

The BMT Newsletter
http://www.bmtnews.org

All issues of the BMT newsletters are online, as well as the book *Bone Marrow Transplants: A Book of Basics for Patients*.

Bone Marrow Donors Worldwide
http://BMDW.LeidenUniv.NL/

The National Marrow Donor Program
http://www.marrow.org

Medical journals

Numerous medical journals are on the World Wide Web. If you do not have access to a medical library, the Web may be your best bet for finding abstracts from technical journals.

American Medical Association Home Page
http://www.ama-assn.org

Allows access to current and past issues of the Journal of the American Medical Association (JAMA), as well as other journals published by the AMA.

British Medical Journal
http://www.bmj.com

Links to sites of medical interest.

The Multimedia Medical Reference Library
http://med-library.com/medlibrary/Medical_Reference_Library/

Provides links to many medical journals.

The New England Journal Online
http://www.nejm.org

Contains full text of editorials, opinion pieces, and letters, but has only abstracts of most other articles.

Medical institutions

HospitalWeb
http://neuro-www.mgh.harvard.edu/hospitalweb.shtml/

A list of hospital sites on the Internet.

Emotional support

Babcock, Elise NeeDell. *When Life Becomes Precious: A Guide for Loved Ones and Friends of Cancer Patients.* New York: Bantam Books, 1997. Written by a counselor with over two decades of experience helping cancer patients, this book is full of practical advice for caregivers of cancer patients. It explains with great warmth how to be supportive, handle special occasions, explain cancer to children, and take care of yourself.

Family Portrait: Coping with Childhood Cancer. Videotape. Twenty-five minutes. VHS. Purchase from: Films for the Humanities and Sciences, P.O. Box 2053, Princeton, NJ 08543. (800) 257-5126. Videotape of five family portraits covering issues such as guilt, sibling rivalry, divorce, the adopted child, and involvement of other family members in the care of the child. Introduction and closing by Bob Keeshan (Captain Kangaroo).

Leukemia Society of America. *Emotional Aspects of Childhood Leukemia.* To obtain a free copy, call (800) 955-4LSA. Thirty-four-page booklet covers feelings of parents, ill child, and siblings from diagnosis through end of treatment or death. Includes many parent experiences.

Mr. Rogers Talks with Parents About Childhood Cancer. 1990. Videotapes (2) guide-book, pamphlet. Forty-seven minutes. VHS. Available from American Cancer Society. (800) ACS-2345. The first tape consists of interviews with parents which illustrate ways to deal with emotions during diagnosis and treatment. The second tape sensitively deals with bereavement.

Sourkes, Barbara M., PhD. *Armfuls of Time: The Psychological Experience of the Child with a Life-Threatening Illness.* Pittsburgh: University of Pittsburgh Press, 1995. Written by a psychologist at the Dana-Farber Cancer Institute and Children's Hospital in Boston, this eloquent book features the voices and artwork of children with cancer. It clearly describes the psychological effects of cancer on children as well as explains the power of the therapeutic process. Highly recommended.

Support groups

American Psychological Association. *Finding Help: How to Choose a Psychologist.* To obtain a free brochure, send a self-addressed stamped envelope to *Finding Help* APA Public Affairs Office, 750 First St. NE, Washington, DC 20002-4242. The brochure provides information about psychotherapy, the types of problems that people take into therapy, and how to choose a therapist.

Bogue, Erna-Lynne, ACSW, and Barbara K. Chesney, MPH. *Making Contact: A Parent-to-Parent Visitation Manual.* Bethesda, Maryland: The Candlelighters Childhood Cancer Foundation, 1987. To obtain, call (800) 366-CCCF. Step-by-step guide on planning and running a parent-to-parent visitation program for parents of children with cancer. Includes guidelines for selection of parent visitors, training to improve parent-visitor contact, developing referral systems, and support resources.

Chesler, Mark A., PhD, and Barbara Chesney. *Cancer and Self-Help: Bridging the Troubled Waters of Childhood Illness.* Madison: The University of Wisconsin Press, 1995. Written for and about the parents of children with cancer, this book provides explanations of how self-help groups are formed, how they function and recruit, and why they are effective. The authors explain how, through self-help groups, parents improve their coping abilities and become better advocates for their child in an increasingly complex healthcare system.

National Cancer Institute. *Taking Time: Support for People with Cancer and the People Who Care About Them.* NIH Publication No. 88-2059. To obtain a free copy, call (800) 4-CANCER. Sixty-one-page booklet includes sections on sharing feelings, coping within the family, and when you need assistance.

Pizzo, Philip A., MD, and David G. Poplack, MD. *Principles and Practice of Pediatric Oncology.* Philadelphia: Lippincott-Raven, 1997. Chapter 47, "Psychiatric and Psychosocial Support for the Child and Family." Chapter 48, "The Other of Side of the Bed: What Caregivers Can Learn from Listening to Patients and Their Families."

Speigel, David, MD. *Living Beyond Limits.* New York: Random House, 1993. Dr. Speigel devised the landmark study which showed that support groups for women with breast cancer not only lowered rates of depression, but significantly increased their life spans. This book is an excellent guide for coping with cancer, strengthening family relationships, controlling pain, dealing with doctors, and evaluating alternative medicine claims. This book is out of print, but may be available from your local library.

Online support

ACOR, The Association of Cancer Online Resources, Inc.
http://www.acor.org

ACOR is currently offering 79 information and support electronic groups to patients, caregivers, or anyone looking for answers and support about cancer and related disorders. ACOR hosts several pediatric cancer discussion groups, including PED-ONC (a general pediatric cancer discussion group) and PED-ALL (pediatric leukemia).

ALL_KIDS Childhood Acute Lymphoblastic Leukemia
http://www.all-kids.org/mailing_lists/

ALL_KIDS is an unmoderated discussion group for parents, siblings, and friends of children up to age seventeen diagnosed with Acute Lymphoblastic Leukemia. Members discuss clinical trials, chemotherapies, coping, and any issue surrounding the care of a child with ALL. Members also provide support, resources, and their personal experiences.

Sickkids Mailing List
Email: *listserv@maelstrom.stjohns.edu*

Moderated (with adult supervision) email support group for children under eighteen who have serious illnesses. The children share information, establish friendships, ask questions, and exchange humor. There is a team of children who serve as discussion managers. To subscribe, leave the subject line blank. Message: subscribe SICKKIDS <your first and last name> (if you have a signature, delete it). Although adults may not participate in the group, they can email questions or concerns to an adult advisor at: *sickkids-request@maelstrom.stjohns.edu*.

SpeciaLove
http://www.speciallove.org

A resource devoted to parents and children with cancer to facilitate networking. This resource is oriented to the family aspects of childhood cancer. SpeciaLove, Inc. was started in 1983 by Tom and Sheila Baker, who lost their thirteen-year-old daughter to leukemia.

Touchstone Support Network
http://www-med.stanford.edu/touchstone/

A nonprofit, nonsectarian, completely volunteer organization that provides emotional and practical support services for children with chronic and life-threatening illnesses. They help seriously ill children and their families cope with the day-to-day stresses of their overwhelming situations to help them maintain as much stability as possible at home, school, work, and in the community.

Commercial online services

Most commercial online services offer a number of health-related topics for which there are support groups, speaker forums, databases, and other services.

If you subscribe to America Online, for example, click on the Health channel. You can access MedLine under "Medical Reference." As of March 1999, the following support groups were active:

Sunday, 7 p.m. EST: Living with Cancer: Self Help Group

Sunday, 10 p.m. EST: Parents of Kids with Cancer

Monday, 7 p.m. EST: Kids and Cancer

Monday, 9 p.m. EST: Compassionate Friends

Monday, 10 p.m. EST: Cancer Survivors Mutual Support

Consult the "Help" feature of your service to find what is offered.

Siblings

Faber, Adele, and Elaine Mazlish. *Siblings Without Rivalry: How to Help Your Children Live Together So You Can Live Too.* New York: Avon Books, 1998. Required reading for parents with fighting siblings. Offers dozens of astonishingly simple yet effective methods to reduce conflict and foster a cooperative spirit.

Leukemia Society of America. *Emotional Aspects of Childhood Leukemia.* To obtain a free copy, call (800) 955-8484. Thirty-two-page booklet deals with the gamut of emotions experienced by all members of the family, including siblings.

Murray, Gloria, and Gerald Jampolsky, eds. *Straight from the Siblings: Another Look at the Rainbow.* Millbrae, California: Celestial Arts, 1982. Written by sixteen children who have brothers and sisters with a life-threatening illness who met at the Center for Attitudinal Healing. A must read for both parents and siblings. Contains beautiful artwork by the children as well as wise words from the heart about reactions to the news, feelings, facing death, making choices, being part of a group, and thoughts for other siblings in a similar situation.

Feelings, communciation, and behavior

Faber, Adele, and Elaine Mazlish. *How to Talk So Kids Will Listen... and Listen So Kids Will Talk.* New York: Rawson, Wade Publishers, 1995. The classic book on developing new, more effective ways to communicate with your children, based on respect and understanding. Highly recommended.

Kurcinka, Mary Sheedy. *Raising Your Spirited Child: A Guide for Parents Whose Child Is More Intense, Sensitive, Perceptive and Energetic.* New York: Harper Collins, 1992. Reassuring guide for how to effectively parent children who are more intense, sensitive, perceptive, persistent, energetic, or uncomfortable with change than average children. Many of the strategies are very effective for children stressed by cancer treatment.

National Cancer Institute. *Talking with Your Child About Cancer.* (800) 4-CANCER. Excellent sixteen-page booklet on talking with your child about diagnosis. Full of helpful hints on how to answer many commonly asked questions.

Nelsen, Jane. *Positive Discipline.* New York: Ballantine Books, rev. ed. 1996. Written by a psychologist, educator, and mother of seven, this book teaches parents how to promote self-discipline and personal responsibility.

Practical support

Finances

Leeland, Jeff. *One Small Sparrow: The Remarkable Real-Life Drama of One Community's Compassionate Response to a Little Boy's Life.* Sisters, Oregon: Multnomah Books, 1995. Written by the father of a baby with leukemia, this heartwarming true story describes how a community raised the entire cost of a successful bone marrow transplant. Contains numerous ideas for methods to raise funds. Christian perspective.

Peterson, Sheila. *A Special Way to Care.* 1988. Available from: Friends of Karen, Box 217, Croton Falls, NY. 10519. Free guide for those who wish to provide financial/emotional support for families of ill children. Discusses how to differentiate between interference and advocacy. Explains how to organize, manage, and perpetuate a support fund. Excellent resource.

Pizzo, Philip A., MD, and David G. Poplack, MD, eds. *Principles and Practice of Pediatric Oncology.* Philadelphia: Lippincott-Raven, 1997. Chapter 53, "Financial Issues in Pediatric Cancer."

Nutrition

Bohannon, Richard, and others. *Food for Life: The Cancer Prevention Cookbook.* Contemporary Books, 1998. Written by an oncologist, a chef, and a writer, this book follows American Cancer Society guidelines. Contains many tasty recipes.

National Cancer Institute. *Managing Your Child's Eating Problems During Cancer Treatment.* To obtain, call (800) 4-CANCER. Thirty-two-page booklet which covers how cancer treatments affect eating, how to cope with side effects, and how to serve more protein and calories.

National Cancer Institute. *Eating Hints for Cancer Patients.* To obtain, call (800) 4-CANCER. Ninety-six-page booklet covers eating well during cancer treatment, managing eating problems, special diets, family resources, and recipes.

Pizzo, Philip A., MD, and David G. Poplack, MD, eds. *Principles and Practice of Pediatric Oncology.* Philadelphia: Lippincott-Raven, 1997. Chapter 42, "Nutritional Supportive Care."

Wilson, J. Randy. *Non-Chew Cookbook.* Wilson Publishing, Inc., 1986. P.O. Box 2190, Glenwood Springs, CO 81602. (303) 945-5600. Contains recipes for patients unable to chew due to the side effects of chemotherapy and/or radiation.

School

American Cancer Society. *Back to School: A Handbook for Parents of Children with Cancer.* To obtain a free copy, call (800) ACS-1234. Sixteen-page introductory booklet covers school reentry, classroom presentations, the importance of advocates, legal issues, IEPs, and special needs.

Anderson, Winifred, Stephen Chitwood, and Deidre Hayden. *Negotiating the Special Education Maze: A Guide for Parents and Teachers.* Bethesda, Maryland: Woodbine House, 3rd ed. 1997. Excellent, well-organized text which clearly explains the step-by-step process necessary to obtain help for your child. Has up-to-date resource list and a comprehensive bibliography. Essential reading for parents of children with special educational needs. If you only read one book, this should be the one.

Deasy-Spinetta, Patricia, and Elisabeth Irvin. *Educating the Child with Cancer.* Candlelighters Childhood Cancer Foundation. Single copies free to families of children with cancer, all others $7.50 per copy. Call (800) 366-CCCF for an order form. This 137-page book discusses all aspects of educating the child with cancer including educational issues, peer relationships, school reentry, liaison programs, classroom presentations, cognitive late effects, preparing for college, college alternatives, legal aspects, and siblings. Includes a bibliography.

Candlelighters Childhood Cancer Foundation Canada. *School Reentry Resource Manual.* 1992. Write to: CCCFC, 10 Alcorn Ave., Suite 200, Toronto, Ontario M4V 3B1, Canada or call (416) 489-6440. Sections for parents, educators, and healthcare professionals regarding siblings, adolescence, survivor's quality of life, programs, bereavement, and grief.

Chai Lifeline. *Back to School: A Handbook for Educators of Children with Life-threatening Diseases in the Yeshiva/Day School System.* 1995. Write to: 48 West 25th St. New York, NY 10010 or call (212) 465-1300. Covers diagnosis, planning for school reentry, infection control in schools, needs of junior and senior high school students, children with special educational needs, and saying good-bye when a child dies. Includes a bibliography and resource list.

Gliko-Braden, Majel. *Grief Comes to Class: A Teacher's Guide.* Centering Corporation, 1531 N. Saddle Creek Rd., Omaha, NE 68104. (402) 553-1200. Comprehensive guide to grief in the classroom. Includes chapters on grief responses, the bereaved student, teen grief, developmental changes, sample letter to parents, sample teacher/parent conference, and suggestions for dos and don'ts.

Hairballs on my Pillow. CARTI. P.O. Box 55050, Little Rock, AR 72215. (800) 482-8561 or (501) 664-8573. Videotape interviews children with cancer and their friends about friendship and returning to school. $35 for video and newsletters for students, exercises and activities for students, and a teacher's notebook of information about cancer, its treatment, and dealing with returning students.

Levine, Mel, MD. *All Kinds of Minds.* Cambridge, Massachusetts: Educator's Publishing Service, Inc., 1993. Highly readable book about different learning styles. Written for grade-school-aged children, but parents benefit from reading it, too.

Levine, Mel, MD. *Keeping a Head in School: A Student's Book About Learning Abilities and Learning Disorders.* Cambridge, Massachusetts: Educator's Publishing Service, Inc., 1991. Book about different learning styles for junior high and high school students.

Peterson's Guides. *Peterson's Guides to Colleges with Programs for Learning Disabled Students or Attention Deficit Disorders.* Princeton, NJ: Peterson's Guides, 5th ed. 1997. Excellent reference, available at most large libraries.

Pizzo, Philip A., MD. and David G. Poplack, MD, eds. *Principles and Practice of Pediatric Oncology.* Philadelphia: Lippincott-Raven, 1997. Chapter 51, "Educational Issues for Children with Cancer."

Silver, Larry, MD. *The Misunderstood Child: Understanding and Coping with Your Child's Learning Disabilities.* Times Books, 3rd ed. 1998. Comprehensive discussion of positive treatment strategies that can be implemented at home and in the school to help children with learning disabilities. Excellent chapters on psychological, social, and emotional development, evaluation, and treatment.

The Compassionate Friends. *Suggestions for Teachers and School Counselors.* P.O. Box 3696, Oak Brook, IL 60522. (630) 990-0010.

Practical support online
Air Care Alliance
http://www.aircareall.org

A nationwide association of humanitarian pilots who help needy patients travel to facilities for necessary treatment.

Patient Advocacy Numbers
http://infonet.welch.jhu.edu/advocacy.html

Federal agencies
Food and Drug Administration
http://www.fda.gov

For information on specific drugs, telnet to *fdabbs.fda.gov* and login as "bbs."

National Institutes of Environmental Health Sciences
http://www.niehs.nih.gov

The US Environmental Protection Agency (EPA)
http://www.epa.gov/children/eleven1.htm

The US Environmental Protection Agency (EPA) has a Children's Health Resources branch that maintains publications on children's health topics, information on hotlines, and links to Internet resources.

Americans with Disabilities Act information available on electronic bulletin boards
The following are telephone numbers of electronic bulletin boards from which ADA documents can be downloaded if you have a computer with a modem.

US Department of Justice (202) 514-6193
Disability Law Foundation (205) 854-9074
(205) 854-2308
(205) 854-0698

Compuserve Disability Forum: Call (800) 635-6225 for your local access number.

GEnie Disability Round Table: Call (800) 638-9636 (GEnie subscribers only) for your local access number.

Project Enable: (304) 755-7842

Washington State access to self-help: (206) 767-7681

After treatment ends
Hoffman, Barbara, JD, eds. *A Cancer Survivor's Almanac: Charting Your Journey.* National Coalition for Cancer Survivorship, 1998. Comprehensive guide to the issues of cancer survivorship. Includes sections on dealing with doctors and hospitals; the mind/body relationship; support services; peer support; employment,

insurance, and money matters; dealing with the family; appendix on survivor resources.

Harpham, Wendy Schlessel. *After Cancer: A Guide to Your New Life*. HarperPerrennial, 1995. Written in a question and answer format, doctor/cancer survivor Harpham addresses the medical, psychological, and practical issues of recovery.

Keene, Nancy, Wendy Hobbie, and Kathy Ruccione. *Childhood Cancer Survivors: A Guide to the Future*. Sebastopol, California: O'Reilly & Associates, 2000. A user-friendly, comprehensive guide on late effects of treatment for childhood cancer. This book, full of stories from survivors of all types of childhood cancer, also covers emotional issues, insurance, jobs, relationships, and ways to stay healthy.

Leukemia Society of America. *Coping with Survival*. To obtain a free copy, call (800) 955-4LSA. Thirty-two-page booklet includes information on diagnosis, communicating with physicians, treatment, life after treatment, and services and support.

Pizzo, Philip A., MD, and David G. Poplack MD, eds. *Principles and Practice of Pediatric Oncology*. Philadelphia: Lippincott-Raven, 1997. Chapter 50, "Late Effects of Childhood Cancer and Its Treatment." Chapter 54, "Pediatric Cancer: Advocacy, Legal, Insurance, and Employment Issues." Chapter 57, "Preventing Cancer in Adulthood: Advice for the Pediatrician."

Terminal illness and bereavement

Callanan, Maggie, and Patricia Kelley. *Final Gifts: Understanding the Special Awareness, Needs, and Communications of the Dying*. New York: Bantam Books, 1997. Written by two hospice nurses with decades of experience, this book helps families understand and communicate with terminally ill patients. Compassionate, comforting, and insightful, *Final Gifts* movingly teaches us how to listen to and comfort the dying. Highly recommended.

Modlow, D. Gay, and Ida M. Martinson. *Home Care for the Seriously Ill Child: A Manual for Parents*. 1991. $7.95 from Children's Hospice International (703) 684-0330. Helps parents explore the possibility of home care for the dying child. It contains practical information on what to expect, methods for pain relief, and control of medical problems. There are appendices on medications, bibliographies, and dos and don'ts for helping bereaved parents.

Pizzo, Philip A., MD, and David G. Poplack, MD, eds. *Principles and Practice of Pediatric Oncology*. Philadelphia: Lippincott-Raven, 1997. Chapter 52, "Care of the Dying Child."

Parental grief

Bereavement: A Magazine of Hope and Healing. Founded in 1987 by a bereaved mother to provide support for those grieving, it allows direct feedback from the bereaved to helping professionals, and helps the nonbereaved learn what helps and what hurts. For a free copy or to subscribe, write or call: Bereavement Publishing, Inc., 8133 Telegraph Drive, Colorado Springs, CO 80920. (719) 282-1948.

Bernstein, Judith R. *When the Bough Breaks Forever: After the Death of a Son or Daughter*. Kansas City, Missouri: Andrews & McMeel, 1997.

Kubler-Ross, Elisabeth, MD. *On Children and Death*. New York: Macmillan, 1983. In this comforting book, Dr. Kubler-Ross offers practical help in living through the terminal period of a child's life with love and understanding. She discusses children's knowledge about death, visualization, letting go, funerals, help from friends, and spirituality.

Morse, Melvin, MD. *Closer to the Light: Learning from Near Death Experiences of Children.* New York: Villard Books, 1990. Dr. Morse, a pediatrician and researcher into children's near-death experiences, writes about the startlingly similar spiritual experiences of children who almost die.

Rando, Therese, PhD, ed. *Parental Loss of a Child.* Champaign, Illinois: Research Press, 1986. Thirty-seven articles cover death from serious illness; guilt; grief of fathers, mothers, siblings, single parents; professional help; advice to physicians, clergy, funeral directors; support organizations.

Wild, Laynee. *I Remember You: A Grief Journal.* San Francisco: HarperCollins, 1994. A journal for written and photographic memories during the first year of mourning. Beautiful book filled with quotes and comfort.

Sibling grief (adult reading)

Doka, Kenneth, ed. *Children Mourning, Mourning Children.* Hemisphere Publications, 1995. A collection of chapters (first presented at the Hospice Foundation of America conference) written by many healthcare professionals who work with grieving children. Topics include children's understanding of death, answering grieving children's questions, the role of the schools, and many others. To obtain, write: Taylor and Francis, 1900 Frost Road, Suite 101, Bristol, PA 19007. $14.95 plus $2.50 for shipping and handling.

Grollman, Earl. *Talking About Death: A Dialogue Between Parent and Child.* Boston: Beacon Press, 1990. One of the best books for helping children cope with grief. It contains a children's read-along section to explain and explore children's feelings. In very comforting language, this book teaches parents how to explain death, understand children's emotions, understand how children react to specific types of death, and know when to seek professional help. It also contains a resource section.

Schaefer, Dan, and Christine Lyons. *How Do We Tell the Children?: A Step-by-Step Guide for Helping Children Two to Teen Cope When Someone Dies.* New York: Newmarket Press, updated ed. 1993. If your terminally ill child has siblings, read this book. In straightforward, uncomplicated language, the authors describe how to explain the facts of death to children and teens and show how to include the children in the family support network, laying the foundation for the healing process to begin. Also includes a crisis section, for quick reference on what to do in a variety of situations.

Sibling grief (young child reading)

Buscaglia, Leo. *The Fall of Freddy the Leaf: A Story of Life for All Ages.* New York: Holt, Rinehart and Winston, 1982. This wise yet simple story about a leaf named Freddy explains death as a necessary part of the cycle of life. This book is out of print, but may be available in your local library.

Hickman, Martha. *Last Week My Brother Anthony Died.* Abingdon, Tennessee: 1984. Touching story of a preschooler's feelings when her infant brother dies. The family's minister (a bereaved parent himself) comforts her by comparing feelings to clouds—always there but ever changing.

Mellonie, Bryan, and Robert Ingpen. *Lifetimes: The Beautiful Way to Explain Death to Children*. New York: Bantam Books, 1983. Beautiful paintings and simple text explain that dying is as much a part of life as being born.

Sibling grief (school-aged children)

Houston, Gloria. *My Brother Joey Died*. New York: J. Messner, 1982. Simple, caring book describes one child's journey through grief after the death of her sibling. Describes the sister's feelings about the funeral, the changed family, her parents' grief, her grandparents' role, and the comfort of a support group.

Temes, Roberta, PhD. *The Empty Place: A Child's Guide Through Grief*. Far Hills, New Jersey: New Horizon Press, 1992. To order, call (402) 553-1200. Explains and describes feelings after the death of a sibling, such as the empty place in the house, at the table, in a brother's heart.

White, E.B. *Charlotte's Web*. New York: Harper, 1952. Classic tale of friendship and death as a part of life. (The videotape is widely available to rent.)

Sibling grief (teenagers)

Gravelle, Karen, and Charles Haskins. *Teenagers Face to Face with Bereavement*. Englewood Cliffs, NJ: J. Messner, 1989. The perspectives and experiences of seventeen teenagers comprise the heart of this book, which focuses on teens coping with grief.

Grollman, Earl. *Straight Talk About Death for Teenagers: How to Cope with Losing Someone You Love*. Boston: Beacon Press, 1993. Wonderful book that talks to teens, not at them. Discusses denial, pain, anger, sadness, physical symptoms, and depression, as well as charts methods to help teens actively work through their feelings at their own pace.

Audio/video

Drying Their Tears. Produced by CARTI, Communication Division, Markham University, P.O. Box 55050, Little Rock, AR 72215. For information, call (800) 482-8561 or (501) 660-7614. Ask for Mary Machen. Video and manual to help counselors, teachers, and other professionals help children deal with the grief, fear, confusion, and anger that occur after the death of a loved one. There are three segments: training facilitators, a section for children aged five to eight, and one for ages nine to teens. Each includes interviews with children and video from children's workshops.

Mr. Rogers Talks with Parents About Childhood Cancer. Videotapes (2), guidebook, pamphlet. Forty-seven minutes. VHS. Available from the American Cancer Society. (800) ACS-2345. The first tape consists of interviews with parents about ways to deal with emotions during diagnosis and treatment. The second tape includes sensitive interviews with three bereaved parents.

The Healing Path. The Compassionate Friends sibling video addresses concerns of surviving siblings, such as sadness, pain, anger, and fear. The video explores eight topics: facing the reality of death, who will listen, changed family life, special days, visiting the cemetery, parental overprotection, feelings and expectations, and looking to the future. For information, call (630) 990-0010 or fax (630) 990-0246.

Glossary

Absolute neutrophil count (ANC); also known as absolute granulocyte (AGC)
Total count of the neutrophils in the blood, which provides an indication of a person's ability to fight infection. To calculate the ANC, add the percentages of seg neutrophils and band neutrophils, divide by 100, and multiply by the total white blood count.

ALL (acute lymphoblastic leukemia)
An acute form of leukemia occurring predominantly in children, characterized by the unrestrained production of immature lymphoblasts (a type of white cell) in the blood-forming tissues, particularly the bone marrow, spleen, and lymph nodes.

AML (acute myeloid leukemia)
An acute form of leukemia characterized by a massive proliferation of mature and immature abnormal granulocytes (a type of white cell).

Allogeneic transplant
Type of bone marrow transplant in which the marrow is donated by another person.

Alopecia
Hair loss; a common side effect of chemotherapy.

Anemia
Condition in which there is a reduction in the number of circulating red blood cells.

Anesthesia
Partial or total loss of sensation, with or without loss of consciousness, induced by the administration of a drug.

Anorexia
Loss of appetite.

Anesthesiologist
A doctor who specializes in the study and administration of anesthesia.

Attending physician
Doctor on the staff of a hospital who has completed medical school, residency, and fellowship.

Acute lymphoblastic leukemia (ALL)
An acute form of leukemia occurring predominantly in children, characterized by the unrestrained production of immature lymphoblasts (a type of white cell) in the blood-forming tissues, particularly the bone marrow, spleen, and lymph nodes.

Asymptomatic
Without symptoms.

Autologous
From the same person. An autologous bone marrow transplant is a procedure in which bone marrow that has been removed from a patient is given back to that patient.

B cells
Type of lymphocyte (white cell) that helps produce antibodies that destroy foreign substances.

Basophil
Type of granulocyte (white cell) that plays a special role in allergic reactions and helps in the healing of inflammations.

Blast cell
An undifferentiated normal cell in an early stage of development; also means a leukemic cell of indeterminable type.

Blood-brain barrier
A network of blood vessels located around the central nervous system with very closely spaced cells that make it difficult for potentially toxic substances— including anticancer drugs—to enter the brain and spinal cord.

Blood type
Identification of the proteins in a person's blood cells so that transfusions can be given with compatible blood products. Examples of blood types are A+, A-, B+, B-, AB+, AB-, O+, O-.

Bone marrow
Soft, inner part of large bones that makes blood cells.

Bone marrow aspiration
Process in which a sample of fluid and cells is withdrawn from the bone marrow using a hollow needle.

Bone marrow biopsy
The removal of a sample of solid tissue from the bone marrow.

Bone marrow transplant
A procedure in which doctors replace bone marrow that has been destroyed by high doses of chemotherapy and/or radiation.

CBC (complete blood count)
Measurement of the numbers of white cells, red cells, and platelets in a cubic millimeter of blood.

CML (chronic myelogenous leukemia)
A disease that progresses slowly and is characterized by increased production of granulocytes in the bone marrow. It is usually associated with a specific chromosomal abnormality called the Philadelphia chromosome.

CNS (central nervous system)
The brain, spinal cord, and nerves.

Cancer
A term for diseases in which abnormal cells divide without control.

Carcinogen
> A substance or agent that produces cancer.

Centigray
> Measurement of radiation-absorbed dose; same as a rad.

Central nervous system
> Brain, spinal cord, and nerves.

Cerebrospinal fluid (CSF)
> Fluid that surrounds and bathes the brain and spinal cord and provides a cushion from shocks.

Children's Cancer Group (CCG)
> An organization that designs and monitors pediatric clinical trials.

Chemotherapy
> Treatment of disease with drugs. The term usually refers to cytotoxic drugs given to treat cancer.

Chromosome
> A structure in the nucleus of a cell that contains genetic material. Normally, 46 chromosomes are inside each human cell.

Chronic myelogenous leukemia (CML)
> A disease that progresses slowly and is characterized by increased production of granulocytes in the bone marrow. It is usually associated with a specific chromosomal abnormality called the Philadelphia chromosome.

Clinical trial
> A carefully designed and executed investigation of a drug, drug dosage, combination of drugs, or other method of treating disease. Each trial is designed to answer one or more scientific questions and to find better ways to prevent or treat disease.

Consolidation
> Portion of the protocol which consists of new combinations of drugs to destroy any cancer cells that survived induction.

Cytomegalovirus (CMV)
> One of a group of herpes viruses that can cause fatal infections in immunosuppressed patients.

Cytotoxic
> Causing the death of cells.

Delayed intensification
> Portion of treatment that comes after the initial induction, consolidation, and interim maintenance. The purpose of this phase is to destroy any remaining cancer cells.

Differentiation
> The process by which cells mature and become specialized.

Echocardiogram
> A diagnostic test that uses ultrasound to visualize the interior of the heart and determine how effectively it is functioning.

Electrocardiogram (ECG, EKG)
A graphic record of the electric current produced by the contraction of the heart.

Electromagnetic fields
Magnetism produced by electrical fields.

Eosinophil
A type of white cell that responds to allergic reactions as well as foreign bacteria.

Erythrocytes
Red blood cells.

External catheter
Indwelling catheter in which one end of the tubing is in the heart and the other end of the tubing sticks out through the skin, for example, a Hickman catheter.

Fellow
A physician who has completed four years of medical school and several years of residency, and is pursuing additional training in a specialized field.

Finger poke
When a laboratory technician pricks the fingertip to obtain a small sample of blood.

Graft
Tissue taken from one person (donor) and transferred to another person (recipient or host).

Graft-versus-host disease
A condition that may develop after allogenic bone marrow transplantation in which the transplanted marrow (graft) attacks the patient's (host's) organs.

Granulocytes
A type of white cell that destroys foreign substances in the body such as viruses, bacteria, and fungi.

Hepatitis
Inflammation of the liver by virus or toxic origin. Fever and jaundice are usually present, and sometimes the liver is enlarged.

Hematocrit
The measurement of the proportion of cells to plasma in a sample of blood. Sometimes called packed cell volume (PCV).

Hematologist
Physician who specializes in the diagnosis and treatment of disorders of blood and blood-forming tissues.

Hemoglobin
The protein found in red blood cells that carries oxygen.

Hemorrhagic cystitis
Bleeding from the bladder, which can be a side effect of the drug cytoxan.

Heparin solution
An anticoagulant injected into indwelling catheters between uses to prevent clots.

Hickman catheter
An indwelling catheter that has one end of the tubing in the heart and the other end outside the body.

HIV (human immunodeficiency virus)
The virus that causes AIDS.

Host
In bone marrow transplantation, the person who receives the marrow.

Human leukocyte antigens (HLAs)
Proteins on the surface of cells that are important in transplantation and transfusion. For BMTs, the HLAs on white cells of the patient and potential donor are compared. A perfect HLA match occurs only between identical twins.

Infusion pump
A small, computerized device which allows drugs to be given at home through an IV or indwelling catheter.

Immune system
Complex system by which the body is able to protect itself from foreign invaders.

Immunosuppression
When the immune system is suppressed, leaving the body susceptible to infection.

Induction
The first part of the chemotherapy protocol for treating some types of leukemia in which several powerful chemotherapy drugs are given to kill as many cancer cells as possible.

Institutional Review Board (IRB)
Group made up of scientists, clergy, doctors, and citizens from the community, which approves and reviews all research taking place at an institution.

Intern
Recent medical school graduate who is receiving his/her first year of supervised practical training in medical and surgical care of patients in hospitals.

Intrathecal
Injecting drugs into the cerebrospinal fluid during a spinal tap.

Intravenous-access line (IV)
A hollow metal or plastic tube which is inserted into a vein and attached to tubing, allowing various solutions or medicines to be directly infused into the blood.

Leukemia
Disease characterized by the unrestrained growth of abnormal white cells in the bone marrow, and often in the spleen and liver; these cancerous cells usually appear in the peripheral blood and may also invade other organs.

Leukocytes
White blood cells.

Leukopenia
A below-normal number of white cells.

Lidocaine
> Drug most commonly used for local anesthesia.

Lumbar puncture (LP; spinal tap)
> Procedure in which a needle is inserted between the vertebrae of the back to obtain a sample of cerebrospinal fluid and/or inject medication.

Lymph
> A clear, colorless fluid found in lymph vessels throughout the body, which carries cells to fight infection.

Lymph nodes
> Rounded bodies of lymphatic tissues found in lymph vessels.

Lymph system
> A system of vessels and nodes throughout the body which helps filter out bacteria as well as performs numerous other functions.

Lymphocytes
> Type of white cell, formed in the lymphoid tissues, that prevents infection and helps provide immunity to disease.

Maintenance
> Part of a leukemia protocol for treating ALL. It follows the intensive induction and consolidation phases and helps destroy any remaining cancer cells.

Medical student
> Student who has completed four years of college and is enrolled in medical school.

Monocytes
> Type of white blood cell.

Neurotoxic
> Substance which is poisonous to the brain, spinal cord, and/or nerve cells.

Neutropenia
> Condition when the body does not have enough neutrophils (a type of infection-fighting white cell).

Neutrophils
> The most numerous of the granulocytic white cells, which migrate through the bloodstream to the site of infection, where they ingest and destroy bacteria.

Nutritionist
> A professional who analyzes nutritional requirements and gives advice on how to eat an appropriate diet for any condition.

Oncologist
> Doctor who specializes in the treatment of cancer.

Oncology
> Study of cancer.

Pancreas
> A gland situated behind the stomach which has two vital functions: it secretes enzymes into the intestines which aid in the digestion of food, and it produces and secretes insulin, a hormone essential for regulating carbohydrate metabolism by controlling blood sugar levels.

Pancreatitis

Inflammation of the pancreas which can cause extreme pain, vomiting, hiccoughing, constipation, and collapse.

Pathologist

Doctor who specializes in examining tissue and diagnosing disease.

Pediatrician

Doctor who specializes in the care and development of children and the treatment of their diseases.

Pediatric Oncology Group (POG)

An organization which designs and monitors pediatric clinical trials.

Petechiae

Small, reddish spots under the skin caused by hemorrhage.

Plasma

The liquid part of the lymph and the blood.

Platelet

Disc-shaped blood cell which aids in blood clotting.

Port-a-cath

Indwelling catheter which has a small portal under the skin of the chest attached to tubing which goes into the heart.

Prognosis

Expected or probable outcome.

Prophylaxis

An attempt to prevent disease.

Protocol

The "recipe" for a child's cancer treatment. Outlines the drugs that will be taken, when they will be taken, and in what dosages. Also includes the dates for procedures (e.g., bone marrow aspiration schedule).

Rad

Radiation absorbed dose. A unit of measurement of the absorbed dose of radiation.

Radiation

High-energy rays which are used to kill or damage cancer cells.

Radiologist

Doctor who specializes in using radiation and radioactive isotopes to diagnose and treat disease.

Randomized

Chosen at random. In a randomized research project, a computer chooses which patients receive the experimental treatment(s) and which patients receive the standard treatment.

Relapse

A return of the cancer after its apparently complete disappearance.

Remission

Disappearance of detectable disease.

Resident
> Physician who has completed four years of medical school and one year of internship, and who is continuing his or her clinical training.

Right atrial catheter
> Indwelling catheter with tubing that extends into the heart which provides access for drawing blood and injecting medication.

Side effect
> Unintentional or undesirable secondary effect of treatment.

Somnolence syndrome
> Syndrome which can occur from three to twelve weeks after cranial radiation. It is characterized by drowsiness, prolonged periods of sleep (up to twenty hours a day), low-grade fever, headaches, nausea, vomiting, irritability, difficulty swallowing, and difficulty speaking.

Spinal tap
> Procedure in which a needle is inserted between the vertebrae of the back to obtain a sample of cerebrospinal fluid and/or inject medication. Also called a lumbar puncture (LP).

Staphylococcus epidermidis
> Bacteria normally present on the skin which can infect the blood through an indwelling catheter.

Stem cells
> Cells from which all blood cells develop.

Streptokinase
> Enzyme sometimes used to dissolve blood clots in catheter tubing.

Stroke
> Loss of consciousness and paralysis caused by bleeding into the brain or clotting that blocks blood flow to a portion of the brain, causing injury or death to brain tissue.

Subcutaneous port
> Type of indwelling catheter comprised of a portal under the skin of the chest attached to tubing leading into the heart.

Systemic
> Affecting the body as a whole.

T cell
> Type of lymphocyte (white cell), derived from the thymus, that attacks infected cells, foreign tissue, and cancer cells.

Thrombocytes
> Platelets.

Thymus
> Small gland located behind the breast bone and between the lungs that plays a major role in the immune system.

Tumor board
> A meeting held at a hospital, attended by oncologists, pathologists, radiologists, fellows, and residents, where complicated cases are discussed to develop a treatment plan.

Urokinase
Enzyme sometimes used to dissolve clots in catheter tubing.

Vancomycin
Antibiotic commonly used to treat infections in indwelling catheters.

Vital signs
Term that describes a patient's pulse, rate of breathing, and blood pressure.

White blood cells
Cells that help the body fight infection and disease.

X-ray
High-energy electromagnetic radiation used in low doses to diagnose disease or injury and in high doses to treat cancer.

X-ray technician
Certified technician who positions patients for x-rays, monitors equipment, and takes x-rays of the body.

Index

Bloom's syndrome, 16
bone marrow aspiration, 46–48
bone marrow donors/donation, 377–379, 383–384
bone marrow transplantation. *See* transplantation
books, lists of, 450–471
Broviac catheters, 121
    See also catheters
busulphan, 28

C

camps, 154–155
Canadian Human Rights Act/Commission, 356
cardiovascular disorders, 346–347
catheters, 121–137
    adhesives used with, 135–137
    Broviac catheters, 121
    choosing/choosing not to use, 133–135
    comparison of (chart), 134
    external, 121–125
    Hickman catheters, 121
    indwelling, defined, 121
    infections, 123–124, 129, 132
    Medi-port, 121
    PICC line (peripherally inserted central catheter), 121, 130–133
    Port-a-cath, 121
    removal of at end of treatment, 336–337
    risks of, 123–125, 129–130, 132–133
    subcutaneous port, 125–130
CBCs (complete blood counts), 197–198, 433 (chart)
celebrations at end of treatment, 337–339
central line, 121
    See also catheters
central venous catheter, 121
    See also catheters
cerebrospinal fluid (CSF), 22
Cerubidine, 166

chemotherapy
    administration, methods of, 158
    antinausea drugs used during, 180–183, 197
    blood counts during, 432
    colony-stimulating factors, 179–180
    defined, 157–158
    dosages, calculation of, 159
    drug types, 158
    guidelines for calling doctor during, 160
    high-dose, 179, 371–372, 384
    intrathecal, 22, 25–26, 158
    pain relief during, drugs for, 183–188
    prior to transplantation, 384
    questions for doctor about, 160
    side effects, possible, 159, 193–215, 248–251, 345–350
    as treatment for
        acute lymphoblastic leukemia (ALL), 21–23
        acute myeloid leukemia (AML), 25–27
        acute promyelocytic leukemia (M3), 25
        chronic myelogenous leukemia (CML), 28–29
        chronic myelomonocytic leukemia (CMML), not generally used, 30
    See also side effects; *specific names of chemotherapeutic drugs*
Chesler, Naomi
    advice for parents and siblings, 305–307
chicken pox (varicella zoster), 201–203, 275, 389
child-life programs and specialists, 38–39, 139–140
chloroma/chloroma biopsies, 18–19
chronic myelogenous leukemia (CML), 27–29
    phases, 28
    Philadelphia chromosome, 28
    treatments and stages in treatments, 28–29

food and meals (*continued*)
    increasing appeal and fun of, 255–256
    for mouth/throat sores, 213
    during nausea and vomiting, 196–197
    snacks, 258–259
    See also nutrition
food supplements, commercial, 263–264
free air services, 447
friends. *See* family and friends
funerals, other rituals, and services, 403–405

G

genetic factors, 16–17, 28
glossary, xiii, 473–481
graft-versus-host disease (GVHD), 374–377, 390–391
grandparents, 74–76
    See also family and friends
granisetron, 181
granulocyte colony-stimulating factor (G-CSF), 26, 179–180
granulocyte-macrophage colony-stimulating factor (GM-CSF), 26, 179–180
granulocytes, 15, 197–200, 435
grief. *See* sadness and grief
growth, effect of treatments on, 229, 392
guilt, 6–7, 291–292
GVHD (graft-versus-host disease), 374–377, 390–391

H

hair loss, 193–195, 226
headwear and wigs, 194
health insurance. *See* insurance
Health Insurance Portability and Accountability Act of 1996, 359
heart problems, 346–347
helplessness, 7–8
hematocrit (packed cell volume (PCV)), 432–434
hemoglobin (Hgb), 432

hepatitis, 53, 54, 351
herpes simplex, 389
herpes zoster (shingles), 202–203, 275
Hexadrol, 172, 180–181
Hickman catheters, 121
    See also catheters
high-dose chemotherapy, 179, 371–372, 384
    See also chemotherapy
HIV/AIDS, 53, 54, 351
HLA (human leukocyte-associated) antigens, 373
Holt, Joanne
    on alternative learning activities, 269
hope, importance of, 10–11
hormones, 158
hospice care, 399–400
hospitals and hospitalization
    billing and billing errors, 237–241
    choice of hospital, 3, 19, 98
    coping with, 112–120
    financial assistance, sources of, 82–83, 244–247, 446–447
    food, 114
    parents as advocates during, 116–118
    parking arrangements, 114–115
    play areas, 118–120
    rooms, 112–114
    siblings' concerns about, 294
    social workers, 139–140
    staff of, 3, 94–97
    transplant centers, 379–381
    See also doctors; insurance
human leukocyte-associated (HLA) antigens, 373
hydrocortisone, 22
hydromorphone, 185–186
hydroxyurea, 169
Hypafix, 135–136
hypnosis, 41, 188

I

imagery, 41–42, 188
immobilization devices, 219–221

immune system, 388–390
  See also blood counts; infections;
    side effects; under specific
    names of chemotherapeutic
    drugs
immunizations, 199, 202–203, 351, 389
immunotherapy, 26
Individual Education Plans (IEPs), 281–
  285
Individuals with Disabilities Act (IDEA),
  279–281
induction/reinduction, 21, 23, 25–26
indwelling catheters. See catheters
infections
  from catheters, 123–124, 129, 132
  chicken pox (varicella zoster), 201–
    203, 275, 389
  and colony-stimulating factors, 179
  cytomegalovirus (CMV), 53, 54,
    389
  detection of, 198–200
  Epstein Barr virus, 377
  following transplantation, 388–390
  hepatitis, 53, 54, 351
  herpes simplex, 389
  herpes zoster (shingles), 202–203,
    275
  HIV/AIDS, 53, 54, 351
  immunizations, 199, 202–203, 389
  interstitial pneumonitis, 389
  from pets, 203–204
  pneumocystis pneumonia (PCP),
    178–179
  pneumonia, 200–201
  prevention of, 198–200, 274–275,
    351–352, 389–390
  sexually transmitted, 351–352
  shingles (herpes zoster), 202–203,
    275
  varicella zoster (chicken pox), 201–
    203, 275, 389
informed consent, 65–66
insurance, 241–244
  Americans with Disabilities Act
    (ADA), 355–357
  challenging claims, 243–244
  COBRA (Comprehensive Omnibus
    Budget Reconciliation
    Act), 358

contact person helpful, 242
and employment discrimination,
  358–359
ERISA (Employee Retirement and
  Income Security Act), 359
financial assistance, sources of,
  244–247
Health Insurance Portability and
  Accountability Act of
  1996, 359
Medicaid, 245
negotiating benefits, 242–243
SSI (Supplemental Security
  Income), 245
understanding policies, 241–242
  See also financial assistance; record-
    keeping
intensification, 26
Internet, use of for information and
  support, 144–145, 450–
  471
interstitial pneumonitis, 389
intrathecal chemotherapy, 22, 25–26,
  158
intravenous (IV) feeding, 249, 264–265
intravenous (IV) lines, starting, 49–50

J

jealousy, 291
Johnson, F. Leonard
  on challenges of childhood
    leukemia, vii–ix

K

ketamine, 44
Komp, Diane
  long term survivors in medical
    profession, 355
Kytril, 181

L

L-ASP/L-asparaginase, 162–163
lactose intolerance, 250

neutropenia, 26
See also blood counts
neutrophils, 15, 197–198, 434
See also blood counts
Numby Stuff, 188
nurses, terms used to distinguish, 96–97
nutrition, 248–265
appetite, changes in, 248–250
balanced diet, 251–253
eating problems as side effects of
treatment, 215, 226, 248–
251
lactose intolerance, 250
supplements, commercial, 263–264
vitamin supplements, 254
See also food and meals

O

oncologists. *See* doctors
Oncovin, 176–178
ondansetron, 182
online sites, lists of, 450–471
overindulgence/overprotection of
children, 322–323
oxycodone, 187
oxycotin, 187

P

pain
acupuncture, 43, 189
biofeedback, 43
distraction from, 42–43
drugs for, 43–45, 183–188
hypnosis, 41
imagery, 41–42
management and relief of during
procedures
pharmacological method, 43–
45
psychological method, 40–43
relaxation, 43
parent-to-parent programs, 147–148
parenting stressed children, checklist
for, 330
parents. *See* family and friends
PCP (pneumocystis pneumonia), 178–
179

PDQ (Physician Data Query), 24, 27
PEG-asparaginase, 162–163
Pentamidine, 178–179
Percoset, 187
peripheral blood stem cell transplants,
376
peripherally inserted central cathethers/
PICC lines, 121, 130–133
See also catheters
pets, 203–204
pharmaceuticals. *See* chemotherapy;
drugs
Phenergan, 183
Philadelphia chromosome, 28
physicians. *See* doctors
PICC lines, 121, 130–133
pill-taking, 54–57
placental blood stem cell transplants,
376–377
plasma, 14
platelet counts, 435
platelet transfusions, 54
platelets, 14–15
pneumocystis pneumonia (PCP), 178–
179
pneumonia, 200–201
Port-a-cath, 121
See also catheters
ports. *See* catheters
postremission therapy, 26
See also chemotherapy;
transplantation
prayer, 189
See also religious support
prednisone, 172–175
procedures
adjunctive therapies during, 40–43
pain relief during, 40–45
planning for, 37–40
presence of parents at, 39
questions before, 46
specific types of
blood draws, 51–52
blood transfusions, 52–53
bone marrow aspiration, 46–
48
catheters, 52, 121–137
echocardiograms, 58
finger pokes, 52

procedures
    specific types of (*continued*)
        ntravenous (IV) lines, starting,
            49 50
        MUGA scan, 59
        pill-taking, 54–57
        platelet transfusions, 54
        spinal taps (lumbar puncture/
            LP), 48–49
        subcutaneous injections, 50–
            51
        temperature-taking, 57
        urine specimens, 58
prochlorperazine, 183
promethazine, 183
prophylactic antibiotics, 178–179
propofol, 44
protocols, 66–68
psychological counseling. *See* emotional
            responses; support and
            self help
puberty, effect of treatments on, 229–
            230, 393
Purinthenol, 169–170

R
radiation oncologists, 218
radiation simulation, 222–223
radiation therapists, 218–219
radiation treatments
    cranial radiation treatment, 223–
        224
    description and types of, 216, 222–
        226
    immobilization during, 219–222
    masks, immobilization, 219–220
    not prescribed for all leukemias,
        217
    oncologists, therapists, 218–219
    questions to ask about, 217–218
    sedation during, 221–222
    side-effects
        coping with, 193–215, 226
        long-term, 227–230, 345–350
        short-term, 226–227
    simulation, 222–223
    testicular radiation treatment, 224–
        225

total body irradiation (TBI), 225–
        226, 392–393
treatment centers, choice of, 218
as treatment for
        acute lymphoblastic leukemia
            (ALL), 21, 23
        acute myeloid leukemia
            (AML), 25
        chronic myelogenous leukemia
            (CML), 29
    when given, 217
radiotherapy. *See* radiation
record-keeping
    blood counts, chart for, 437
    calendars/journals, use of for, 232–
        234
    computers/tape recorders, use of
        for, 234–235
    financial records, 235–241
    medical records, 231–235
    special education records, 286
recurrence after transplant, 392
    See also relapse
red blood cells (RBCs), 14–15, 52–53,
        434
    See also blood counts
relapse
    emotional responses, 365–366
    recurrence after transplant, 392
    signs and symptoms of, 362–365
    treatment plans, 367–370
relaxation therapy, 43
religious support, 83–84, 148–149
resource organizations, 439–449
right atrial catheters, 121
    See also catheters
Rubex, 167–168
Rubidomycin, 166

S
sadness and grief
    at diagnosis, 10–11
    of parents, 414–419
    of siblings, 292–293, 412–414
    See also death and bereavement;
            emotional responses

schools
communication with, 267–269
infections, avoiding at, 274–275
learning disabilities
acceptance of, 286–288
accommodations and services
for, 278–286
identification of, 278–279
Individual Education Plans
(IEPs), 283–285
Individuals with Disabilities
Education Act (IDEA),
279–281
infants and preschoolers,
services for, 285–286
legal rights to, United States and
Canada, 279–281
for preschoolers, 276, 285–286
returning to, 270–274
schoolwork, keeping up with, 269
siblings' needs at, 270
teachers and classmates, role of,
268–269
and terminal illness, 276–278
second opinions, 5, 106–107, 367, 372
secondary malignancy, 230, 394
sedation. *See* anesthesia and sedation
self help. *See* support and self help
Septra, 178
sexual activity, post-treatment, 351–
352, 393
SGOT (serum glutamic oxaloacetic
transaminase), 436
SGPT (serum glutamic pyruvic
transaminase), 435
shingles (herpes zoster), 202–203, 275
siblings, 289–311
coping, helping with, 307–311
emotional responses of, 92, 289–
295, 311
grief and responses to death, 403,
412–414
hospitalization, concerns about,
294
individual experiences of, 295–305
parental anger at, 9
parents, concerns about, 294–295
parents not spending enough time
with, 323–324

polio immunization of, 199
positive outcomes for, 311
schools, needs at, 270
telling about diagnosis, 35–36
and transplantation, 387
ways to help with, 79–80
See also family and friends
side effects
of antinausea drugs, 180–183
of chemotherapy
bed wetting, 209–211
cardiovascular (heart)
disorders, 346–347
constipation, 206–207
dental problems, 211–212,
347–348
diarrhea, 204–206
eating problems, 215, 248–
250
fatigue and weakness, 207–
209, 348–349
fertility/sterility issues, 345–
346
hair loss (alopecia), 193–195,
226
heart problems, 346–347
learning disabilities, 215
low blood counts, 197–204
nausea and vomiting, 180–
183, 196–197
skin and nail problems, 214–
215
sores in mouth and throat,
212–213
taste and smell, changes in,
213–214
long-term, 227–230, 278–279,
345–350, 391–394
of prophylactic antibiotics, 178–
179
of radiation, 226–230
of transplantation, 387–394
See also blood counts; late effects;
*specific names of drugs and
treatments*
signs and symptoms of leukemia, 1–3,
362–365
skin and nail problems, 214–215, 226
sleepiness, 226–227

smell, changes in, 213–214, 226, 250–251

smoking, 351

social workers, 139–140, 150–151

somnolence syndrome, 226–227

sores, mouth and throat, 212–213

Sourkes, Barbara
    effect of cancer on sense of control, 315
    psychotherapy important for ill child, 154
    understanding question before answering, 34–35

spinal taps (lumbar puncture/LP), 48–49

spiritual support, 83–84, 148–149

SSI (Supplemental Security Income), 245

stem cell transplantation, 371–372, 376–377
    See also transplantation

sterility, 225, 345–346, 393

stress. See emotional responses

subcutaneous injections, 50–51

subcutaneous ports, 121, 125–130
    See also catheters

substance abuse, 4, 324

sulfamethoxazole, 178

sun, limiting exposure to, 199, 214

supplemental feeding, 264–265
    enteral nutrition, 265
    intravenous (IV), 249, 264–265
    total parenteral nutrition (TPN), 265
    tubes used for, 249, 264–265
    See also nutrition

support and self help
    camps, 154–155
    child-life programs and specialists, 38–39, 139–140
    clergy and religion, 83–84, 148–149
    continued need for during bereavement, 405–412
    counseling, individual and family, 149–154

groups
    for children with cancer, 145–146
    continued need for during bereavement, 411–412
    on Internet, 144–145
    for parents, 140–145
    for siblings, 146

hospital social workers, 139–140

organizations providing, 439–449

parent-to-parent programs, 147–148

See also family and friends

swollen glands, 226

syngeneic bone marrow transplants, 375–376

T

tantrums, 316–317

taste, changes in, 213–214, 226, 250–251

Tegaderm, 135–136

telling children and teens about diagnosis, 31, 33–36

temper, loss of, 316–317, 321–322

temperature-taking, 57

testicular radiation treatment, 224–225

tests. See procedures

therapists. See counseling and counselors; emotional responses; social workers; support and self help

throat sores, 212–213

thrombocytes, 15

thrombocytopenia, 14

thyroid function, 393

total body irradiation/radiation, 225–226, 392–393

total parenteral nutrition (TPN), 265

transfusions, blood, 52–53

transfusions, platelet, 54

transplant centers, choosing, 379–381
    See also hospitals and hospitalization

About the Author

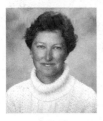 Nancy Keene, the author of *Childhood Leukemia: A Guide for Families, Friends & Caregivers, Second Edition,* is one of the original developers of the Patient-Centered Guides series. She has been involved with the medical world for over two decades, both as a caregiver and as a patient. Nancy's daughter Kathryn was diagnosed with high-risk acute lymphoblastic leukemia when she was three years old. Nancy supported and advocated for Kathryn during the two years she underwent intensive treatment. Kathryn is now eleven years old.

Nancy was one of the first five people appointed as patient advocates to the Children's Cancer Group (CCG), a research organization consisting of pediatric cancer specialists from Canada, the United States, and Australia. She attends CCG meetings and facilitates communication between CCG investigators and the patient community.

In addition to *Childhood Leukemia: A Guide for Families, Friends & Caregivers, Second Edition,* Nancy has also written *Your Child in the Hospital: A Practical Guide for Parents, Working with Your Doctor: Getting the Healthcare You Deserve,* and, with Honna Janes-Hodder, *Childhood Cancer: A Parent's Guide to Solid Tumor Cancers.* She is now working on a book about late effects of cancer treatment, *Childhood Cancer Survivors: A Practical Guide to the Future,* with Kathy Ruccione and Wendy Hobbie.

Nancy lives in Washington state and is busy writing and raising her two daughters. She spends her limited free time volunteering in school, talking with parents of children newly diagnosed with cancer (in person, on the telephone, and on the Internet), reading an eclectic mix of books, and dreaming of travel.

Colophon

Patient-Centered Guides are about the experience of illness. They contain personal stories as well as a combination of practical and medical information. The faces on the covers of our Guides reflect the human side of the information we offer.

Edie Freedman designed the cover of *Childhood Leukemia: A Guide for Families, Friends & Caregivers, Second Edition,* using Adobe Photoshop 5.0 and QuarkXPress 3.32 with Onyx BT and Berkeley fonts from Bitstream. The cover photo is from Rubberball Productions and is used with their permission. Kathleen Wilson prepared the cover mechanical.

Nancy Priest, Edie Freedman, and Alicia Cech designed the interior layout for the book. The interior fonts are Berkeley and Franklin Gothic. Mike Sierra prepared the text using FrameMaker 5.5. Some of the photographs in Appendix A are reprinted with permission from the following: Lifetouch, J.C. Penney's at Southcenter, and Olin Mills Studio. Nancy Keene's photo is © Donette Studio, Bellingham, Washington.

The book was copyedited by Lunaea Hougland and proofread by Kristin Barendsen. Abigail Myers, Sarah Jane Shangraw, and Sheryl Avruch conducted quality assurance checks. Katherine J. Wilkinson wrote the index. The illustrations that appear in this book were produced by Robert Romano, Rhon Porter, Chris Reilley, and Martha Deller using Macromedia Freehand 8 and Adobe Photoshop 5. Interior composition was done by Claire Cloutier LeBlanc and Anna Snow.

Patient-Centered Guides™

Questions Answered
Experiences Shared

*We are committed to empowering individuals to evolve
into informed consumers armed with the latest information and
heartfelt support for their journey.*

When your life is turned upside down, your need for information is great. You have to make critical medical decisions, often with what seems little to go on. Plus you have to break the news to family, quiet your own fears, cope with symptoms or treatment side effects, figure out how you're going to pay for things, and sometimes still get to work or get dinner on the table.

Patient-Centered Guides provide authoritative information for intelligent information seekers who want to become advocates of their own health. They cover the whole impact of illness on your life. In each book, there's a mix of:

- **Medical background for treatment decisions**
  We can give you information that can help you to intelligently work with your doctor to come to a decision. We start from the viewpoint that modern medicine has much to offer and also discuss complementary treatments. Where there are treatment controversies we present differing points of view.

- **Practical information**
  Once you've decided what to do about your illness, you still have to deal with treatments and changes to your life. We cover day-to-day practicalities, such as those you'd hear from a good nurse or a knowledgeable support group.

- **Emotional support**
  It's normal to have strong reactions to a condition that threatens your life or changes how you live. It's normal that the whole family is affected. We cover issues like the shock of diagnosis, living with uncertainty, and communicating with loved ones.

Each book also contains stories from both patients and doctors — medical "frequent flyers" who share, in their own words, the lessons and strategies they have learned when maneuvering through the often complicated maze of medical information that's available.

We provide information online, including updated listings of the resources that appear in this book. This is freely available for you to print out and copy to share with others, as long as you retain the copyright notice on the print-outs.

http://www.patientcenters.com

Other Books in the Series

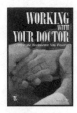

Working with Your Doctor
Getting the Healthcare You Deserve
By Nancy Keene
ISBN 1-56592-273-5, Paperback, 6" x 9", 382 pages, $15.95

"*Working with Your Doctor* fills a genuine need for patients and their family members caught up in this new and intimidating age of impersonal, economically-driven health care delivery."
—*James Dougherty, MD, Emeritus Professor of Surgery,*
Albany Medical College

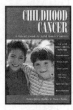

Childhood Cancer
A Parent's Guide to Solid Tumor Cancers
By Nancy Keene
ISBN 1-56592-531-9, Paperback, 6"x 9", 544 pages, $24.95

"I recommend [this book] most highly for those in need of high-level, helpful knowledge that will empower and help parents and caregivers to cope."
—*Mark Greenberg, MD, Professor of Pediatrics,*
University of Toronto

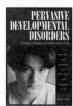

Pervasive Developmental Disorders
Finding a Diagnosis and Getting Help
By Mitzi Waltz
ISBN 1-56592-530-0, Paperback, 6" x 9", 592 pages, $24.95

"Mitzi Waltz's book provides clear, informative, and comprehensive information on every relevant aspect of PDD. Her in-depth discussion will help parents and professionals develop a clear understanding of the issues and, consequently, they will be able to make informed decisions about various interventions. A job well done!"
—*Dr. Stephen M. Edelson, Director,*
Center for the Study of Autism, Salem, Oregon

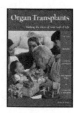

Organ Transplants
Making the Most of Your Gift of Life
By Robert Finn
ISBN 1-56592-634-X, Paperback, 6" x 9", $19.95, 320 pages
"*This book is factual, easy to read and intelligently written ... a wonderful job.*"
—*Joan Miller, RN,*
Department of Cardiothoracic Surgery,
Stanford University School of Medicine

Patient-Centered Guides
Published by O'Reilly & Associates, Inc.
Our products are available at a bookstore near you.
For information: 800-998-9938 • 707-829-0515 • info@oreilly.com
101 Morris Street • Sebastopol • CA • 95472-9902

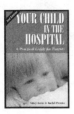

Your Child in the Hospital
A Practical Guide for Parents, Second Edition
By Nancy Keene and Rachel Prentice
ISBN 1-56592-573-4, Paperback, 5" x 8", 176 pages, $11.95

"When your child is ill or injured, the hospital setting can be overwhelming. Here is a terrific 'road map' to help keep families 'on track.'"

—*James B. Fahner, MD, Division Chief,*
Pediatric Hematology/Oncology, DeVos Children's Hospital,
Grand Rapids, Michigan

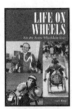

Choosing a Wheelchair
A Guide for Optimal Independence
By Gary Karp
ISBN 1-56592-411-8, Paperback, 5" x 8", 192 pages, $9.95

"I love the idea of putting knowledge often possessed only by professionals into the hands of new consumers. Gary Karp has done it. This book will empower people with disabilities to make informed equipment choices."

—*Barry Corbet, Editor,* New Mobility Magazine

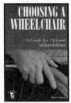

Life on Wheels
For the Active Wheelchair User
By Gary Karp
ISBN 1-56592-253-0, Paperback, 6" x 9", 576 pages, $24.95

"Gary Karp's *Life On Wheels* is a super book. If you use a wheelchair, you cannot do without it. It is THE wheelchair-user reference book."
—*Hugh Gregory Gallagher, Author,*
FDR's Splendid Deception

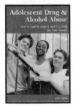

Adolescent Drug & Alcohol Abuse:
How to Spot It, Stop It, and Get Help for Your Family
By Nikki Babbit
ISBN 1-56592-755-9, Paperback, 6"x9", $17.95, 304 pages

"The clear, concise, and practical information, backed up by personal stories from people who have been through these problems with their own children or clients, will have readers keeping this book within easy reach for use on a regular basis."

—*James F. Crowley, MA*
President, Community Intervention, Inc.
Author, Alliance for Change:
A Plan for Community Action on Adolescent Drug Abuse

Patient-Centered Guides
Published by O'Reilly & Associates, Inc.
Our products are available at a bookstore near you.
For information: **800-998-9938** • **707-829-0515** • **info@oreilly.com**
101 Morris Street • Sebastopol • CA • 95472-9902

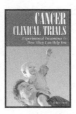

Cancer Clinical Trials
Experimental Treatments and How They Can Help You
By Robert Finn
ISBN 1-56592-566-1, Paperback, 5" x 8", 216 pages, $14.95

"I highly recommend this book as a first step in what will be for many a difficult, but crucially important, part of their struggle to beat their cancer."

—From the foreword by Robert Bazell, Chief Science Correspondent for NBC News and Author, Her-2: The Making of Herceptin, a Revolutionary Treatment for Breast Cancer

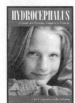

Hydrocephalus
A Guide for Patients, Families & Friends
By Chuck Toporek and Kellie Robinson
ISBN 1-56592-410-X, Paperback, 6" x 9", 384 pages, $19.95

"Toporek, a medical editor, and wife Robinson, a writer and hydrocephalus patient, fill a void of information on hydrocephalus (water on the brain) for the lay reader. Highly recommended for public and academic libraries."

—Library Journal

"In this book, the authors have provided a wonderful entry into the world of hydrocephalus to begin to remedy the neglect of this important condition. We are immensely grateful to them for their groundbreaking effort."

—Peter M. Black, MD, PhD, Franc D. Ingraham Professor of Neurosurgery, Harvard Medical School, Neurosurgeon-in-Chief, Brigham and Women's Hospital, Children's Hospital, Boston, Massachusetts

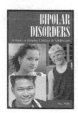

Bipolar Disorders
A Guide to Helping Children & Adolescents
By Mitzi Waltz
ISBN 1-56592-656-0, Paperback, 6" x 9", 450 pages, $24.95

"As bipolar disorders are becoming more commonly diagnosed in children and adolescents, a readable, informative guide for these youths and their families is certainly needed. This book certainly fits the bill. It covers all of the major topics that are of greatest importance to guide parents and families on the topic of pediatric bipolarity ..."

—Robert L. Findling, MD, Director, Division of Child and Adolescent Psychiatry, Co-director, Stanley Clinical Research Center, Case Western Reserve University/University Hospitals of Cleveland

Patient-Centered Guides
Published by O'Reilly & Associates, Inc.
Our products are available at a bookstore near you.
For information: **800-998-9938** • **707-829-0515** • **info@oreilly.com**
101 Morris Street • Sebastopol • CA • 95472-9902